3RD EDITION

HEALTH PROMOTION

Principles and practice in the Australian context

MARY LOUISE FLEMING
& ELIZABETH PARKER

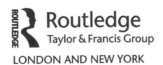

Routledge
Taylor & Francis Group

LONDON AND NEW YORK

First published 1995 by Allen & Unwin

Published 2020 by Routledge
2 Park Square, Milton Park, Abingdon, Oxon OX14 4RN
605 Third Avenue, New York, NY 10017

Routledge is an imprint of the Taylor & Francis Group, an informa business

National Library of Australia
Cataloguing-in-Publication entry:

Fleming, Mary Louise.
  Health promotion : principles and practice in the
  Australian context.

  3rd ed.
  Bibliography.
  Includes index.
  ISBN 1 74175 017 2.

  1. Health promotion – Australia. 2. Health education –
  Australia. 3. Public health – Australia. I. Parker,
  Elizabeth (Elizabeth Anne), 1945- . II. Title.

613.0994

Index by Russell Brooks
Set in 11/14 pt Minion by Midland Typesetters, Australia

ISBN-13: 9781741750171 (pbk)

Contents

Figures and tables

FIGURES

TABLES

Contributors

Peter Anderson, Dominique Bird, Michael Hardie, Beryl Meiklejohn, Brian
Oldenburg and Tricia Willis
School of Public Health
Queensland University of Technology
Brisbane, Queensland

Robert Friedman
Boston University School of Medicine
Massachusetts, USA

John Mendoza
Chief Executive Officer
Mental Health Council of Australia
Canberra, Australian Capital Territory

Elvia Ramirez and Rita Prasad-Ildes
Queensland Transcultural Mental Health Centre

Sue Smyllie
Formerly Queensland Health

Katrina Walton
Wellness Coordinator
Greenslopes Private Hospital, Queensland

Jillian Woolmer
Formerly the Healthy Lifestyle Coordinator
Curtin University of Technology
Perth, Western Australia

Foreword

There has been a clear and very impressive decline in preventable mortality in most developed countries, including Australia, since the 1960s. While inferring precise causal relationships is always difficult, preventive activities and health promotion have undoubtedly contributed to this decline. For example, health promotion programs and activities have certainly contributed to the decline in the number of deaths due to circulatory diseases, unintentional accidents, injuries and poisonings, infectious diseases and some cancers. Australia is recognised internationally for many of its health promotion programs and preventive activities, as well as its contribution to research in this field.

The strength of health promotion practice and research in countries like Australia has come about as a result of several factors. First, there is a generally well developed infrastructure for, and commitment to, health promotion and prevention at all levels of government in Australia. Second, there has been an increase in the funding of public health programs, as well as the research and evaluation efforts that underpin these activities. Finally, there is an increasingly well trained and differentiated public health and health promotion workforce.

All of this progress notwithstanding, the global and other challenges confronting health promotion and public health professionals in this new millennium are still substantial, and we need to continue learning from the lessons of the past and to improve further on our practice in the future. The skills required of health promotion practitioners are many and varied, and the knowledge base is expanding daily. This book provides an excellent introduction to the theory and practice of health promotion in a developed country such as Australia. It identifies the position of health promotion with respect to public health, and the steps and skills required for effective health promotion practice. Most importantly, though, the book tells us in a very practical, down-to-earth fashion how to plan, implement, manage and evaluate health promotion programs in a variety of settings: workplaces, schools, rural and remote areas, and elsewhere in the community. This third edition of *Health Promotion: Principles and practice in the Australian context* will make a substantial contribution to the skill level of practitioners.

Professor Brian Oldenburg
School of Public Health
Queensland University of Technology

Acknowledgments

We would like to thank the many people who collectively or individually assisted us in the writing of this third edition of the book.

We are grateful to the contributors of the case studies; their programs highlight health promotion in practice in Australia. Beryl Meiklejohn, from the Faculty of Health, Queensland University of Technology, provided helpful feedback on Indigenous health for Chapter 8. A special thank you to Trish Gould, who worked tirelessly to assist us to provide up-to-date contemporary research information for this third edition.

To Elizabeth Weiss of Allen & Unwin we offer many thanks for her assistance throughout the project and her ongoing faith in our ideas and ability. We also thank those other staff from Allen & Unwin who assisted in bringing this third edition to fruition.

The support, encouragement, patience and sheer endurance of our families need to be acknowledged and applauded.

Introduction

If we look back over the centuries, we see that the process of maintaining and enhancing general community health has evolved through a shifting array of theories and public health practices. With each new era, new methods have been sought to address the most common causes of mortality and morbidity in society. In recent years the need for a fundamental change in public health strategy has arisen, one in which health promotion has a vital part to play because of the impact of human behaviour and the social milieu on health. Health promotion has emerged as a multidisciplinary approach to tackling current causes of mortality and morbidity and to advancing the public's health.

Stimulated by the World Health Organization's activities since the 1970s, health promotion in Australia has flourished at both national and state levels where government bodies have been structured, health promotion foundations established and, in universities, health promotion teaching programs introduced. This has meant that students, teachers and practitioners need to keep up with advances in the theory, skills and practice of health promotion in Australia. Practitioners and practitioners-to-be need to understand the roots of health promotion within the realm of public health, to become skilled in program planning and evaluation, and to be able to manage programs. In addition, practitioners can develop their repertoire from studying the application of theory in a range of different settings. This book has been written with these needs in mind. Current approaches in health promotion and the challenges they pose are introduced and analysed using a 'settings' approach. These settings provide readers with an opportunity to reflect on their own practice and to become familiar with the range of contexts in which health promotion takes place.

The book is divided into three parts. *Part I* contains three chapters. Chapter 1 introduces the reader to the social history of public health, including the main phases in the evolution of public health to contemporary times, and provides some examples of early public health developments in Australia. Health promotion within the 'new public health' paradigm is the basis for Chapter 2. International developments in health promotion provide the context for the theory of health promotion and its relationship with health education, along with the emergence of the new paradigm. All of these contemporary developments are considered within a public health framework. Chapter 3 outlines the major social and cultural determinants of health and their impact on the health status of the Australian population. In particular, contemporary national strategies and initiatives designed to improve health are included, together with a discussion of a number of national health policy documents and national health strategies and initiatives, such as the National Public Health Partnership and chronic disease prevention policies.

Chapters 4 and 5 form *Part II* of the book. These chapters focus on the skills needed by health promotion practitioners to plan effective initiatives. Evidence suggests that well-planned and well-evaluated programs are more likely to be successful. Critics of health promotion claim that poorly planned and evaluated programs are the main reasons health promotion fails. In Chapter 4, we address these concerns and offer an introduction to models of program planning and evaluation that can be used as frameworks for health promotion program planning, implementation and evaluation. Chapter 5 introduces the reader to the skills needed to manage health promotion programs. With the growth of health promotion in the non-government, school, workplace, hospital and public sectors, practitioners increasingly are called upon to manage activities at various levels, including small-scale projects, large-scale programs and health promotion departments. An introduction to the modern organisation, to management theory and its application to the manager of a health promotion program, is a central element of this chapter. Discussion of the management skills required of a health promoter and a management 'checklist' are also included in Chapter 5.

Part III of the book deals with practical settings. We draw on the World Health Organization's recognition that health promotion occurs in various settings, and through intersectoral collaboration, in our discussion of the principles of the Ottawa Charter as they relate to health promotion activities. In using these settings to illuminate health promotion in practice in Australia, we bring together theory, policy and application. An example or two illustrates the point. In Chapter 11, we begin with the recognition of the special needs of rural and remote communities, then highlight rural health policies and provide examples of health promotion in action. Similarly, in Chapter 8 we discuss the relationship between indigenous people's culture and health and set the focus of health promotion activity among indigenous people.

National and state initiatives in school health promotion are discussed in Chapter 6. The expansion of traditional classroom health education to include comprehensive health promotion and 'health promoting schools' initiatives offer the school health educator a range of theories and initiatives for consideration.

Chapter 7 focuses on community health promotion and traces the development of community health in Australia through the national Community Health Program to community-based campaigns. Challenges for health promotion practitioners in understanding their role in a community and models of community organisation are explained.

Chapter 8 provides an overview of Aboriginal and Torres Strait Islander health status and the health promotion principles and practices in action in indigenous communities. Ethical guidelines for research within communities and initiatives for training indigenous health workers are highlighted.

Health promotion in the workplace has witnessed an array of program initiatives, particularly in the United States and in Australia. What are the effective models of workplace health promotion? What is the role of the health promoter in the workplace? These questions and a discussion of contemporary health management practice form the basis of Chapter 9.

Chapter 10 deals with health care settings—for instance, hospitals and community health centres—as a site of health promotion. The notion of primary health care is discussed, and initiatives in health promotion in health care settings are analysed and discussed.

Policies and programs in rural and remote health promotion are addressed in Chapter 11. The recent recognition of the impact of social conditions and isolation on rural and remote health is highlighted, national policies are identified, and health promotion programs are analysed and profiled.

PART I

BACKGROUND

Three chapters set the background for health promotion principles and practice.

Chapter 1 traces the history and impact of public health in early European Australia. The different eras of public health and the evolution of health promotion and its development as a legitimate public health endeavour are discussed.

Chapter 2 profiles the social and cultural determinants of health status in Australia, as well as outlining the leading mortality and morbidity profile of Australians. The impact of contemporary Australian policies on health promotion is discussed.

Chapter 3 looks at health promotion within the context of national and international developments of the 'new' public health. An ecological public health model and its implications for health promotion are considered, and health promotion initiatives in Australia are highlighted.

1

A social history of public health

- *Defining public health*
- *Health promotion and public health*
- *Concepts of health and disease*
- *The origins of public health*
- *Public health in Australia*
- *The emergence of contemporary public health*

This chapter presents a brief history of public health and identifies the main historical phases that have led to the emergence of what is termed the 'new public health'. The range of social, economic, political, administrative and lifestyle factors considered to have played a part in influencing developments in public health throughout its history are described and analysed. In addition, some of the significant developments taking place in public health, both within Australia and internationally, are highlighted. Thus, the chapter provides a framework with which to analyse developments leading to the emergence of a contemporary public health perspective.

Measures to improve the health of the public were evident in both Greek and Roman societies. Roman aqueducts, Greek and Roman bathing spas, and the swamp-draining projects are examples of early town planning and public health measures. Some medieval monasteries had proper water supplies, as well as heating and ventilation systems, but most developing European cities had great difficulty in supplying safe water (Terris 1987).

DEFINING PUBLIC HEALTH

Over the centuries, the term 'public health' has been defined by various players in the public health field. Historically, the definitions have given us word pictures of the evolution of the field. For example, early definitions were limited essentially to sanitary measures designed to guard against nuisances and health hazards and as protective measures for the community. Decisions about whether a problem fell within the realm of public health were initially based on the criteria of insanitation and, later, communicability. Emphasis on the prevention of disease in the individual appeared later with the emergence of germ theory and the bacteriological and immunological discoveries of the late nineteenth and early twentieth centuries.

The extensions of the definition of public health were created by shifts in values occasioned by particular circumstances. For example, by the end of the nineteenth century the substantial improvements in adult and child mortality were being contrasted with unchanged *infant* mortality rates. This concern with infant health remained dominant for the whole of the first half of the twentieth century.

The discipline basis of public health developed from an early focus on sanitary science to a latter-day perspective that incorporated medical science (Pickett & Hanlon 1990).

In 1920, C.E.A. Winslow, a professor of public health at Yale University, defined public health as:

> . . . the science and art of preventing disease, prolonging life, and promoting physical health and efficiency through organized community efforts for the sanitation of the environment, the control of community infections, the education of the individual in principles of personal hygiene, the organization of medical and nursing service for the early diagnosis and preventive treatment of disease, and the development of the social machinery which will ensure to every individual in the community a standard of living adequate for the maintenance of health. (Winslow 1920, p. 3)

Winslow's broad definition of public health represented an invitation for debate. The endeavours of public health proponents to make all of these activities their own inevitably led to discord between the medical profession and the proponents, as well as disharmony between public health authorities and other institutions. Starr (1982) suggested that much of the history of public health is a record of struggles over the limits of its mandate. These disputes have long antecedents, but the conflict was intensified by an historical convergence between medicine and public health.

Gordon defined public health as 'the collective measures which a community takes to prevent disease. This means that the agents practising this form of prevention usually are: the federal government; state governments; and local authorities' (1976, p. 797). Commenting on the future of public health in the late 1970s, Gordon established its boundaries by suggesting that public health had a bright future if it maintained its interest in the whole rather than the separate parts—in other words, if it left the clinical mystique to the clinicians wherever possible. He went on to suggest that the public health world should be training assessors, planners and people who critically contemplate medicine in its social background. Its sphere, according to Gordon, might be seen as including: fact-finding; specific prevention (for example, food and drug regulation, and occupational and environmental health legislation); health education (other than at the level of the individual patient); education of specialists in public health; and overall planning and administration. Meanwhile, Beaglehole et al. define public health as 'collective action for sustained population-wide health improvement' (2004, p. 2084).

The account of public health given by Last (1997, p. 6) defines its role in a broad societal context: 'Public health activities change with changing technology and social values, but the goal remains the same—to reduce the amount of disease, premature death, and disease-produced discomfort and disability in the population'. The Public Health Association of Australia (1997) similarly defines public health as:

> . . . a combination of science, practical skills, and beliefs that is directed to the maintenance and improvement of the health of all people. It is one of the efforts organised by society to protect, promote and restore the people's health through collective or social actions.

These contemporary definitions of public health have evolved from a social health perspective, one that focuses on the social, economic and environmental determinants of health and disease (Beaglehole et al. 2004). Additionally, they highlight the broad-ranging characteristics of public health practice: those that emphasise collaborative and comprehensive actions and initiatives, embedded in their social context.

One of the most significant contributions to the evolution of public health in more recent times has been the *Ottawa Charter for Health Promotion*, formulated at an international conference on health promotion held in Ottawa, Canada, in 1986 (Figure 1.1). It has become one of the focal points in the work of the World Health Organization (WHO) in advocating a comprehensive approach to public health and health promotion practice. The charter emphasises the role of healthy public policy, the social and physical aspects of the health environment, community education in health advocacy and action, and the development of individual skills in health advocacy. It reinforces the need to reorient community services towards prevention. The formulation and international adoption of the Ottawa Charter marked the emergence of a framework for action in public health practice that includes five equally essential components:

- consideration of healthy public policy
- creating supportive environments
- educating communities in health advocacy and action
- developing individual skills in health advocacy
- reorienting health services towards implications of preventive strategies.

Figure 1.1: The Ottawa Charter for Health Promotion

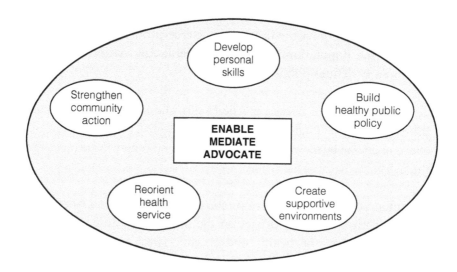

Source: World Health Organization (1986a)

The charter has made a significant contribution to the way in which public health is defined and to the range of strategies employed in protection, promotion and restoration of the public's health. The charter is discussed in greater depth in Chapter 2 (see 'Principles of health promotion').

Contemporary definitions of public health extend Gordon's (1976) and Last's (1983) notions of collective community measures to prevent disease, by focusing on a multidisciplinary approach that draws on a broad social base.

What has emerged under the title of 'new public health' is an approach that brings together environmental change and personal preventive measures with appropriate therapeutic interventions, especially for the elderly and the disabled (Ashton & Seymour 1990, p. 21). The 'new public health' is said to go beyond an understanding of human biology to recognise the importance of social aspects of health problems caused by lifestyle. Therefore, many contemporary health problems are seen as being social, rather than solely individual, problems; underlying them are concrete issues of local and national policy. What is needed to address these problems are multisectoral policies that support the promotion of health. The following case study illustrates the utility of wide-ranging policies, strategies and guidelines in addressing one of the factors contributing to health problems.

GOVERNMENT PRIORITIES FOR PUBLIC HEALTH AREAS: SMOKING

Although smoking rates have been declining over the last 30 years in Australia, especially in men, smoking is still the greatest single risk factor for chronic diseases and the single most preventable cause of death (AIHW 2002a). However, there have been improvements: over the past fifteen years, the rates and patterns of smoking have changed, as has tobacco-related morbidity and mortality.

In 1991, the proportion of the Australian population aged fourteen years and over who were daily smokers was 24 per cent (AIHW 2005g); whereas by 2004, this proportion had declined, to 17.4 per cent (2.9 million). In 2004, except for the 14–19-year-old age group, the rate of daily smoking was higher for males than females (AIHW 2004e).

These improvements are, to some extent, attributable to Commonwealth, state and territory legislation prohibiting, restricting or regulating access to or use of tobacco products. Policies, legislation and strategies include:

Demand reduction strategies
Marketing and promotion
- anti-smoking advertisements
- sponsorship prohibited or restricted by legislation
- value-added promotions
- minimum pack size

Education
- health warning labels
- telephone help services
- media campaigns
- school-based programs
- cessation services

Supply reduction strategies
- reducing vending machine numbers in public places
- passive smoking reduction through reducing access to cigarettes
- retailer compliance campaigns

Pricing mechanisms
- Excise (Commonwealth Department of Health 2004).

More recently, public health has aligned itself with the ecological movement and framed public health activities within an 'ecological public health' paradigm.

HEALTH PROMOTION AND PUBLIC HEALTH

One of the key concepts in this expanded contemporary vision of public health is health promotion. Health promotion—as a means of achieving 'Health For All'—is seen as a process of enabling people to increase control over and improve their health. Health itself is regarded as a 'resource for everyday life, not the objective of living' (WHO 1986a).

At a general level, health promotion has come to represent a unifying concept for those who recognise the need for change, in the ways and conditions of living, in order to promote health. In this socio-ecological approach the *basic* resources for health are identified as income, shelter and food. Improvements in health require a secure foundation in these basics, but they also require information on life skills, opportunities for making healthy choices among goods, services and facilities, and favourable social and cultural conditions—a 'total' environment that enhances health. Labonte has suggested that health promotion in practice aims to extend the boundaries of medically defined, institutionally controlled forms of 'programming'. In this new paradigm:

> . . . empowerment, or the capacity to define, analyse and act upon problems in one's life and living conditions, joins treatment and prevention as important health professional and health agency goals. Psychology, political science and social theories join educational, marketing, policy and medical theories in developing program actions. (Labonte 1992a, pp. 6–7)

How has health promotion been defined, specifically? The Ottawa Charter defined it as:

> . . . the process of enabling individuals and communities to increase control over the determinants of health and thereby improve their health. It has come to represent a unifying concept for those who recognise the basic need for change in both the ways and conditions of living in order to promote health. Health promotion represents a mediating strategy between people and their environments, combining personal choice with social responsibility for health to create a healthier future. (WHO 1986a)

Health promotion involves techniques which enable:

- public policies and programs to be thoroughly evaluated for their beneficial, neutral and harmful health impacts;
- the reinforcement of the capacity of communities to undertake advantageous action at a local level;
- the development of the capacity of health care systems to undertake prevention and health education, and to enhance the informal care given by family;
- the provision of support to people so that they can control and enhance their health through behaviour and lifestyle changes, in addition to

learning how to be more astute consumers of preventative measures and health care services (Mittelmark 2000).

In light of these contemporary developments, we need to consider the nature and scope of health promotion as a political, social and economic process and as a set of strategies for improving the nation's health. The contemporary public health sphere recognises health promotion as an important element in such strategies.

CONCEPTS OF HEALTH AND DISEASE

No introduction to the history of public health and the role of health promotion is complete without some consideration of definitions of health and disease themselves. The occurrence of death and disease can only rarely be described as a matter of chance. They are influenced by a number of determinants, including the social and spatial organisation of a population; the individual's genetic endowment and exposure to a range of risk factors; the physical environment; patterns of relationships and mobility, and access to health services (Perdiguero et al. 2001; Scott 2004). Therefore, to promote health and preclude disease, we must shift our focus from disease itself and expend more of our energies fostering the multifaceted socio-ecological communities to which we belong (Waltner-Toews 2000).

As the nineteenth century became a turbulent battleground for public health reform, theories about the causes of disease continued to be hotly debated. A number of disease theories formed the framework for this debate. The germ (or contagion) theory held that for every disease there was a corresponding pathogen. From a modern point of view, it is difficult to understand that the phenomenon of contagion was not recognised with the first contagious disease. The first clear statement on the existence of micro-organisms was produced by scientist Girolamo Fracastoro of Verona in 1546 (Veith 1982). It was only in the nineteenth century that this theory began to make a decisive impact, when the theory of micro-organisms could be substantiated with the aid of suitable apparatus. By contrast, the environmental theory supported the sanitary reforms that represented the first great revolution in public health. Unfortunately, that support was based on the erroneous belief that illness was a sign of dirty air, or miasma. The theory of divine retribution suggested that a person's illness was a punishment for sinning. Disease as a personal defect was another prominent theory.

As is evident from the discussion above, not all of these theories of disease supported the development of public health interventions. The germ theory tended to support the development of scientific medicine and treatment of the individual, although, with the recognition of contagious diseases, public health measures such as quarantine were introduced. The divine retribution and personal defect theories cited the cause of illness as either spiritual or the individual's class or behaviour. Only the environmental theory of disease can be clearly linked with sanitary reform measures. However, into the early nineteenth century, even though this type of public health strategy improved the health of the population, its use was based on incorrect assumptions about the cause of disease.

The most persistent theory of the nineteenth century—the personal defect theory—had as its core the notion of individual responsibility for illness. While British utilitarian Edwin Chadwick supported the environmental theory of disease and pushed for sanitary reform, the culture of nineteenth-century Britain gave him the opportunity to write about the poor as the population group most often exposed to disease. They were 'less susceptible to moral influences, and the effects of education are more transient than with a healthy population; these adverse circumstances tend to produce an adult population short-lived, improvident, reckless and intemperate, and with habitual avidity to sexual gratification . . .' (Pickett & Hanlon 1990, p. 28).

Despite the persistence of the personal defect theory of disease, by far the most volatile debates during the nineteenth century occurred between the germ theorists and the environmental theorists. Analysis of changing patterns of mortality and morbidity indicates that significant decreases in the rate of death due to infectious diseases can be attributed, in part, to sanitary reforms. In addition, the militancy of the nineteenth-century working class resulted in improved wages and working conditions, along with improved living standards and nutritional status, which significantly heightened people's resistance to micro-organisms in air, food and drinking water. The interrelationship between the two theories of disease is evident when one considers that clean water and proper sewerage are environmental changes that work, in part, because they reduce or eliminate exposure to microbes and, as well, because they make for a generally healthier population.

The ways in which health and illness were defined depended upon a number of different factors. For example, the ways in which professionals define health and illness are different from the ways in which other members of society define them. Across time and cultures, depending on people's concerns, there have always been varied conceptions of health and illness (Waltner-Toews 2000). Although the models of health and illness may vary, these concepts play a defining role, indicating what should, and what should not, be the objects of public health concern. According to Engelhardt (1981, p. 31), the concepts are ambiguous, operating as both explanatory and evolutionary notions. Health and disease are normative as well as descriptive terms. For example, they describe states of affairs, factual conditions, while at the same time presenting them as good or bad. Moreover, health must be defined in regard to particular goals, which raises the question of who selects the goals (Waltner-Toews 2000).

THE ORIGINS OF PUBLIC HEALTH

The public health movement is said to have had its origins in a fundamental change in values that accompanied new concepts of State responsibilities—concepts that preceded the French Revolution (1789–99) and became institutionalised by it (Susser 1981). It was not until the late eighteenth century that public health and disease prevention came into being as a broadly institutionalised practice.

However, measures to protect the health of the public can be traced to much earlier times. For example, in eleventh- and twelfth-century England, laws were passed making it an offence to pollute drinking water. In 1185 Paris became the first city to pave its streets to make it easier to wash away the human waste from the streets and gutters. Early in the fifteenth century, several German cities outlawed hog pens within city limits. Unfortunately, most of these measures failed to significantly curb the epidemics of infectious diseases that periodically swept Europe (Tesh 1982). A forward-thinking perspective on the nature of public health came from the German theorist Ludwig von Seckendorff, who in the 1660s proposed to the German government that a health program be established that would concern itself with:

> . . . the maintenance and supervision of midwives, care of orphans, appointments of physicians and surgeons, protection against plague and other

contagious diseases, excessive use of tobacco and spirituous beverages, inspection of food and water, measures for cleaning and draining towns, maintenance of hospitals, and provision of poor relief. (Pickett & Hanlon 1990, p. 24)

Susser (1981) argued that the rationalising philosophy of the early public health movement in nineteenth-century Britain flowed from a utilitarian philosophy mixed with the liberal idea of 'the maximum good for the maximum number'. For example, the Poor Law of 1832 contained the stringent condition of 'less eligibility', whereby charitable support should always be less attractive to individuals than support acquired by their own labour. The architect of that law was the utilitarian Edwin Chadwick, who was also the executive architect of the early public health movement.

Aside from philosophical debates, other more practical examples from history point to the barriers to effective public health intervention. For example, the ineffectiveness of Britain's original Boards of Health, created during the plague-afflicted fourteenth to seventeenth centuries, in controlling infectious disease was partly due to the limited strategies they had at their disposal. Treatment options were minimal and often dangerous to the patient, and prevention consisted primarily of quarantine. These quarantine measures were resented by the merchants, who understandably wanted to retain the flow of goods and customers. The religious orders also resented the Boards and their powers to ban public congregations during an epidemic.

Thus, it could be argued that the justifications for the shifts in values that occurred in the early public health movement were not just altruistic, although public health was of necessity a reformist and sometimes a radical movement. Certainly, the public health movement was essential for the survival of the burgeoning cities created by nineteenth-century industrial capitalism (Susser 1981). Public health was nevertheless radical in a real sense. The pursuit of community health at a population level was new, and the assumption of State responsibility for maintaining community health was equally so (aside from acute emergencies such as plague or other epidemics). The originality of public health was to attack disease and poverty in the community at large at their perceived source in the environment. Inevitably, conflict arose between the *new ethic* implicit in a definition of health that included public health and the *old ethic* implicit in the one-to-one responsibilities of physicians for individual patients.

Three phases of public health activity

In Europe and North America, three distinct phases of public health activity can be identified over the last 160 years:

- **Public health and environmental change,** as the first distinct phase, began in the industrialised cities of northern Europe in response to high mortality and morbidity rates among the working class. The movement of large numbers of people to the cities, due to the Industrial Revolution, produced a massive change in population patterns and the physical environment. The public health response to this situation was a movement based on the activities of medical officers of health and sanitary inspectors supported by legislation. The focus of the movement was improvements in sanitation and the provision of safe water and food supplies. This public health movement, with its emphasis on environmental change, lasted until the 1870s.
- **Individualism and State involvement,** as the second phase, dated from around 1880 to 1930, represented a more individualistic approach, which was influenced by the development of the germ theory of disease and the possibilities offered by vaccination. As the most pressing environmental problems were brought under control, action to improve the health of the population turned to preventive services such as immunisation and family planning. Later, other initiatives were introduced, including community and school health services. The second phase also represented the increasing involvement of the State through the provision of hospital and clinical services.
- The third phase was the **therapeutic era,** which dated from the 1930s, with the advent of insulin and sulphonamides. The beginning of this era coincided with the decline of infectious diseases and the development of ideas in many developed countries about the welfare state. Historically, it marked a weakening of government departments of public health and a shift of power and resources to hospital-based services. This shift was associated with the impact of diseases on governing elites. A serious infectious disease, such as the bubonic plague, affected the entire population, thus necessitating a greater interest on the part of the middle classes in ensuring protection of the whole population. However, unless directly affected, the middle classes had little interest in the health of the population as a whole (Ashton & Seymour 1990, p. 15).

One of the important factors that sealed the ultimate triumph of a more scientific approach to treatment was its compatibility with the interests of the fast-emerging wealthy classes (Willis 1983). The therapeutic model focused attention on individual pathology and individual therapies designed to cure disease. This biomedical reductionism reinforced the belief that all social problems were caused by illness and that disease had nothing to do with either working conditions or the health hazards associated with poverty. Scientific medicine also promised fast cures for sick workers. As this model came to dominate professional thinking about health, public health practice began to lose most of its vision of social reform. For example, as early as the 1920s, public health messages concentrated on guidelines to healthy living, such as 'don't spit' and 'eat an apple a day'.

Challenges to the therapeutic era

By the 1970s the therapeutic era was increasingly being challenged. The challenge arose from massive increases in health care costs resulting from technological innovation in treatment methods and an apparently limitless demand for medical care. Increases in health care costs were coupled with dramatic demographic changes that were taking place with a very rapid growth in the elderly population. McKeown's (1976) critical analysis of the role of medicine and the medical profession in reducing mortality and morbidity lent support to the growing interest in a reappraisal of priorities.

The decline of infectious diseases in the nineteenth century has been attributed to numerous factors. Scientific medicine, with its discovery of specific germs and development of vaccines and antibiotics, contributed to the decline of some infectious diseases such as smallpox and diphtheria. These diseases, however, were not the leading causes of death in the nineteenth century. Neither were infectious diseases such as cholera and typhoid (apart from periods of epidemic and pandemic) the major or even persistent causes of death. The major causes were tuberculosis, whooping cough, scarlet fever, pneumonia and influenza. The decline of infectious diseases can be attributed also to other factors, such as improved sanitation, better nutrition, improvements in working and living conditions, and family planning. McKeown's (1976) seminal work on the study of death records covering three centuries in the United Kingdom demolished the modern myth that health advances during the nineteenth century could be attributed mainly to medical technology. Szreter's (1988) reanalysis of McKeown's data added a further dimension to our understanding of the social reform, sanitary reform and professional advocacy dimensions that contributed to the decline of infectious diseases.

The rising cost of medical treatment has been critically examined as it no longer provides a significant return in terms of improvements in a population's health status. The increasing intervention of governments in the management and financial support of the health care 'system' has meant that funding of health care inevitably competes with other demands for public spending. It is from this context of cost containment, it is often argued, that the 'healthy lifestyle' movement emerged (see Chapter 2, 'Lifestyle phase').

PUBLIC HEALTH IN AUSTRALIA

The emergence of organised efforts to protect the health of the population (particularly the contribution of governments) presents a picture of the modern history of public health. That picture began with a focus on nineteenth-century Europe and the role of public health in the aftermath of the Industrial Revolution. In Australia, a somewhat different picture emerged, as the first phase of public health intervention, between European settlement and the early 1800s, was marked by British administration of a colony fighting for its survival (O'Connor 1991).

Colonial Australia

The establishment of the British colony in New South Wales, according to Lord Sydney, took place for two primary reasons. First, there was the potential threat of escape of large numbers of prisoners from the overcrowded prisons in England; and second, there was the danger of the breakout of 'infectious distempers' (Historical Records of New South Wales 1892, p. 14). The proposition that the British government established a colony in New South Wales as a dumping ground for its criminals is not the only explanation suggested by Australian historians. Two further propositions can be identified: first, the availability of materials useful to the navy in its activities in the Indian Ocean; and second, that the colony was founded to promote trade with nearby China.

The debate over the reasons for the establishment of the colony clearly demonstrated the multiple roles of the State from the settlement's first conception. It has often been suggested that the State played a particularly important role in Australian history. However, the State that established the first settlement in the late 1700s and the State of the 1850s was not the same institution. The British State was not simply transplanted into the colonies as they developed. While the resources of the British State were obviously involved, and many of its features formed a model for future development, the colonial State departed from the British model in a number of ways. First, departure from the model was evident in the nature of force applied to control the convicts and the Aborigines. Second, it was evident in the degree of power vested in the military, a factor that permeated all aspects of the colony. The reconstruction of the British State in New South Wales and the impact of new environmental and social conditions, dominated by the penal nature of the colony, had a unique impact on patterns of mortality and morbidity.

A complex range of factors contributed to rises and falls in patterns of mortality and morbidity in the colonial population. Biological factors, such as transmissibility of infections, increased population density, and the creation of a permanent infectious disease 'pool' impacted on patterns of colonial mortality and morbidity. Furthermore, the introduction of 'new diseases' decimated segments of the population, for example Indigenous Australians, who were more susceptible to diseases to which their communities had not previously been exposed. Resistance levels among the colonists also fluctuated, particularly those of infants and children (O'Connor 1991, p. 402). However, biology was not the direct determinant of the health of the colonial population; it was mediated by the colonial society's social organisation, its administration and economic development, and colonial beliefs about disease causation and the actions needed to promote health.

Influences on public health development

There have been several important influences on the development of public health in Australia. Lewis (1989) articulates six major influences at the national level. These are similar to general themes identifiable in public health development overseas, but are modified by the fact of Australian society having commenced its life as a convict colony.

The first of Lewis's influences was the existence of an ideology in which State promotion of national efficiency and national development figured prominently in the late nineteenth and early twentieth centuries. Efficiency, although not easily defined, meant something like the purposeful application of expert or scientific knowledge to economic, social and political spheres of national life in order to advance the power and effectiveness of the nation in a world of competitive nation-states and empires. Many believed that basic to this entire endeavour was the 'physical efficiency' of the population. A more positive government, guided and promoted by an elite group of experts, was advocated if the nation was to survive class conflict at home and international conflict abroad.

Bureaucratic ascendancy in Australian society was the second major influence on public health development. Like all modern societies, Australia experienced the inexorable growth of bureaucracy consequent upon the expansion of State functions. The uniqueness of the Australian situation was that ascendancy was established in the colonial period well before the political centralisation resulting from the Second World War. In colonial Australia the lack of a leisured middle class ready to give time to public affairs meant that reliance was placed on bureaucrats for rule-making and arbitrative functions. Since colonial times, highly successful bureaucrats have both created and administered policy in public health (Lewis 1989).

The third influence was the structure of the Australian government and the constitutional division of powers between the federal and state governments. During the ten years following federation of the Australian colonies the Commonwealth was obliged, under the Constitution, to give back to the states three-quarters of its revenue, thus greatly retarding the growth of its own administration. State jealousies and the difficulty of constitutional amendment blocked formal legal extension of Australian government functions, including health-related activities. However, in the relatively prosperous 1920s some growth of functions—notably in health, scientific research and overseas marketing—took place via extra-constitutional and bureaucratic means.

The fourth influence on public health development was the existence of a well organised and politically sophisticated medical profession, devoted to private practice of medicine and to professional independence from the State. However, the profession was ready to sanction State intervention, not only in the traditional public health sphere but also in health care, if the intervention was on terms it found acceptable.

The existence of a reformist Labor Party, struggling in a capitalist economy with a government policy of collective responsibility and equitable access in health matters, was the fifth major influencing factor. At the same time, conservative parties were emphasising individual responsibility in a contributory insurance approach to health.

The advance of scientific knowledge in medicine and public health was Lewis's sixth influence. The prominence of bacteriology in the last two decades of the nineteenth century shifted the focus of public health from the sanitary environment to the identification of infectious disease in the individual and to control by isolation and later by mass vaccination.

The evolution of new disciplines in modern laboratory-based medicine, the development of powerful new diagnostic techniques and the production of new therapeutic agents gave curative medicine in the early 1920s totally unpredicted effectiveness. However, new technologically intensive medicine was much more costly and increasingly sited in the hospital. At the same time that the new, more effective preventive medicine was pushing the State towards responsibility for the health of all individuals, more effective but more expensive curative medicine was creating conditions requiring greater State intervention to finance hospitals and the technological infrastructure needed for the new therapies.

As noted above, most of the themes identified by Lewis within Australia were also evident at an international level. Certainly, the fundamental stages in the development of public health and the emergence of conflict between public health activity and the activities of curative medicine were evident in Australia as in other developed countries.

Phases of public health development

The phases of development delineated by Gordon (1976) and Lewis (1989) represent the significant eras in public health in Australia over the past 200 years. While Gordon outlined six phases and Lewis four, their analyses are similar. For example, both authors identified a colonial period, followed by a second period marked by the introduction of legislative and quarantine procedures, and periods that saw the development of Australian government and state departments of health. Both Gordon and Lewis commented on periods of development marked by the provision of preventive health services, education on prevention and the creation of a national health service. Baum's (2004) analysis is similar to that of both Gordon and Lewis, with the exception of the inclusion of an 'Indigenous era'. These phases are summarised below.

PHASES IN PUBLIC HEALTH DEVELOPMENT IN AUSTRALIA

Gordon's six phases

One: Colonial medical officers. Quarantine and vaccination.

Two: Health Acts based on *English Act* of 1875. Part-time local authority medical officers of health, and health inspectors at local authority level.

Three: Infectious disease outbreaks lead to government action. Expert medical officers in public health. Public health commissioners employed by states.

Four: New public health activities—for example, support for breastfeeding, scientific inspection of food, general examinations for schoolchildren, VD clinics. Public health commissioners appointed. Limited local authority involvement. Local councils' environmental sanitation and infectious disease control, supervised by health commissioners.

Five: State health departments. Medical officers involved in preventive clinical activities. School health and VD clinics; maternal and child welfare in early 1920s, voluntary agencies involved from early twentieth century. Advisers in industrial medicine appointed from US after First World War. Massive campaign against tuberculosis in 1940s and 1950s. Education on prevention of communicable diseases, nutrition, antenatal care.

Six: State-developed child guidance clinics and geriatric services. Education about prevention—for example, heart disease, cancer and road accidents.

Source: Adapted from Gordon (1976)

Lewis's four phases

One: Public health measures in the Australian colonies, providing a backdrop to developments at the national level involving activities of the colonial government.

Two: Federation. Quarantine up to First World War. Public health as pursued by the states focuses on prevention and control of disease in individuals and concerns itself, albeit in a way that does not trespass on the preserves of private practice, with the health of particular groups of signal importance to the productive and reproductive health of the community—essentially mothers and children and, to a lesser extent, industrial workers.

Three: Establishment and growth of Federal Health Department, First World War to 1930s. (Federal government persuaded by J.H.L. Cumpston to create the department; on the narrow constitutional base of quarantine power, the aim is to promote national public health development through the device of 'cooperative federalism'.)

Four: Creation of a national health service. During Second World War, attempts made to translate notions of greater collective responsibility for health care into concrete schemes. Public health doctor/bureaucrats put forward a plan for a national health service which is State-financed, provides for universal access, and integrates preventive and curative medicine, but does not eliminate private practice.

Source: Adapted from Lewis (1989)

Baum's six phases

One: Indigenous era: connections to the land, spirituality and the integration of health and life highlighted. The practice of traditional healers is an established part of the culture.

Two: Colonial era: control of infectious diseases, and the provision of safe water, and sanitation, which is enforced by public health and quarantine acts.

Three: Nation-building era: establishment of Commonwealth Department of Health. Organised exercise programs, medical examinations for children, hygiene advice for the population.

Four: Affluence, medicine and infrastructure: State intervention in 'non-health' sectors that influence health; growth of hospitals and technologies. Limited emphasis on public health.

Five: Lifestyle era: focus on chronic disease, and lifestyle factors and individual behaviour, and concomitant lifestyle interventions.

Beginnings of women's, Aboriginal and community health movements.

Six: New public health era: led by WHO policies, with an emphasis on poverty and equity. Growth of healthy public policy and legislation. Development of 'settings' approaches.

Source: Adapted from Baum (2004)

For the public health and health promotion practitioner, the importance of recognising these phases relates to developing an understanding of the changing and expanding nature of Australian public health activity over some 200 years. Public health students should appreciate the significant factors that have helped to shape contemporary public health activity. Components of many of these phases continue in present-day public health practices. Some components, such as legislative and policy initiatives, have re-emerged as prominent aspects of contemporary public health activity.

Although the various phases of public health activity in Australia have had some unique features, such as colonialism and the role of the State in the administration and provision of health services, overall the public health initiatives of developed countries have displayed a number of common themes. These themes are explored in the final section of this chapter as an introduction to the competing approaches that influence contemporary public health and health promotion.

THE EMERGENCE OF CONTEMPORARY PUBLIC HEALTH

The changing nature of public health roles and responsibilities, particularly over the past 160 years, has inevitably led to conflict between public health authorities and a range of other institutions and groups. For example, the authorities have met opposition from religious groups and others holding 'moral' objections to State intervention, and there has been opposition to public health measures from business circles anxious to protect their financial interests.

At the end of the nineteenth century, both the moral and economic boundaries of public health were at issue as public health agencies intruded into activities that the medical profession believed to be rightly its own.

This conflict has long antecedents, but it was intensified by an historic convergence between medicine and public health (Starr 1982).

The impact of scientific development further intensified the conflict between medicine and public health. As public health authorities gradually developed a more precise conception of the sources and models of transmission of infectious diseases and concentrated on combating particular pathogenic organisms, attention shifted from the environment to the individual. This meant that public health exponents increasingly came to rely on the techniques of medicine and personal hygiene (Starr 1982, p. 181). The shift in attention and priorities towards mothers and children and the reproductive process greatly sharpened the conflict between public health and individual medical practice. This was because it led to the intrusion of public health into individual care through antenatal and well-baby clinics (Susser 1981, p. 102).

Such shifts in priorities towards preventive care for mothers and their children entailed a change in the *type* of operations that were considered legitimate for public health—not just a change in the targets of these operations. An ethical justification became available for public health action in personal as well as community health. The road was open for action directed towards health that had as its central concern the personal behaviours of individuals. These personal behaviours became the subject of scientific judgments about the protection of the public's health.

Three contemporary approaches

While conflict between the various interest groups involved in public health seems a constant, at least three different contemporary approaches to public health can be described. These approaches provide an insight into the changing face of the politics of health. They have been described as the 'individual responsibility' model, the 'old public health' model and the 'new public health' model (Legge 1989). They are contentious theoretical descriptions, and many commentators on public health have argued that all three paradigms are essential to improve and maintain the public's health (McMichael 1993). A similar set of theoretical paradigms used to describe health promotion activity is covered in Chapter 2 (see 'The role of health promotion in public health'); here, a brief introduction to each model will set the scene for later discussion. The models are not discussed in any chronological order, as each continues to play a role in contemporary public health.

The 'individual responsibility' model focuses on the extent to which the individual looks after his or her health, and to a lesser degree on the chance influences affecting the individual's health. Caring for one's health then becomes largely a matter of personal choice—or parental or carer choice in the case of children and the elderly. Access to adequate food and shelter, sufficient knowledge about healthy behaviours, and public health protection are considered to be widely available to the majority of the population. Legge (1989, p. 472) suggested that the model 'overlooks', or assumes as inevitable, the economic and social inequalities that affect health chances. One of the consequences of focusing on individual responsibility is that other people's health is not seen as the concern of the individual, thus denying any level of collective responsibility for health. The most likely setting for this model lies within the culture of the clinic and the hospital (Legge 1989).

The 'old public health' model is based on the discipline of epidemiology and the subject matter of the biomedical and behavioural sciences (Holman 1992). It analyses causes of disease in terms of 'factors' in the individual and in the social and physical environments. Strategies are aimed at interrupting the 'chain of causation', with the traditional tools being education, the provision of services and legislation (Legge 1989).

At first the major concerns—and the greatest triumphs—of public health occurred in relation to the physical environment and occupational hazards (for example, water, sewage, food, working conditions and housing) associated with the Industrial Revolution of the nineteenth century. The main concern of public health activities over the last century has often been said to encompass strategies to counter the development of 'lifestyle diseases'. Public health interventions dealing with such diseases have demonstrated success in reducing mortality and morbidity. For example, clinical, educational, policy and legislative strategies have combined to achieve reduced mortality from cardiovascular disease over the last three decades—although evidence is scant as to the level of contribution of each strategy to the overall reduction in mortality.

The strengths and limitations of the 'old public health' model are evident when compared with the 'individual responsibility' model. For example, the former focuses on both collective and individual responsibility for illness prevention—the factors that determine the boundary between collective and individual responsibility being determined mainly on the basis of the risks and cost to the rest of the community.

Legge's critique of the 'old public health' is based on its three key issues: the knowledge–action gap; social isolation and the limits of support services; and economic inequalities in health. Legge argued that health education, as one of the three key strategies in the 'old public health', makes important assumptions about knowledge as a precondition of behaviour change. He suggested that a political science of health should account for the knowledge–action gap (Legge 1989, p. 475). Others have argued that this analysis is a simplistic representation of health education and that it has always recognised multifactorial influences on health behaviour (Green & Raeburn 1988, 1990).

The second key issue in Legge's critique of the 'old public health' is the relationship between social isolation and a range of illnesses. He believed that the 'old public health' failed to provide a framework for 'understanding social isolation and lack of support within a broader economic and cultural framework'. Further, it failed to address the underlying structural issues, as well as compensating for lack of social support (1989, p. 476).

The third key issue centred on the limited recognition given to the contribution of economic inequalities to ill health—inequalities that require a health policy response. Legge suggested that, to a large degree, the observed inequalities in health in the 'old public health' are not directly attributable to lack of economic resources. Paradoxically, he suggested, the effectiveness of public health campaigns conducted over thirty years have actually exacerbated existing inequalities. He argued for 'a framework for understanding inequalities in health within a broader political context, and for addressing the underlying structural issues' (1989, p. 477).

The 'new public health' model represents a significant paradigm shift when compared with the 'old public health' model (Kickbusch 1989a). In particular, it shifts the focus from behaviour change to a healthy public policy, and it replaces the lifestyle approach with the notion of enhancing life skills (McPherson 1992) (see Chapter 2, 'Defining the new public health—and beyond').

Holman has identified five 'new public health' movements, which he argues should coexist in a comprehensive approach to program planning and professional training in public health. These five movements (and, therefore, five strategic approaches) to health advancement are described as health protection, preventive medicine, health education, healthy public policy and community empowerment (Holman 1992, p. 4).

Holman suggested that the dichotomy between the 'old public health' and the 'new public health' 'is a poor substitute for a wealth of history that underlies current public health theory and practice' (1992, p. 9). Holman offered an alternative concept of 'total public health', a comprehensive approach representing 'an organised and fully integrated application of all effective knowledge and skills' (1992, p. 10).

While there continues to be critical debate about the 'old public health' and the 'new public health', placing public health within a broader social framework has also been advocated. Both of these public health models have been compared and contrasted with more generally oriented community development and social change movements. In these social movements, health advancement is located outside a public health framework and within a more general set of human goals (Catford 1991; Labonte 1992a; Nutbeam 1993b).

The comprehensive approach advocated by Holman clearly challenges public health practitioners to work towards a single set of goals using a wide range of available strategies and approaches. It remains to be seen how important the ultimate goals are to public health practitioners and just how deep the differences between proponents of 'traditional' public health and the 'new public health' have become. It also remains to be seen how broadly these social movements can influence public health approaches.

The future success of public health will be determined by developments that enhance public health approaches and acknowledge that individual and population wellbeing is dependent on the total health of our environment—that is, ecological public health, which offers an holistic framework, encompassing the environmental and economic determinants of health, and the sustainable use of resources (WHO 1998).

REVIEW

This chapter covered a wide range of issues that have affected contemporary public health practice. The multiplicity of factors contributing to the history of public health and the phases marking its evolution were discussed. Substantial changes in the way in which public health has been defined over the centuries were highlighted. Changes in values about advancement of the public's health and the consequent redefinitions of public health activity instigated the new phases. In many instances, public health interventions have been justified in terms of altruistic appeals to health needs, but they have often harnessed forces far from altruistic in nature. Judgments about the nature and role of public health activity are constantly being made through a choice of priorities compatible with our definition of health.

In Australia and other developed Western nations, common themes have appeared in the history of public health. These themes include the sanitary revolution, the change towards an individualistic approach to health and health care, and the so-called therapeutic era. In contemporary discussions about public health a new paradigm has emerged that integrates environmental change and personal preventive measures with appropriate therapeutic interventions. In our dealing with the inevitable periods of conflict in the evolution of public health, Holman (1992) encourages us to use all available strategies in a comprehensive approach to program planning and professional training.

REVISION

Consider the main issues addressed in this chapter. Review each of these points in light of your understanding of the history of public health and the emergence of the 'new public health' and 'ecological public health'.

1. How do concepts of health and disease influence public health practice, and what is the relationship between these concepts and definitions of public health?
2. What are the main themes in the history of public health, both internationally and in Australia?
3. How has public health evolved, and where does the notion of the 'new public health' fit in?
4. What are the three main models of public health, and how has each model contributed to the history of public health?
5. What is 'ecological public health' and what new aspects/issues does it support?

2

Ecological public health and health promotion

Is there a 'new public health'? If so, how can it be defined? How does it differ from the 'old public health'? What role does health promotion play in the new public health, if any, and how can it play a role in achieving 'Health For All in the 21st century'? Have we gone beyond the new public health into what McPherson (1992) described as an 'ecological public health' phase? These questions are the focus of this chapter.

As we saw in Chapter 1, the term 'old public health' refers to a world view developed in the nineteenth century, one that has continued to provide the context for much of the research and public health initiatives. The classification of this tradition as 'old' arises because of the increasing development towards what has been termed the 'new public health' and, more recently, 'ecological public health' (Baum 2004; Catford 2004).

INTERNATIONAL DEVELOPMENTS

The World Health Organization (WHO) has played a leading role in articulating and promoting the new public health. This movement has gathered momentum since the 1970s with the WHO providing a substantial international forum for the broad concept of 'Health For All' (McPherson 1992, p. 119) and associated new public health and health promotion initiatives.

McPherson (1992, p. 120) neatly classified the WHO initiatives since 1977 into four conceptual phases: the **primary health care phase** of the late 1970s, marked by the Declaration of Alma-Ata; the 'health field concept' and the **lifestyle phase** of the early 1980s, with an important role for health education and a recognition of the mediating role between the social and physical environment and the health of the individual; the **new public health phase** of the mid to late 1980s; and the **ecological public health phase** from the late 1980s to the present time. In this section, we consider the first two of McPherson's phases. In the following section, 'Defining the new public health—and beyond', the nature and scope of the new public health and the emergence of an ecological public health phase are addressed.

Primary health care phase

In Geneva in 1977, the WHO indicated that 'the main social targets of governments and the WHO in the coming decades should be the attainment by all the citizens of the world, by the year 2000, of a level of health that will permit them to lead a socially and economically productive life' (1981, p. 9). Acknowledging the unacceptably high levels of poor health of millions of people in the world, the WHO called for a new approach to health and health care in order to achieve a more equitable distribution of health resources (WHO/UNICEF 1978). In 1978, the WHO and UNICEF held a major international conference on primary health care attended by representatives from 134 nations. The outcome of the conference was the Declaration of Alma-Ata. A year later, the World Health Assembly formally adopted the Declaration of Alma-Ata. Subsequently, governments and health groups throughout the world employed the slogan 'Health For All by the Year 2000'.

The Declaration recognised that inequalities in health are deeply embedded in the way society works—economically, politically and culturally—and called for collaboration across sectors as part of a new vision of primary health care (Legge 1989). The Declaration contained a number of important principles that provide cornerstones for action within the new public health. In particular, principles such as equity and social justice, intersectoral collaboration, community participation and empowerment, and health promotion and disease prevention were highlighted.

The 'Health For All' slogan attempted to draw attention to inequalities in health and to the goal of bringing health within the reach of everyone. It is clear that the determinants of health are extremely complex and deeply embedded within society. This means that attempts to reduce inequalities in health will involve, by necessity, social, economic and political intervention, as well as public health measures.

Lifestyle phase

One of the most substantial contributions to the transformation in thinking about health in the past thirty years has been the document *A New Perspective on the Health of Canadians* (Lalonde 1974). The Lalonde Report, as it is known, has been both praised and criticised; it has been criticised because it focused too much on lifestyle and not enough on the influence of social, economic and political environments on the health of the population. The lifestyle approach, with its focus on individual behaviours, led to blaming of the victim and failed to address the question of why unhealthy behaviours and lifestyles occurred in the first place (McPherson 1992, p. 121). In order to counter this focus on the individual as the source of ill health, the WHO European member countries redefined 'lifestyle' as 'patterns of behaviour choices made from alternatives that are available to people according to their socioeconomic circumstances and to the ease with which they are able to choose certain ones over others' (Kickbusch 1986b, p. 118).

Despite its emphasis on lifestyle, the Lalonde Report was the first major government initiative to acknowledge publicly that the health care system was not the most important factor in determining health status. The 'health field' concept, as it came to be known, with its concern with lifestyle, environment, socioeconomic factors and the health care system, was subsequently developed at a conference held in Toronto in 1984. This event moved the concept towards a clearer recognition of the relationship between health and environment (McPherson 1992, p. 112).

The concept of the 'health field' has been widely copied, modified and expanded. Similar national health reports were later published in the United States, Great Britain, Sweden and elsewhere. Hancock, commenting on major achievements in advancing the health of Canadians since the Lalonde Report and on its far-reaching international impact, concluded:

> More sophisticated and comprehensive models of the determinants of health are available; national health goals and strategies have been developed in a number of countries; our concepts of health promotion have moved well beyond 'victim blaming' lifestyle approaches to multi-faceted, community-based approaches; there is increasing interest in the health implications of public policy in non-health policy sectors and a more positive vision of health has been articulated. (1986, p. 93)

DEFINING THE NEW PUBLIC HEALTH—AND BEYOND

The main concern of the First International Conference on Health Promotion (Ottawa, Canada, 1986) was the move towards a new public health. The meeting produced a charter for action to achieve 'Health For All by the Year 2000'—and beyond. The Ottawa Charter specified essentials for health including freedom from war, a stable ecosystem, equity and resources such as education and income. Important strategies to improve health included building healthy public policy, creating supportive environments, strengthening community actions, developing personal skills and reorienting health services (WHO 1986a). Consequently, the charter emphasised the role of systems, institutions and communities, in addition to individual abilities and behaviours, in producing options and possibilities for the attainment of health. The conference and the resulting charter built on the progress made through the declaration of primary health care at Alma-Ata, through the WHO's *Targets For Health For All* document (WHO 1986b), and through the debate at the abovementioned World Health Assembly on intersectoral action for health.

The new public health

The Ottawa Charter (1986a) has been described as the first document to articulate the agenda for the new public health (Ashton et al. 1986). As we saw in Chapter 1, some authors have argued that the dichotomy between the 'old' and the 'new' public health disregards the wealth of history that underlies current theory and practice and prevents due attention being given to a comprehensive approach to public health theory and practice (Holman 1992, p. 9). McPherson defined the changing focus of public health activity in the 1980s in the following way:

> Known as the new public health, policy replaced behaviour as the centre of attention, and the lifestyle approach was replaced by the notion of enhancing life skills. It has regained the political base, which it had in its sanitary phase at the turn of the century, and its focus now includes the socioeconomic factors that impinge on people. It has rejoined its environmental base and the focus is on social systems in which people live. (McPherson 1992, p. 123)

The Second International Conference on Health Promotion (Adelaide, 1988) explored in greater depth 'building healthy public policy' as a key action area of the Ottawa Charter, and reaffirmed the principles of primary health care. As a context for health promotion action encouraging healthier lifestyles, healthy public policy occupies a unique position: it provides a framework within which strategic advances can be made in relation to personal development, public participation and healthy environments. Public policies in all sectors have some bearing on health and are an important agency for decreasing social and economic injustice, for example by facilitating equal access to resources, in addition to health services. The conference produced the Adelaide Recommendations, which necessitate a commitment to health by all sectors. Four priority areas for action were identified: supporting the health of women; improving food security, safety and nutrition; cutting tobacco and alcohol use; and creating supportive environments for health (WHO 1988).

Further developments in the new public health emerged from the Third International Conference on Health Promotion, entitled *Supportive Environments for Health* (Sundsvall, Sweden, 1991). This conference continued the link—established in the first conference in Canada—with the sequence of events that began with the WHO's commitment to the goals of 'Health For All' (WHO/UNICEF 1978). One of the four priority areas identified for action at the second conference, 'creating supportive environments for health', was the focus of the third international conference. The conference identified war, fast population growth, insufficient food, being deprived of the instruments of self determination, and the destruction of natural resources as some of the factors detrimental to wellbeing. The Sundsvall conference brought together a wide range of people to consider the interface between the environment and health. While no binding agreements were reached at Sundsvall, Nutbeam (1993b) argued that the conference statement clearly articulated a focus on public health and health promotion. The statement highlighted the international community's need to take action to create supportive environments for health—to relieve the crushing impact of social and economic conditions and the degradation of the physical environment on people in developing and developed countries alike (WHO/United Nations Environment Program 1991).

The Fourth International Conference on Health Promotion (Jakarta, Indonesia, 1997) had partnerships and settings as prominent themes. Building new alliances for health, including those with private sector partners, was a major theme. The private for-profit sector had a strong presence in Jakarta and there was considerable disquiet among some delegates about the lack of opportunity to discuss some of the ethical and other issues associated with involving the for-profit sector (Baum 1998). On a positive note, the conference reaffirmed the principles of the Ottawa Charter and set out a series of priorities for health promotion in the 21st century. These included promoting social responsibility for health, increasing investments for health development in all sectors, consolidating and expanding partnerships for health, increasing community participation and empowering the individual, and securing an infrastructure for health promotion (Baum 1998).

The Fifth Global Conference on Health Promotion—entitled *Health Promotion: Bridging the Equity Gap* (Mexico City, 2000)—extended the developments of the preceding four conferences, especially advancing the priorities of the fourth conference (WHO 2000). Equity issues became central to the health promotion concept and were also a theme of the previous conferences. Insight as to the basis of health inequities had advanced considerably; nevertheless, social and economic inequalities persisted. Accordingly, the fifth conference concentrated on reducing this disparity, both within and between countries (WHO 2000). The conference brought together politicians and other key decision-makers from both health and non-health sectors; representatives from development agencies, non-governmental organisations, community-based organisations and the private sector; and professionals from various fields, representing the diverse sectors of society that are accountable for, or have an effect on, the determinants of health (WHO 2000). Member States and societies as a whole were exhorted to implement the following action principles:

- strengthen the evidence base for health promotion
- increase investments for health development
- promote social responsibility for health
- increase community capacity and empower individuals and communities
- secure an infrastructure for health promotion
- reorient health systems and services with health promotion criteria (WHO 2000).

The Charter of the Sixth Global Conference on Health Promotion (WHO 2005a) identified actions and undertakings requisite to addressing the determinants of health in a globalised world. The main aims of the charter are summed up as follows: 'The Bangkok Charter affirms that policies and partnerships to empower communities, and to improve health and health equality, should be at the centre of global and national development' (WHO 2005a, p. 1). The Bangkok Charter built on the health promotion philosophies and strategies instituted by the Ottawa Charter (WHO 1986a), and sought to involve people, groups and organisations vital to the achievement of health, including:

- governments and politicians at all levels
- civil society
- the private sector
- international organisations
- the public health community.

The conference delegates reiterated that every person has a basic right to attain the highest possible standard of health. At the conference it was determined that health promotion is founded on this key human right, and the charter advocated a constructive and comprehensive view of health as a determinant of the quality of life. A core mission of public health was established as health promotion and the part it plays in controlling threats to health. It was recognised that the worldwide milieu for health promotion had considerably altered since the Ottawa Charter. Major factors now influencing health included:

- increasing inequalities within and between countries
- new patterns of consumption and communication
- commercialisation
- global environmental change
- urbanisation.

The conference identified additional influences on health, comprising demographic, social and financial transformations that influence employment, educational settings, family arrangements, and community mores. The marginalisation and powerlessness of women, children, disabled and indigenous peoples was noted as having increased. Globalisation was seen to introduce innovative possibilities for collaboration to advance health, including improved information and communication systems. To handle the problems of globalisation, the delegates laid down that policy needs to be consistent through all levels of governments, United Nations bodies, and other organisations, including the private sector (WHO 2005a).

The Bangkok Charter laid out that to improve the application of these policies, it is essential for all sectors and settings to:

- **advocate** for health based on human rights and solidarity
- **invest** in sustainable policies, actions and infrastructure to address the determinants of health
- **build capacity** for policy development, leadership, health promotion practice, knowledge transfer and research, and health literacy
- **regulate and legislate** to ensure a high level of protection from harm and enable equal opportunity for health and wellbeing for all people
- **partner and build alliances** with public, private, non-governmental and international organisations and civil society to create sustainable actions (WHO 2005a).

In examining the historical evolution of the new public health, it is clear that healthy public policy is the cornerstone of the new movement. According to Palmer and Short (1989, p. 50), this 'social' movement links traditional public health concerns (which tended to focus on physical aspects of the environment such as clean air and water, food, infection control, and occupational health and safety legislation) with broader social, environmental and economic factors. The new public health movement emphasises both the need to draw on knowledge from different perspectives and the importance of a social movement as a stimulus, support and base. This means that healthy public policy is not solely a health activity conducted by professionals. The loose network of groups and individuals that share the healthy public policy philosophy tend to emphasise health promotion, community participation and intersectoral collaboration. An intersectoral approach requires coordination of policies and actions in trying to achieve the maximum positive impact on the health of a community. It requires cooperation between governments, government departments, the private sector and non-government organisations in developing healthy public policies.

The new public health, as promoted by the WHO, represents a signifi-cant paradigm shift vis-à-vis the old public health. It remains, however, essentially health-centred, justifying initiatives such as those contained in the Ottawa Charter and the Jakarta Declaration on the grounds of the health outcomes they are expected to produce. When we compare and contrast these public health models with more generally oriented com-munity development and social change movements, we see that health advancement can be located within a broader set of human goals (Legge 1989, p. 482). When health advancement is thus located, the justification for health initiatives may not always rest on the basis of health outcomes but rather on the basis of broader objectives such as social change.

AN ECOLOGY OF PUBLIC HEALTH

In concert with these international health promotion conferences, there has been a growing public concern over threats to the global environment. McPherson suggests that this linking of the public health 'together with the concept of sustainable development, recognises that development must operate within the parameters of available resources and the productive potential of the ecosystem' (1992, p. 124).

The World Commission on the Environment and Development (WCED), in its report *Our Common Future* (1987), clearly focused on the need to develop an understanding of the imperative of sustainable develop-ment. It defined sustainable development as 'meeting the needs of the present generation without compromising the ability of future generations to meet their own needs' (WCED 1987). In more recent times, it has become clear that an economic imperative can quickly reduce the gains made by the environmental movement. For example, the United Nations Conference on the Environment and Development—the Earth Summit— held in Rio de Janeiro in 1992 clearly produced a commitment on the part of governments to a range of actions to protect and repair the physical environment. However, it was notable that several prominent nations failed to support proposed broad-based changes to protect the environ- ment (Nutbeam 1993b). It is clear that in working for supportive environments for health we must utilise a model of public health advocacy that does more than articulate the problem. Any such model should provide solutions that mediate between the conflicting interests of health, the environment and the economy (Nutbeam 1993b).

Catford (1991), however, cautions health promoters to be wary of emphasising environmental health issues only because of their impact on human health. He argues that we need to share and understand the issues raised by professionals and activists in other fields who have a concern for the preservation of the environment for reasons other than health if we are to form broad coalitions of mutual support and action. Other authors have discussed the degradation of the global environment as the third major challenge for health promotion (Brown et al. 1992, p. 219). Meeting this challenge, according to Brown et al. (1992, pp. 226–8), will mean a radical reorientation of the field of health promotion in terms of the contri- bution that health promotion can make to environmental management. The authors argue for the use of existing health promotion strategies, such as protection, prevention, resilience and adaptation, as options for managing environmental change (1992, p. 228).

In Australia, the revised *National Health Goals and Targets* (Nutbeam et al. 1993c) contains a section on creating 'healthy environments'. In that section, six environments are separately considered: the physical environ- ment; transport; housing; work; schools; and health care settings. The authors of the report indicate that in developing targets for change and improvement in these environments, they have tried first to reflect existing strategies and priorities and then identified opportunities for health advancement within such a framework (Nutbeam et al. 1993c).

Linking sustainable development with healthy public policy, Kickbusch (1989a, p. 12) described public health as 'ecological in perspective, multi- sectoral in scope and collaborative in strategy'. With the emergence of an ecological model of health, which recognises the inextricable links between people and their environment (Catford 2004), the practice of public health has shifted further towards recognition of the social, political and economic realities.

A fundamental aspect of ecological public health is environmental health and the provision of basic requirements for life. For example, the public health impact of natural disasters and, therefore, their management have been recognised as an important priority of the public health system. The health needs of populations immediately following natural disasters are urgent and significant, with the two main areas of priority for health requirements being:

- the provision of adequate safe drinking water, basic sanitation facilities, waste disposal and adequate shelter;
- the provision of food protection measures, instituting or continuing vector control procedures (for example mosquito control) and the promotion of personal hygiene (PAHO 2000).

The following case study illustrates the necessity of providing fundamental services immediately following such a disaster.

THE INDIAN OCEAN TSUNAMI, 2004

On 26 December 2004, an earthquake measuring 9.0 on the Richter scale caused a tsunami that devastated twelve countries* surrounding the Indian Ocean, and affected many more. With so many people still unaccounted for, the death toll for the whole area is likely to be more than 286 000 (COEDMHA 2005). The tsunami displaced more than one million people and left five million people without essential services.

Following the tsunami, cholera and other waterborne diseases became a considerable threat (AusAID 2005), and it was feared displacement and overcrowding would lead to an increase in the risk of measles, tuberculosis, meningitis and respiratory diseases (WHO 2005c).

The infrastructure that existed before any such disaster affects both the magnitude of destruction and the ability to recover afterwards (World Vision Resource Centre 2005). When such a disaster occurs, the loss of life is much higher in developing countries than in developed countries, and many more people could die due to the breakdown and/or lack of infrastructure and the consequent lack of access to basic services. In addition, malnutrition is of increasing concern, as people whose nutritional status is already inadequate are more at risk from infectious disease and its associated mortality (WHO 2005c). The high priority needs are for preventative public health measures (including sanitation and clean water), medical care, food, shelter and clothing (WHO 2005c).

Following such a disaster, it is essential that aid organisations are able to assess needs, act quickly and coordinate their efforts with each other, in order to provide rapid and appropriate assistance to those in need.

The tsunami has had a considerable impact on the most vulnerable populations such as children, women, the elderly, the sick and disabled, the poor, and those in more remote areas (Clay 2005; WHO 2005c).

Catastrophic natural disasters are more likely to gain people's attention and eclipse the less dramatic long-term development work. While responding to the urgent needs of the affected populations was seen as crucial, it was also viewed as critical that longer-term reconstruction, development and rehabilitation begin (Clay 2005; United Nations 2005), and the tsunami's effect on the longer-term Millennium Development Goals (MDGs) be alleviated (United Nations 2005). The Millennium Declaration, launched in 2000, is an agenda for global development that sets out a plan for halving global poverty by 2015. The Millennium Declaration has eight measurable goals, comprising issues such as hunger, gender equity, safe drinking water, and sanitation. All 191 member States of the United Nations have endorsed these goals (United Nations 2005).

Disaster aid should consider the requirements of long-term community development whenever feasible. This means developing approaches that will address the emergency needs of communities, as well as improving their resilience and capacity to recover and flourish in the long term (World Vision Resource Centre 2005).

* Bangladesh, India, Indonesia, Kenya, Malaysia, Maldives, Myanmar, Seychelles, Somalia, Sri Lanka, Tanzania, Thailand

THE AUSTRALIAN PERSPECTIVE

'Health For All by the Year 2000' was first discussed at the national level at the 1983 Conference of Australian Health Ministers—although, as a signatory to the Declaration of Alma-Ata, Australia had formally committed itself to the concept in 1981. National developments presented below are discussed chronologically.

Advancing Australia's health

In 1984 the Australian federal and state governments prepared a draft national strategy document titled *Advancing Australia's Health: Towards national strategies and objectives for health advancement*. The document included sections on overall health goals, priority areas for action, strategies and measures, and management information considerations. The nature and extent of contemporaneous problems were used to identify priority subject areas for examination. Measures for prevention and promotion were also identified, as were targets and policy options to achieve 'Health For All' by the year 2000.

The Better Health Commission

Developments at the national level saw the establishment of the Better Health Commission by the Australian government in 1985. The commission's report (1986) set out to identify national health goals for Australia. The commission was established to investigate and report on the current health status of the Australian population, to identify factors underlying health problems, and to formulate recommendations on ways to address these (Nutbeam et al. 1993c, p. 7). The commission recommended national health goals for cardiovascular disease, nutrition and injury (Better Health Commission 1986).

Health For All Australians

A Health Targets and Implementation Committee was subsequently established by the Australian Health Ministers' Advisory Council. In 1988, the committee produced a report, *Health For All Australians*. The committee's mandate was setting national health goals and the development of an administrative mechanism to implement prevention and health promotion policy. The report set goals and targets in three general categories: population groups; major causes of illness and death; and risk factors. There were five priority areas for action:

- control of high blood pressure
- improved nutrition
- injury prevention
- health of older people
- prevention of cancer, particularly lung, skin, breast and cervical cancers (Health Targets and Implementation Committee 1988).

The report proposed the establishment of a national program for better health that would plan, implement and manage strategies for achievement of the nominated goals and targets. It also proposed a close examination and reorientation of major structural areas of the health system to allow the recommended changes to take place.

Since its publication, a number of strengths and weaknesses of *Health For All Australians* have been identified and discussed. Its main strength lay in its recognition of the economic and social barriers to better health and the existence of a health care system focused more on illness than on the advancement of health. Furthermore, it marked the first time in this country that a set of national goals and targets for health had been developed and documented.

The weaknesses of *Health For All Australians* can be classified into three main areas. First, the report approached the task of setting goals and priorities using a biomedical model of health, even while acknowledging the wide range of factors that influence the health of Australians. Brown (1988, cited in Wass 1994, p. 18) argued that targets were set for disease categories, while no targets were set for population groups or for 'conditions which severely limit people's health but which have not been categorised as a disease—for example, chronic back pain'. Second, defining of targets was limited to areas where substantial health statistics existed. Third, the conceptual framework within which the goals and targets were developed did not fully reflect the social view of health that had informed the analysis (see Nutbeam et al. 1993c, p. 8). For the authors of *Goals and*

Targets for Australia's Health in the Year 2000 and Beyond the experience of working with the goals and targets set out in *Health For All Australians* provided three important lessons. First, there was a need for a broader framework for action; second, mechanisms for accountability and effective monitoring needed to be clearly defined; and third, there was a need to engage the health sector in the whole process (Nutbeam et al. 1993c, pp. 8–9).

In 1989, after the release of *Health For All Australians*, the National Better Health Program was established and resulted in a range of projects. It provided funding for health promotion activity, with a particular focus on the five priority areas outlined above (see also Australian Institute of Health 1990, p. 81). A strategic plan set a broad framework for action at the national level, and participating states established Health For All committees to develop action plans based on the national framework (McPherson 1992, p. 127). The National Better Health Program was evaluated in 1992 and the evaluation report, *Towards Health For All and Health Promotion* (Department of Health, Housing and Community Services 1993), contained among its recommendations the establishment of a national Health For All Strategy, to be supported by legislation. Until the mid 1990s, the responsibility for funding health promotion programs was administered through the National Health Advancement Program (Wass 1994, p. 19).

The National Health Strategy

Established in 1990, the National Health Strategy was set up to identify ways of improving the effectiveness and efficiency of the health system, with particular emphasis on examining the financing of health services (Nutbeam et al. 1993c, p. 4). The National Health Strategy's terms of reference included the social impact of health costs, the wide range of social institutions involved in health care, the conflicts existing between interest groups, and the need for improved preventive services (Macklin 1990).

Discussing contemporary directions for policy in health, Brown (1992, pp. 113–14) highlighted two initiatives: first, the directing of economic policy towards sustainable development, with the subsequent potential to maximise social and environmental wellbeing; and second, the national health strategy process.

Goals and targets for Australia's health

Goals and Targets for Australia's Health in the Year 2000 and Beyond (Nutbeam et al. 1993b) was the second major report in a decade that attempted to set measurable objectives for the health status of the Australian population. The terms of reference covered three broad areas (Nutbeam et al. 1993b, p. 247):

- a comprehensive review of the current set of national health goals and targets, including the development of an improved framework and categories, and new goals and targets;
- refinement and incorporation of the Interim National Aboriginal Health Goals and Targets; and
- examination of options and making of recommendations on the use of the goals and targets in policy, program development and resource allocation, together with their monitoring and review.

Three important observations about inequalities in health status substantially influenced the approach taken by the team to goal- and target-setting. First, improving the health of all Australians requires action at both an individual and a community level. Second, much of this 'social action' requires close consideration of the health impact of decisions taken outside the health sector. Third, the health system itself has an important role to play in redressing health inequities in terms of the range and direction of services provided (Nutbeam et al. 1993b, p. 13).

The authors said that goals, in the context of this report, 'are general statements of intent and aspiration' designed to indicate the 'direction and desired pace of change in pursuing improvements in the health of the population', and should reflect the values of the community in general and the health sector in particular regarding a healthy society (Nutbeam et al. 1993b, p. 5). Targets, on the other hand, were seen to be specific and measurable.

Nutbeam et al. proposed around 400 targets across the areas of preventable morbidity and mortality, healthy lifestyles and risk factors, health literacy and life skills, and healthy environments (1993b, pp. 15–16). Consideration was given to 'challenges for the health care system', but no goals and targets were set, although the authors stated 'there is a respectable body of international opinion that [states] setting goals and targets related to service delivery and performance in the health care system could be an effective mechanism for ensuring the maximum health benefit from invest-ment' (Nutbeam et al. 1993b, p. 237).

O'Brien (1994) suggested that there was limited discussion in the literature about the substance of the *Goals and Targets for Australia's Health in the Year 2000 and Beyond* report, and about monitoring progress towards the goals and targets. Channon (1993) criticised the report for its focus on mortality, morbidity and risk factors before other considerations and because it did not identify community participation as a major goal.

Concerning the shortcomings of the 1993 *Goals and Targets* report, the authors did emphasise the potential pitfalls facing them at the outset of the task. Nutbeam et al. (1993c, p. 5) concluded that 'goal and target setting is as much a strategic approach to planned change as it is a tech-nical exercise in predicting future trends in health status indicators'. The report certainly set an agenda for health promotion principles and strat-egies to be diffused throughout the health care system and the broader public health arena.

The Australian Health Ministers' Advisory Council decided on further action in four focus areas: cardiovascular health; mental health; cancer control; and injury prevention and control. The Commonwealth Depart-ment of Human Services and Health developed national policies in these four areas, as well as an overview report, *Better Health Outcomes for Australians* (Better Health Commission 1994), which drew together the common threads and challenges facing the health care system in the four focus areas. In addition to these reports, 'activity scans' were undertaken on the four focus areas. These activity scans identified and mapped levels of activity, involvement and investment in each focus area. The federal government undertook a process of consultation on these activity scans in early 1994, and final reports for each of the four focus areas were presented to the health ministers in June 1994. Diabetes mellitus, asthma, arthritis and dementia have since been added to the National Health Goals, now known as the National Health Priority Areas.

National Public Health Partnership

In 1995, chief health ministers from states around the country discussed the need for a national approach to public health. A proposal for a formalised partnership was sent to a number of government and non-government organisations, ultimately leading to an agreement by Australian health ministers in 1996 to enter into a National Public Health Partnership (NPHP News 1997). State, territory and Commonwealth ministers for health agreed to work collaboratively on a broad public health agenda to improve collaboration and coordination in public health efforts across the country. The priority work areas for the Partnership included:

- public health information
- public health legislation reform
- public health research and development
- public health workforce development
- public health planning and practice improvement
- coordination of national public health strategies
- initiatives—environmental health, food safety, mental health promotion and strategic inter-governmental nutrition alliance.

The objectives of the Partnership were to:

- improve the health status of all Australians—in particular, population groups most at risk;
- improve collaboration on the national public health effort;
- develop better coordination and increase sustainability of public health strategies;
- strengthen public health infrastructure and capacity nationally;
- facilitate the contribution of public health services, such as local government, public health research and education programs, and relevant agencies from the states and territories and Commonwealth;
- establish two-way exchange with key professionals, community, consumer, educational and industry interests on the development of national public health priorities and strategies; and
- enhance the capacity of states and territories to respond to local priorities.

In 1999, research conducted by the NPHP found that there was a significant consensus on the broad range of functions of public health, including:

- research, monitoring and assessment of health status and determinants
- ensuring healthy and safe environments
- health education and community development
- public health policy development and implementation
- public health education and training
- public health management
- prevention, surveillance and control of communicable diseases
- prevention and surveillance of non-communicable diseases
- prevention and surveillance of injuries
- healthy growth and development programs and services
- programs and services directed at specific population groups and individuals.

The objective of the study was to work towards a national statement of public health functions as the basis for defining, measuring and building capacity in public health (NPHP News 1999).

The federal government continues to promote partnerships between a range of organisations, including all levels of government, communities, non-government organisations (NGOs) and industry. For example, the National Drug Strategy (2004) embraces a far-reaching approach to drugs, which includes the misuse of alcohol, tobacco and prescription drugs, in addition to illicit drugs. This strategy includes the sponsorship of partnerships between, specifically, the Commonwealth, state and territory health, law enforcement and education sectors, NGOs, research organisations, communities and private industry (Ministerial Council on Drug Strategy 2004).

THE ROLE OF HEALTH PROMOTION IN PUBLIC HEALTH

The early 1980s were a time of overriding concern about public expenditure on health. Major issues concerning the future of the welfare state, the private/public mix, and social and individual responsibility for health were discussed without the call for health promotion being heard (Kickbusch 1989a). This lack of attention can be contrasted with the substantial focus of the late 1980s on primary environmental care and an ecological strategy for health (Kickbusch 1989a; Labonte 1992a).

The medicalisation of public health led to investments in diagnosis and cure with little emphasis on prevention. Many of the major social movements of the 1980s, such as the ecology movement, have set health agendas but they have not managed to create a joint public health lobby to impose public accountability for health matters on those in power. A strong role for the public in health is even more necessary because of the complex forces and interaction of political and economic interests. This is why health promotion concentrates on advocacy about formulation and implementation of healthy public policy.

The debate that surrounds the renaissance of public health is often couched in adversarial terms between prevention and treatment (Ashton & Seymour 1988, p. 26). In recent years, debate over public health has seen a revival of the argument over the responsibility for health, with a modern 'victim blaming' view still attracting support from those who continue to argue in favour of treatment as the main mechanism for dealing with health problems. The issue is complicated by a widespread move against paternalistic forms of administration and services, as part of a more general move towards participative as opposed to representative democracy (Ashton & Seymour 1988, p. 27).

Historical and more contemporary developments highlighting the range of factors impacting on the health of the population demonstrate that the public health movement as a whole will not have any lasting impact on the advancement of the public's health without intersectoral collaboration. Furthermore, there must be a willingness on the part of public health practitioners to form broad coalitions of mutual support and action. Arguably, this type of collaborative effort is where health promotion offers the greatest possibility for advancing health.

A good starting point for our discussion about the nature and extent of health promotion activity is to consider some of the theoretical approaches that have marked significant paradigm shifts in public health activity. The following box presents an overview of four general approaches to health education and health promotion that have shaped, to a greater or lesser extent, contemporary practice (Labonte 1992a, pp. 3–5; WHO 1998).

FOUR GENERAL APPROACHES TO HEALTH EDUCATION AND HEALTH PROMOTION

1. **Medical approach.** For much of the last century our dominant concept of health has been influenced by the 'disease-treatment'

model. The model is dominant in the sense that it is the one imbued with scientific, professional and institutional authority. Many prevention efforts focused on medically defined or physiological risk factors, such as hypertension, lack of immunisation, early cancer detection or, more recently, high cholesterol or lipids levels. Regardless of the setting for health care, the emphasis remained on treating or preventing disease by correcting problems in the mechanical functioning of the body.

2. **Behavioural approach.** The early 1970s saw the introduction of a behavioural (lifestyle) approach (Lalonde 1974). This change in thinking about determinants of health occurred for many reasons, including the increased role of chronic degenerative diseases (such as heart disease and cancers) as leading causes of mortality and morbidity. Health, from the behavioural risk factor perspective, moved beyond disease prevention by incorporating notions of promoting physical and emotional wellbeing. 'Health determinants' became synonymous with 'healthy lifestyle'. Program actions added educational, behavioural, social marketing and policy theories alongside medical theory.

3. **Socio-environmental approach.** The expansion of health thinking in the 1980s led to the incorporation of a sociological and environmental analysis of health and disease. One of the reasons for this shift was a recognition that most lifestyle improvements occurred principally among better educated, more privileged members of society. Research indicated that healthier lifestyles were often low priorities for people living in poverty. Furthermore, health education campaigns were accused of 'victim blaming' both in their content (for example, bad eating habits) and, indirectly, in their focus on personal behaviours at the expense of a broader consideration of social and environmental contexts in which personal behaviours are embedded.

4. **Ecological approach.** The ecological public health paradigm developed in response to global environmental problems, such as the destruction of the ozone layer, pollution and global warming, and their impact on health. As early as the mid 1980s there was discussion about the complex relationship between people and their environment, and the need to conserve the

environment (WHO 1986a). Ecological public health highlights the relationship between accomplishing the best possible health outcomes for populations, equity in health and the sustainable use of resources (WHO 1998).

PRINCIPLES OF HEALTH PROMOTION

In 1984, a new program of health promotion was established in the WHO European Regional Office, and a working party met to discuss 'Concepts and Principles in Health Promotion'. The resulting document was released in 1985, followed by a glossary of health promotion terms in 1986 and frameworks for research, training and ethics in health promotion in 1988. The concepts and principles were developed on the basis of a conception of 'health' as the extent to which an individual or group is able, on the one hand, to realise aspirations and satisfy needs and, on the other hand, to change or cope with the environment (Health Promotion International 1986, p. 73). The concepts and principles included the following:

- Health promotion involves the population as a whole in the context of their everyday life, rather than focusing on people at risk for specific diseases.
- Health promotion is directed towards action on the determinants or causes of health.
- Health promotion combines diverse, but complementary, methods or approaches, including communication, education, legislation, fiscal measures, organisational change, community development and spontaneous local activities against health hazards.
- Health promotion aims particularly at effective and concrete public participation.
- Health professionals, particularly in primary health care, have an important role in nurturing and enabling health promotion. (WHO/Regional Office for Europe 1986, p. 74)

However, the WHO working party warned of some of the potential political and moral dilemmas in attempting to balance personal and public responsibility for health. These were:

- focusing on a view of health as the ultimate goal encompassing all life;
- the inappropriateness of directing health promotion programs at individuals at the expense of tackling economic and social problems;
- producing resources, including information, in ways that are not sensitive to people's expectations, beliefs, preferences or skills;
- the danger that health promotion might be appropriated by one professional group and made a field of specialisation to the exclusion of other professionals as well as lay people (Health Promotion International 1986, p. 75).

The Ottawa Charter (WHO 1986a) built on these principles and suggested, in particular, the need for health promotion action to take place in five broad areas, as follows:

- **Build public policies that support health.** Health promotion goes beyond health care and makes health an agenda item for policy-makers in all areas of governmental and organisational action. Health promotion requires that the obstacles to the adoption of health-promoting policies be identified in non-medical sectors together with ways of removing them. The aim must be to make healthier choices easier.
- **Create supportive environments.** Health promotion recognises that at both the global and local level, human health is bound up with the way in which we treat nature and the environment. Societies that exploit their environments without attention to ecology reap the effects of that exploitation in ill health and social problems. Health cannot be separated from other goals and changing patterns of life. Work and leisure have a definite impact on health. Health promotion, therefore, must create living and working conditions that are safe, stimulating, satisfying and enjoyable.
- **Strengthen community action.** Health promotion works through effective community action. At the heart of this process are communities having control of their own initiatives and activities. This means that professionals must learn new ways of working with individuals and communities—working *for* and *with* rather than *on* them.
- **Develop personal skills.** Health promotion supports personal and social development through providing information and education for health and by helping people to develop the skills they need to make healthy choices. By doing so, it enables people to exercise more control

over their own health and over their environments, making it possible for people to learn through life, to prepare themselves for all of its stages, and to cope with chronic illness and injuries. This process has to be assisted in the school, at home, at work and in community settings.

- **Reorient health services.** The responsibility for health promotion in health services is shared among individuals, community groups, health professionals, medical care workers, bureaucracies and governments. They must work towards a health care system that contributes to the pursuit of health.

To facilitate effective and efficient health promotion in these five areas, the charter (WHO 1986a) urged the development and application of advocacy, mediation and enabling skills to ensure that people are empowered to gain greater control over their lives.

HEALTH PROMOTION STRATEGIES

Health promotion strategies need to be integrated, intersectoral and participatory. They cannot fall back on concentrating on individual behaviour when they meet powerful vested interests. They must be subject to public debate and serious ethical considerations (Kickbusch 1989a, p. 3). Health promotion best enhances health through integrated action at different levels—economic, environmental, social and personal. In the mid 1980s, the WHO had already begun to articulate a broad range of approaches to health promotion, summarised below:

- The focus of promotion is access to health, to reduce inequalities and to increase opportunities to improve health. This involves changing public and corporate policies to make them conducive to health, and involves reorienting health services toward the maintenance and development of health in the population, regardless of current health status.
- The improvement of health depends upon the development of an environment conducive to health, especially in conditions at work and in the home. Since this environment is dynamic, health promotion involves the monitoring and assessment of technological, cultural and economic influences on health.

- Health promotion involves the strengthening of social networks and social supports. This is based on the recognition of the importance of social forces and social relationships as determinants of values and behaviour relevant to health, and as significant resources for coping with stress and maintaining health.
- The promotion of lifestyles conducive to health involves consideration of personal coping strategies and dispositions, as well as beliefs and values relevant to health, all shaped by lifelong experiences and living conditions. Promoting positive health behaviour and appropriate coping strategies is a key aim in health promotion.
- Information and education provide an informed base for making choices. They are necessary and core components of health promotion, which aims at increasing knowledge and disseminating information related to health. Addressing information and education needs should include: consideration of the public's perceptions and experiences of health; knowledge from epidemiology and social and other sciences on patterns of health and disease and factors affecting them; and descriptions of the 'total' environment in which health and health choices are shaped. The mass media and new information technologies are particularly important (Health Promotion International 1986, p. 74).

As the overriding theme of all public health strategies is improving the health of the entire population—rather than being solely concerned with individuals—it is sensible to explore the use of community development principles in health promotion. In 'Improving Australia's Health: The role of primary health care' (National Centre for Epidemiology and Population Health 1992), the principles and practices of health promotion were reviewed from a primary health care perspective. From this perspective the community should be intimately involved in determining how best to care for and promote its health (see Chapter 7 for further discussion).

Another common theme in approaches to health promotion is collaboration between a range of public and private sectors. This theme was taken up in *Pathways to Better Health* (National Health Strategy 1993b), whose authors used a settings approach to explore health promotion practice. They focused on six areas of intervention: expansion of community-wide programs; strengthening the role of community health centres; supporting healthy schools; advocating the wider role of general practitioners in health promotion; creating 'healthy' hospitals; and developing safe and healthy workplaces (pp. 9–10). All of these areas are covered in Part III of this book, where we examine the range of settings in which health promotion takes place.

The *Pathways to Better Health* authors also pointed out that the approaches to be adopted in health promotion could be both broad and complex. For example, they referred to two possible approaches: the identification of 'individuals at risk' of some health problem, together with efforts to diminish barriers to their access to appropriate information and care, and addressing a large social group or 'population' in its entirety. In the latter case, the risk is likely to be broad-based within the population and thus the intervention is likely to be applicable to a large number of people, regardless of the level of risk. See, for instance, the Australian Government's (2005) *Building a healthy, active Australia*, which is aimed both at addressing obesity and supporting the promotion of healthy lifestyles, as well as assisting in the prevention and management of chronic disease through a range of programs and initiatives. Such programs and initiatives include:

- **National Guidelines for Diet and Physical Activity,** developed and disseminated by the National Health and Medical Research Council (NHMRC);
- **Rural Chronic Disease Initiative** (RCDI), to improve the health of small rural communities by organising activities designed to meet local needs;
- **Clinical Practice Guidelines for the Management of Overweight and Obesity,** evidence-based guidelines and related information resources for the management of excess weight and obesity by general practitioners, developed by the NHMRC;
- **Indigenous adult health checks,** available under Medicare since 2004—Indigenous people aged between fifteen and 54 can have check-ups every two years to help prevent and treat chronic illness (Australian Government 2005).

One of the most important points to be made in any discussion of health promotion strategies is that 'there is a continuum of practice from population-based health promotion running through clinical practice to palliative care—and indeed preventive efforts can feature in all of these settings, as can those seeking health gain' (National Health Strategy 1993b, p. 18).

REVIEW

We have explored two main developments in contemporary public health in this chapter. First, we analysed the nature and extent of the 'new public health'; indeed, we saw that some authors (Holman 1992) cautioned public health professionals not to reinforce the dichotomy between the 'new' and the 'old' public health, when the wealth of historical knowledge about public health practice suggested that various approaches to public health each had a place and a purpose. We also highlighted a number of contemporary developments in public health—a broadening understanding of what constitutes health and the concept of health itself; the dynamic notion of a 'Health For All' movement; public health reinstating itself as a collective effort, using an intersectoral approach to achieve the goal of a 'socially and economically productive life'; and an increasing focus on a positive and active advocacy for health within a framework of ecological sustainability.

Second, in this context, health promotion is not seen as a new or separate discipline, but as a necessary and timely consideration of public health. The work of Kickbusch (1986a, 1989b, 1989c, 1997) and colleagues at the European Regional Office of the WHO has led to the development of a more sophisticated approach to health promotion, recognising that it calls for a community development approach—working with all sectors of the community to create and improve upon the conditions that result in improved health. In this, health promotion involves a strategy of mediation, enabling and advocacy that seeks to develop community support systems and to make health a politically accountable issue.

REVISION

Consider the main issues addressed in this chapter. Review each of these points in light of your understanding of the new public health and the nature and scope of health promotion.

1. *Identify the main factors that have contributed to the emergence of the new public health in Australia. What role have international trends played in its development?*

2. *Compare and contrast the 'new' and the 'old' public health paradigms, and define the concept of an 'ecology' of public health. How does an ecology of public health impact on contemporary health promotion practice?*
3. *Define the dimensions of the 'new public health' and consider some of the significant themes that have emerged since the Declaration of Alma-Ata in 1978.*
4. *Identify the principles and strategies of health promotion, particularly the dimensions of the* Ottawa Charter for Health Promotion.
5. *Briefly describe the range of future challenges for health promotion.*

3

National strategies for promoting health in Australia

- *The state of the nation's health*
- *Developing a national approach*
- *National health policy*
- *Public health and national health policy*
- *Research and health promotion*
- *Establishing intersectoral partnerships for health*
- *Chronic disease*
- *Contemporary issues*

Health policy and strategy gained momentum on the national health agenda in the 1980s and 1990s, thanks to a buoyant political commitment. Consequently, a range of initiatives designed to reduce the burden of ill health and to promote health for all Australians have, since that time, gained prominence.

The Australian Institute of Health and Welfare (AIHW) was established in 1987 (AIHW 1992). The AIHW collaborates with a number of international organisations, including the World Health Organization (WHO) and the Organisation for Economic Cooperation and Development (OECD), to improve the quality of health information (AIHW 2005f). The AIHW publishes biennial reports to illuminate the state of the nation's health and welfare; the reports include the leading causes of death and ill health in Australia, in addition to trends in mortality and morbidity within various subgroups of the population.

This chapter examines the current health status of Australians and the Australian government's policy responses to the challenges our national health profile offers. Health promoters need to understand the dimensions of the policies, be skilled in policy analysis, and reflect on the role research plays in policy development and health promotion practice. They also need to be able to draw on national health policy in the development of strategic and operational plans and in the planning of health promotion programs.

THE STATE OF THE NATION'S HEALTH

Major causes of death

An analysis of trends in mortality illustrates the gains made in the overall health status of Australians. There has been an acknowledged shift away from infectious diseases as the leading cause of death in the early part of the twentieth century—from 12 per cent of all deaths in 1921 to 3.7 per cent in 2002 (AIHW 2004a). Accompanying this shift was an increase in both the age-standardised death rates and the proportion of deaths attributed to diseases of the circulatory system and to cancers.

There was a constancy of mortality rates, especially among males, from the 1940s through to the 1960s. Following a steady increase in mortality from cardiovascular diseases from the early 1900s, a phase of decline started in the late 1960s and has continued to the present day. Thus, contemporary age-standardised death rates for diseases of the circulatory system, in 2002, account for 3 per 1000 for males and 2.1 per 1000 for females (AIHW 2004a). These figures are approximately one-third of those reported for 1971 (AIHW 2004a).

Life expectancy is the average number of years of life remaining to a person; for Australians it has increased dramatically since the early 1900s. An Australian boy born in 2002 can expect to live 77.4 years and a girl to 82.6 years (AIHW 2004a). In the period 1901–10, life expectancy at birth was 55.2 years for boys and 58.8 years for girls (AIHW 2004a). These improvements are mainly attributable to a decrease in infant and child mortality, as well as improvements in the rates of diseases of the circulatory system. The life expectancy at birth for Australian males is higher than in New Zealand, the United Kingdom and the United States, but lower than in Japan, Iceland and Sweden; for Australian females the life expectancy is fifth, after Japan, France, Switzerland and Spain (AIHW 2004a).

Six main causes of death accounted for approximately half of all deaths in Australia in 2002; these were cardiovascular diseases, lung cancer, chronic obstructive pulmonary disease, colorectal cancer, cancer of the prostate and cancer of the breast (AIHW 2004a).

Ill health in Australia

With respect to **communicable diseases**, it is evident that despite reductions in the impact of diseases such as measles, there are still deaths from immu-nisation-preventable diseases, such as whooping cough—four deaths in 2002; *Haemophilus influenzae* type b (Hib)—two deaths in 2002; and meningococcal disease—48 deaths in 2002 (AIHW 2004a). Australia estab-lished a childhood vaccination program in the 1920s; however, data on coverage rates were deficient until the institution of the National Notifiable Diseases Scheme (NNDSS) in 1991, and the Australian Childhood Immunisation Register (ACIR) in 1996 (AIHW 2004a). Initiated in response to a fall in childhood immunisation levels and a rise in preventable child-hood diseases, the ACIR has collected vaccination data since 1 January 1996 for children under seven years of age (Medicare Australia 2005). One of the key successes in health protection has been the Immunise Australia program. In 1995, immunisation coverage rates for children in Australia were as low as 53 per cent; now the rate for twelve-month-old infants is over 90 per cent. Established in 1997, the 'Immunise Australia Program—The Seven Point Plan', built upon the initiatives of 1993's National Immunisation Strategy (Commonwealth Department of Health and Ageing 2004). A Common-wealth, state and territory initiative, it aimed to increase national childhood immunisation rates in order to lessen the morbidity and mortality from vaccine-preventable disease in Australia (Commonwealth Department of Health and Ageing 2004). The core goals of the Immunise Australia program were to achieve:

- a greater than 90 per cent vaccination coverage of children at two years of age for all diseases specified in the schedule;
- near-universal vaccination coverage at school entry; and
- near-universal vaccination coverage of girls and boys under seventeen years of age for measles, mumps and rubella (AIHW 2004a).

Internationally, immunisation programs have been demonstrated to be one of the most cost-effective weapons against disease. Subsidised immunisation for measles since 1970 has averted approximately 4 million cases in Australia for the period 1970–2003. It is estimated that this has saved the government more than $8.5 billion or $155 for every $1 spent on preventing measles, through reduced treatment costs since 1970 (Commonwealth Department of Health and Ageing 2004). The public health benefit from immunisation is the reduction of morbidity and mortality due to vaccine-preventable diseases within the population. In Australia, the ultimate goal is the control, and in some cases elimination, of vaccine-preventable diseases. This goal is unlikely unless childhood immunisation coverage rates increase to the level needed to achieve herd immunity for each of the diseases targeted by vaccination. The goal of the Seven Point Plan, therefore, was to ensure long-term high levels of childhood immunisation coverage in the Australian population. The following case study outlines the strategies contained within the Seven Point Plan and Table 3.1 demonstrates the trend in improved immunisation coverage rates since 1997.

IMMUNISE AUSTRALIA PROGRAM

The strategies contained within Immunise Australia's Seven Point Plan were primarily targeted at parents of children aged up to six years, with immunisation providers being the main secondary target group. The seven principal strategies, arrived at through research and consultation with relevant stakeholders, were:

- **Initiatives for parents.** The Childcare Rebate, Child Care Benefit and Maternity Immunisation Allowance to be paid to parents whose children meet the immunisation requirements—that is, they are up to date with their immunisations or are exempted.
- **A greater role for general practitioners.** The General Practitioner Immunisation Initiative (GPII) was implemented in 1998 to give financial incentives to general practitioners who monitor, promote and provide the scheduled immunisations to children up to six years of age.
- **Monitoring and evaluation of immunisation targets.** This was to be conducted through the Australian Childhood Immunisation Register, which commenced in 1997.

- **Immunisation days.** These were supported with a range of educational materials, with the aim of improving immunisation rates in areas where coverage was low.
- **Measles eradication.** The measles elimination strategy was aimed at increasing measles vaccination coverage, as part of a longer term strategy to eradicate measles from Australia.
- **Education and research.** This was designed to increase community awareness, acceptance and active support for childhood immunisation.
- **School entry requirements.** Parents were required to submit details of children's immunisation histories when they enrolled children for school (Commonwealth Department of Health and Ageing 2004).

Table 3.1: Trends in immunisation coverage rates, 1997–2005

Age	1997[1]	2002[2]	2005[3]
1 year	74.9%	90.5%	91.0%
2 years	63.8%	87.8%	91.7%
6 years[4]	na	80.6%	83.2%

1 AIHW (2002e)
2 AIHW (2004a)
3 Medicare Australia (formerly the Health Insurance Commission) (2005)
4 Vaccination coverage at six years of age was assessed for the first time in 2002 (AIHW 2004a).

In 2003, the National Meningococcal C Vaccination program commenced. Worth $291 million over the four years from 2003 to 2006, the program will ensure over 6 million children are vaccinated against the meningococcal C bacterium. Children and young people up to the age of nineteen will be eligible for the free vaccine (Commonwealth Department of Health and Ageing 2004).

The **AIDS epidemic** is comprised of sub-epidemics in largely separate population groups. There has been a continual decline in the annual number of HIV diagnoses in Australia, from over 2500 in 1985 (AIHW 1998), to 1077 in 1993, and 657 in 1998 (AIHW 2004a). However, there was an increase to 808 in 2002 (AIHW 2004a). In Australia in 2002, there were approximately 13 120 people living with HIV/AIDS; the number of new cases of AIDS is now somewhat stable at 200–250 each year (AIHW 2004a).

The leading cause of **cancer death rates** for women in 2002 was breast cancer (16 per cent of all cancers); lung cancer (15 per cent) and colorectal cancer (13 per cent) followed (AIHW 2004a). In males, lung cancer accounted for 22 per cent of cancer deaths, and prostate and colorectal cancer accounted for 13.3 per cent and 11.5 per cent, respectively (AIHW 2004a). While death rates for males from lung cancer have been falling steadily since the 1980s, lung cancer death rates among women have climbed by 2 per cent per year (AIHW 1998, p. 89). The risk of cancer increases with age in adult life. Males have a higher incidence than females beyond 55 years of age. Females have a higher incidence than males between ages 25 and 54 years, because female-only cancers have an incidence almost seven times that of the male-only cancers in this age range.

Cardiovascular disease (CVD) includes all diseases of the heart and the circulatory system. Ischaemic heart disease was the major cardiovascular cause of death in Australia in 2002, accounting for 20.1 per cent of all male deaths and 18.8 per cent of all female deaths (AIHW 2004a). Stroke accounted for 7.2 per cent of male deaths and 11.7 per cent of all female deaths (AIHW 2004a), while other heart diseases (including heart failure) accounted for 5 per cent of male deaths and 7.2 per cent of all female deaths (AIHW 2004a).

Among Australians of all ages, death from CVD is 1.7 times the rate of death from cancer and 26 times the rate of death from traffic accidents. Indigenous Australians die from CVD at approximately twice the rate of the total Australian population. People of lower socioeconomic status, and people born in Australia, have higher CVD rates than those of higher socioeconomic status and Australian residents who were born overseas (Bennett 1996).

Injury is a significant cause of mortality and morbidity in Australia, accounting for 5.8 per cent of all deaths in 2002. Injury and poisoning accounted for 436 513 hospital admissions in 2001–02, constituting 6.8 per cent of total admissions (AIHW 2004a). Injury mortality can be divided into three main groups: road deaths, suicides and other types of injury. In 2002, 24.4 per cent of all injury deaths were road deaths. In recent years death rates from suicide have gradually decreased, with the rate in 2002 for males aged between 15 and 24 the lowest it has been since

1984 (AIHW 2004a). Suicide deaths account for 30 per cent of all injury deaths (AIHW 2004a). 'Other injury' now accounts for the largest proportion of injury deaths, at 46 per cent in 2002. This is a diverse group including falls (19.4 per cent of injury deaths), fires and 'other unintentional' (9.9 per cent), poisoning (7.2 per cent), homicide (4 per cent) and drowning (3 per cent) (AIHW 2004a). Overall rates hide substantial differences in the injury experience of segments of the population (AIHW 2004a). For instance, injury mortality rates for Indigenous Australians are several times higher than for the population as a whole. In addition, people who live in remote areas—and to a lesser extent, rural areas—have higher rates than do urban residents (AIHW 2004a).

In the past, there has been no reliable information about the number of people in Australia who have a **mental disorder** or the types of disorders that are prevalent in the community. In 1997, the Australian Bureau of Statistics (ABS) conducted the National Survey of Mental Health and Wellbeing. From that survey, it was estimated that 17.7 per cent of Australian adults had experienced the symptoms of a mental disorder at some time during the twelve months prior to the survey. The prevalence of mental disorder generally decreased with age, with young adults aged eighteen to 24 having the highest prevalence of mental disorder. However, mental disorders such as dementia and Alzheimer's disease were not included in the survey results. In 2001, the ABS performed the National Health Survey; compared to the National Survey of Mental Health and Wellbeing (ABS 1997), more people experienced moderate or higher levels of psychological distress (36 per cent) than in 1997 (26 per cent) (ABS 2002b). In 2002, **suicide** rates for men of all ages were substantially greater than for women (AIHW 2004a). Men tend to use violent methods of suicide, such as hanging and shooting, while women tend to use more passive methods, such as poisoning. Suicide rates have declined from 14.7 per 100 000 in 1997 to 11.8 per 100 000 in 2002 (AIHW 2004a).

Diabetes mellitus is a disease in which the body makes too little of the hormone insulin or cannot use it properly. This disturbs the body's main energy processes, especially those involving glucose. The two most common forms of diabetes are type 1 diabetes (insulin-dependent diabetes mellitus) and type 2 diabetes (non-insulin-dependent diabetes mellitus) (AIHW 2004a). Diabetes has a major impact on quality of life. Its long-term effects include a greater risk of heart disease, stroke, impotence, blindness, kidney problems, lower limb amputations and reduced life expectancy. Older people,

Indigenous people and some sections of the overseas-born population are at particular risk of type 2 diabetes (AIHW 2004a). In 2001, 554 200 people (2.9 per cent of the population) reported having been diagnosed with diabetes mellitus and considered themselves to still have the condition, compared with 355 000 (2.4 per cent) in 1995 (ABS 2002c). The prevalence of diabetes has increased more than twofold over the past two decades, and it is among the top 10 leading causes of death in both sexes (AIHW 2004a).

There is wide variation between the principal **causes of hospitalisation** for people at different stages of life. The main causes of admission for children, up to the age of fourteen years, are respiratory illness and injury (AIHW 2004a). For the period 2001–02, young Australians aged twelve to 24 years accounted for 8.5 per cent of total hospitalisations. The single most common reason for hospitalisation for this group was impacted teeth. Hospital admissions were higher for young females aged twelve to 24, due to pregnancy and childbirth; for males, the main cause of hospitalisation was injury (AIHW 2004a). Frequent causes of admission for people aged 45 to 64 years included diseases of the digestive system, genito-urinary disorders and injury, as well as diseases of the circulatory system and cancers. For people aged over 65 years neoplasms, care involving dialysis, circulatory diseases, and diseases of the digestive system were the leading causes of hospitalisation (AIHW 2004a). For women over 75 years, the fifth most common cause of hospitalisation was injury resulting from falls (AIHW 2004a).

Mental disorders were not ranked among the most frequent causes of hospital admissions for this period; however, people with mental disorders had a significantly longer average length of stay than for all other conditions (AIHW 1998).

Population health

Population health is the analysis and evaluation of health and disease in defined populations rather than individuals (WHO 1998; AIHW 2005f). The population health discipline emphasises understanding health and disease in communities, and highlights interventions to improve health status and wellbeing through approaches that focus on the inequities in health status between groups (AIHW 2005f). Australia has three main concerns for health interventions: priority population groups, priority age groups and disease priorities (AIHW 2005f).

There are several population subgroups with poorer health than the general population, due to a range of environmental and socioeconomic factors. For example, there is evidence that medical care in rural and remote Australia is not as accessible as in urban areas and this could have a direct bearing on people's health status. The priority subgroups for health interventions comprise:

- Indigenous people
- those in rural and remote areas
- those who are socioeconomically disadvantaged
- war veterans
- prisoners
- people born overseas (AIHW 2005f).

Ill health in sub-populations

The high standard of health enjoyed by the majority of the Australian population is a recent development; however, concurrent with the improvements in health have come differing levels of health for different sections of the population (AIHW 2004a). The relevance of this sub-population approach is that examination of data from the population as a whole does not clearly indicate the variation in health status between sub-populations. Sub-populations may be defined in terms of several criteria, including socioeconomic, ethnic, racial, religious, geography and disease states (Harper et al. 1994).

In the 40 years between 1950 and 1990, world life expectancy rates improved more than they did during the entire previous span of human history (World Bank 1993). Despite the improvement, some sub-populations have not enjoyed better levels of health. Regarding Australia, five sub-populations are considered here: Aboriginal and Torres Strait Islander peoples; overseas-born persons; mothers and infants; children and young adults; and older people.

Indigenous Australians
The term 'Indigenous Australians' refers to Australian Aborigines and Torres Strait Islanders. According to Thomson, this group is defined as people of Aboriginal or Torres Strait Islander descent who identify

themselves as such and are accepted as such by the community in which they live (2003, p. 508). Indigenous Australians endure more disability and reduced quality of life, and die at younger ages, than do non-Indigenous Australians (ABS & AIHW 2005). In almost all disease categories, Indigenous rates are worse than non-Indigenous rates (Harper et al. 1994; AIHW 2004a; ABS & AIHW 2005). In particular, mortality rates are much higher for Indigenous males than for non-Indigenous males, with those in the 35 to 44 years age group dying at a rate more than five times that of non-Indigenous males (AIHW 2004a).

Life expectancy at birth remains much lower for Indigenous people than for the total Australian population. For the period 1999–2001 the life expectancy for an Indigenous male was 56, compared with 77 for all Australian males; similarly, the corresponding figures for females were 63 and 82 respectively (AIHW 2004a; ABS & AIHW 2005). For a more comprehensive discussion of Indigenous health issues, see Chapter 8.

Overseas-born persons

The 2001 population census (ABS 2003) identified that 4 105 444 (21.9 per cent) of the current Australian population were born over-seas. While migrants can be considered as a group, they are not homogeneous because they come from a range of different ethnic, racial and religious backgrounds (Harper et al. 1994). At the same time, a number of factors have an impact on health status after migration, including standard of living and health in the country of origin, ethnic characteristics, socioeconomic position of communities in Australia, and matters of language and culture.

Immigrants generally enjoy better health than do people born in Australia (AIHW 2004a). This may be due to Australia's immigration policy, which over the years has meant that, on arrival, the overall health of immigrants has been as good as, or better than, that of the general popu-lation. However, as the period of residence increases, overall health declines in many instances (AIHW 1998; AIHW 2002d)—after about twenty years in Australia, the rates for migrant groups are similar to those of Australian-born residents (Harper et al. 1994, p. 47). The following factors contribute to the deterioration of health status among migrants:

• the stress of migration and settlement, particularly for those refugee migrants who have experienced torture or trauma;

- the loss of status, and socioeconomic disadvantage experienced by many migrants on arrival in Australia;
- access to health information and health and community services being severely limited for migrants with little or no skill in English; and
- inadequate services and provisions, often the result of the providers' failure to consult with relevant ethnic communities and organisations (Better Health Commission 1994, p. 12).

For the purposes of the 2001 census, immigrants were grouped into four broad birthplace groups to provide some insight into the diversity within the overseas-born population. These are 'United Kingdom and Ireland', 'Other Europe', 'Asia' and 'other'. Standardised mortality ratios (SMRs) were found to be lower for males and females in all four birthplace groups. When asked in the 1995 National Health Survey about health risk factors, age-standardised percentages for the determinants and risk factors showed marked differences between birthplace groups. A much smaller proportion of Asian migrants reported being overweight, being smokers or having high alcohol consumption than other birthplace groups, but were less likely to walk for exercise, use sun protection, or have regular Pap smear tests or breast examinations. Migrants from the United Kingdom and Ireland provided similar responses to the Australian-born population. It is clear that a commitment to multicultural health means services and programs should be designed and delivered so that they mirror the needs of their non-English-speaking clients.

Mothers and infants
In 2002, the age of mothers in Australia ranged from twelve to 54 years; those at the extremes of this range are more likely to have adverse perinatal outcomes. The mean maternal age increased from 28.2 years in 1993 to 29.4 years in 2002, with the proportion of mothers aged between 20 and 24 years decreasing from 19.9 per cent in 1993 to 15.2 per cent in 2002, and the percentage of mothers aged 35 years and over increasing from 11.8 per cent in 1993 to 18.1 per cent in 2002 (AIHW 2004b). The perinatal death rate has declined markedly in the last two decades, but rose slightly in 1996 to 8.5 deaths per 1000 total births (ABS 1997), and then to 9.8 per 1000 births in 2002 (AIHW 2004b). A key indicator of babies' health is the proportion having a birth weight of less than 2500 grams. These low-birth weight infants have a higher morbidity and mortality risk, and require

longer periods of hospitalisation after birth. In 2002, 16 230 (6.4 per cent) live-born babies had weights of less than 2500 grams. The rate of live-born babies of Indigenous mothers that were of low birth weight was twice that of babies of non-Indigenous mothers (AIHW 2004b; ABS & AIHW 2005). Over one-third (38.4 per cent) of births in the Northern Territory were to Indigenous mothers, and the territory's rate of low birth weight is higher than in the rest of Australia (AIHW 2004b).

Children and young adults

Biological factors, events during pregnancy, and socioeconomic and physical circumstances are some of the factors that affect the health of children. Generally, the health status of boys is worse than that of girls, with boys experiencing higher rates of mortality, hospitalisation and disability (AIHW 2004a). In 2000, the leading cause of death for children aged less than one year was conditions originating in the perinatal period, accounting for 49 per cent of deaths (AIHW 2002c). Other leading causes of death were congenital abnormalities (25 per cent) and sudden infant death syndrome (12 per cent) (AIHW 2002c). For children aged one to fourteen years in 2000, injuries resulting from accidents, poisoning and violence caused more than 45 per cent of deaths (AIHW 2002c). For the period 1999–2000, the largest cause of hospital admissions for boys and girls less than one year of age was conditions originating in the perinatal period, followed by acute respiratory infections. While for children aged one to four years, asthma (unspecified) was the main reason for admission, followed by diarrhoea and gastroenteritis of presumed infectious origin. Chronic tonsillitis was the main reason for hospital admission in the five to fourteen years age group (AIHW 2002c). In 1998, 9.6 per cent of boys and 5.4 per cent of girls aged up to fourteen years were reported to have one or more disabilities (AIHW 2002c).

For people aged twelve to 24 years, mortality is relatively low but morbidity is relatively common. In 2002, the most common cause for hospitalisation for both male and female young persons was impacted teeth (AIHW 2004a). In contrast to children, there were more admissions for females than males in the fifteen to 24 years age group. The higher rate of female admissions relates to pregnancy and childbirth (AIHW 2004a). For males, the second major cause of hospitalisation was injury, which contributed 27 per cent of their total hospitalisations (AIHW 2004a). In 2002, over 70 per cent of the total deaths of young people were due to injury and poisoning, including traffic accidents and suicide. For males aged eighteen to 24 years, the mortality rate was highest, at 91 deaths per 100 000, mostly due to the high rate of suicide in this group (AIHW 2004a).

Older people

In 2001, the life expectancy of Australians aged 65 years was 17.2 years for men and 20.7 years for women (AIHW 2004a). This combined group has around the sixth highest life expectancy in the world. Cardiovascular disease is the leading cause of death in people aged 65 years and over (AIHW 2004a). Arthritis was the most common long-term condition reported in the 1995 National Health Survey by people aged 65 years and over, closely followed by vision and hearing problems. Hypertension was also reported as a major long-term health condition. In the 1995 National Health Survey, the majority of older Australians living in the community rated their health as good, very good or excellent (64 per cent). In the 2004–05 National Health Survey (ABS 2006), sight conditions, arthritis, hearing loss and high blood pressure were the most common conditions in the 65 and over age group. In this age group just under half (49 per cent) reported they had arthritis, 14 per cent reported they had diabetes mellitus, and 18 per cent reported a heart, stroke or vascular disease. In 1993, it was estimated that 3.2 million people in Australia had a disability, with 36 per cent of them aged 65 years or over (AIHW 1998). Of these older people, the most prevalent disabling condition was arthritis, followed by circulatory diseases, musculoskeletal conditions (other than arthritis), nervous system diseases and respiratory diseases. Prevention or remedial treatment of such diseases would result in a significant reduction in disability at older ages. Older Australians have a higher rate of admission to hospital than the general population and tend to stay longer.

While it is clear that Australia's population is ageing, there have been unprecedented improvements in life expectancy at older ages. It thus becomes important to direct research and health systems resources to the prevention and treatment of non-fatal disabling diseases such as dementia, arthritis, hip fracture and loss of vision and hearing (AIHW 1998).

A challenge for practitioners

This analysis of the health status of sub-populations has highlighted the complexity of factors that contribute to the mortality and morbidity of these groups. It is evident that their health status is often negatively influenced by social, educational, environmental, economic, political and personal factors. The challenge for health promotion practitioners is to recognise the particular needs of sub-populations and to develop programs in consultation with the groups concerned. This may mean that public health strategies—including social, structural, health promotion and policy—are needed to improve the health of the sub-populations discussed above.

DEVELOPING A NATIONAL APPROACH

A timeline of significant events

The international impetus for activities to promote the health of Australians came in 1981 with the publication of the World Health Organization's *Global Strategy for Health For All by the Year 2000* (WHO 1981). By 1985, Australia had established the **Better Health Commission** for three main reasons: to investigate and report on the current health status of the Australian population; to identify factors underlying any health problems; and to make recommendations on ways to address health problems (Nutbeam et al. 1993c). The Better Health Commission recommended national health goals for three main problem areas: CVD, nutrition and injury.

In response to the international initiatives and obligations taken under the aforementioned WHO publication, the Australian Health Ministers' Advisory Council (AHMAC) established the **Health Targets and Implementation Committee**, also known as the Health For All Committee. The principal task of the Committee was to develop a set of national goals and targets with the intention of reducing inequalities in health status (Better Health Commission 1994, p. 1). The report of the Committee, *Health For All Australians*, represented an important effort to refocus attention towards a positive vision of what health policy should aim to achieve—better health for all Australians (Nutbeam et al. 1993b, p. 7). In 1988, the Australian Health Ministers' Conference endorsed twenty goals and 65 targets, grouped into three major categories: population health, major causes of sickness and death, and risk factors. The goals and targets were set for major causes of premature death, major risk factors, causes of premature morbidity, and areas in which change had been demonstrated to be feasible. Five major national priority areas were proposed, including improved nutrition, preventable cancers, high blood pressure, injury prevention and the health of older people.

The **National Better Health program**, implemented in 1998, was charged with initiating strategies to achieve the targets in each of these areas. The principles underpinning the original goals and targets were:

- equity in the distribution of health and health care resources;
- greater community involvement in health decision-making;
- development of effective health promotion and illness prevention programs;
- recognition of the importance of intersectoral involvement in the development of healthy public policy;
- recognition of the need for an integrated, accessible and appropriate primary health care system;
- recognition of the need for infrastructures that would ensure the achievement of health promotion and illness prevention goals and targets.

The National Better Health program encountered a number of problems, including inadequate funding, difficulties with communication between the states and the Commonwealth, confusion over roles and principles, a lack of involvement by non-government stakeholders, and a lack of uniformity in establishing priorities and implementing strategies for change.

Nutbeam et al. (1993c) acknowledged the valuable work of the National Better Health program, the Better Health Commission and the National Health Goals and Targets Implementation Committee, but commented on the limitations of the process and on the challenges that faced the authors of the 1993 *Goals and Targets* document referred to below. Nutbeam and his colleagues (1993c, pp. 8–9) articulated three important lessons from the 1988 implementation experience:

- the need for a broader framework for action, with an emphasis on modifying the underlying social and environmental determinants of health and legitimising action to do this;
- the need for mechanisms of accountability and effective monitoring to be clearly defined;
- the importance of engaging the health system in the process.

In 1990, a joint AHMAC/NHMRC (National Health and Medical Research Council) working group was established to select initial focus areas for national agreement and action. Reports from the working groups were produced in the following areas: CVD, cancer, mental health and injury prevention. A new, more comprehensive, set of national health goals and targets was released early in 1993 in a report entitled *Goals and Targets for Australia's Health in the Year 2000 and Beyond*. The report highlighted the need for an optimal balance of services from promotion through to palliative services. It sought to expand the sectors traditionally involved in health promotion and to actively involve the wider health care system and the community in implementing the revised goals and targets (Better Health Commission 1994, p. 9).

Further development of the program culminated in the endorsement by the Australian state and federal health ministers of five National Health Priority Area (NHPA) initiatives in 1996. The NHPAs were cardiovascular health, cancer control, injury prevention and control, mental health and diabetes mellitus. Asthma was added in 1999 and arthritis and musculoskeletal disorders in 2002. The recent addition of dementia brought the number of NHPAs to eight (Commonwealth Department of Health and Ageing 2005c). To improve health outcomes in the priority areas, the NHPA program seeks to:

- monitor health outcomes and progress towards set targets;
- identify the most appropriate and cost-effective points of intervention;
- identify the most appropriate role for government and non-government organisations in fostering the adoption of best practice;
- identify and discourage inappropriate practice;
- investigate some of the basic determinants of health, such as education, employment and socioeconomic status (National Health Priority Action Council 2002, p. 8).

Australian health ministers require a national report to be prepared on each priority area every two years; the first NHPA report was released in 1997, and provided baseline data for the five NHPAs (AIHW/CDH&F 1997). The NHPA reports for cancer control and injury prevention and control were released in 1998. These reports built on the first report as well as outlining strategies for change across the continuum of care for the particular NHPA. Reports on CVD, mental health and diabetes mellitus followed in 1999.

The process of developing strategies to improve the health outcomes of Australians in each of the four areas has highlighted a number of common challenges facing the health system which require further consideration. It is evident that there is a complex interaction of government departments and agencies, non-government bodies and industry groups involved in the provision of health care or activities that impact on health. Furthermore, health services are provided in a range of community and institutional settings without always maximising the opportunities for multidisciplinary care, coordinated referral and follow-up procedures. Widespread variations in treatment practices are a feature of health services in Australia.

The development of a health outcomes approach requires renewed efforts to involve patients and the community in decision-making about health care priorities. Efforts need to be increased in the provision of information to health professionals about the links between treatment and outcomes, and in the promotion of appropriate care guidelines. Finally, strategies to address the health disadvantage of particular population groups need to be developed and adopted with renewed effort.

In recognition of a more systematic, cohesive national approach to identifying and solving public health problems, the Council of Australian Governments (COAG) agreed on a National Public Health Partnership (NPHP), which was endorsed by AHMAC. The Partnership provides a multilateral public health policy framework within which specific bilateral public health outcomes funding agreements should be negotiated (NPHP 1997). The NPHP is implemented through a partnership group, which is constituted as a subcommittee of AHMAC. Five working parties have been established on legislation, information, planning and best practice, research and development, and workforce development. An advisory group with representation from non-government organisations has also been established. The NPHP has adopted the following set of guiding principles.

- Each community or population subgroup should have access to strategies, services and activities which optimise their health status, as determined by access to a healthy and safe environment, including clean air and water, adequate food and housing.
- Public health efforts must proceed in partnership with public health sectors and non-health sectors, and in collaboration with international partners, to optimise population health outcomes.

- A supportive legal and political environment is integral to the public effort.
- Priority setting and decision-making should be based on scientific evidence as far as possible, on optimum capacity to scan and monitor the health determinants, and on criteria that are open to public scrutiny and debate (NPHP 1997).

The work of the NPHP is epitomised in the development of exemplary public health policies—for example, those relating to smoking, and definitions of core public health roles (Baum & Keleher 2002). The NPHP was initially concerned with establishing frameworks to enable state and Commonwealth jurisdictions to respond to threats to public health (Baum 2004). Key players in public health outside the immediate circle of state and Commonwealth public health officials were only accorded advisory status, and stakeholders from other sectors were not formally involved at all. 'The extent to which the NPHP is inclusive of key players,' wrote Baum (2004, p. 53), 'will be one of the main ways in which its success or otherwise will be judged'. In concert with the NPHP, the Commonwealth and state governments have been engaged in bilateral negotiations on a Public Health Outcomes Funding Agreement, which will see funding pooled into a number of 'broad-banded areas'. The initial areas are HIV/AIDS, women's health, alternative birthing, education on female genital mutilation, breast and cervical screening, childhood immunisation and illegal drugs. Baum (2004, p. 54) concludes that the future of public health is at a turning point, with the government committed to reducing expenditure, and privatising and contracting out services. According to Baum (2004), the future of public health remains uncertain. On the one hand, there are the significant gains made by public health in promoting health and preventing disease. On the other, there are threats to public health from rapid globalisation and a deteriorating physical environment (Baum 2004, p. 56). A concerted public health effort will be required.

NATIONAL HEALTH POLICY

In the process of developing a national health policy a number of influences, both international and national, have impacted on policy and strategic developments. These influences are summarised in Figure 3.1.

They do not represent a total picture of the multiplicity of influences on health policy development, but they do highlight the range of key players and significant stages in the development of contemporary health policy in Australia.

In 1993, AHMAC set out the commitment of Commonwealth, state and territory ministers to achieve a level of individual and population health within available resources through a focus on improving health outcomes. AHMAC defined a health outcome as a change in the health of an individual, a group of people or a population that is attributable to an intervention or series of interventions.

At the same time, the health ministers endorsed the concept of setting national goals and targets as a means of making significant improvements in the health status of Australians. The National Health Summit of 1993 agreed that the development of national goals and targets ought to be embedded within the broader framework of a national health policy.

Developing a national health policy

The Commonwealth, states and territories agreed at 1993's National Health Summit to develop a shared policy framework for the Australian health system. This framework has assisted in efforts to restructure the health system, improve data collection, and rationalise roles and responsibilities. Central themes of the National Health Policy are the development of key strategies to improve health outcomes, and of information systems that support an outcomes approach to resource allocation. The fundamental principle underlying the development of a national health policy is that opportunities to achieve better health outcomes for Australians clearly remain. Central to the National Health Policy will be an agreed set of health goals, targets and implementation strategies for major causes of mortality and morbidity. The reports of the implementation working groups referred to below represent the first steps in this process.

The development of a national health policy marks an acknowledgment by governments for the need to reorient policies and programs towards improving *health*, rather than simply health care.

Figure 3.1: Policy and strategies for health advancement

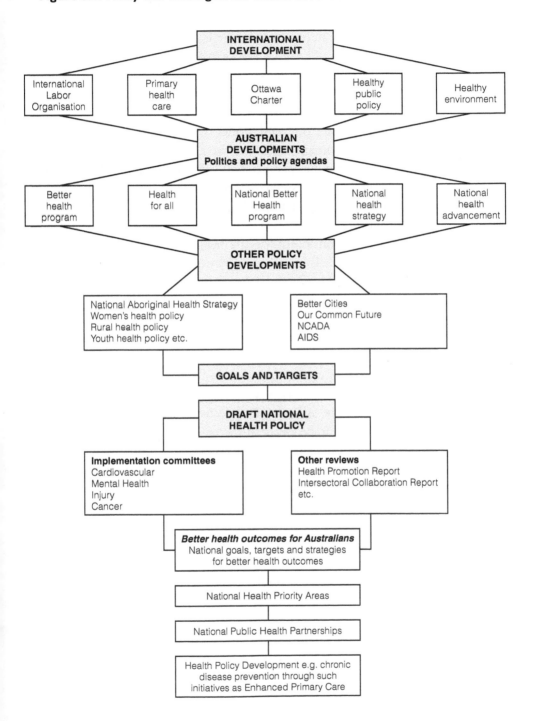

PUBLIC HEALTH AND NATIONAL HEALTH POLICY

Public health policies are necessary, as there is unlikely to be an equitable and competent provision of health services in an uncontrolled and unregulated free market (Scott 2004). Moreover, such policies need to consider equity issues and the broad range of factors that impact on health, including education and employment policies (Vega & Irwin 2004).

The international debate on health policy over the past twenty years has seen a shift from the dominant health service and resource-centred orientation towards a broader policy perspective. This has emphasised the major social, environmental and personal determinants of health and, consequently, priority areas for policy-making (Leppo & Vertio 1986, p. 5). Healthy public policy is typified by a concern for health and equity in all policy spheres, and responsibility for the health impact of policies. The major goal of public policy is to create an environment in which people are facilitated to make healthier choices. In addition, public health policies should enhance social and physical environments. All government sectors, not just the health sector, need to consider health as an important issue when developing policy, and be accountable for the health impacts of their policies (WHO 1988, 1998).

As an intrinsic part of modern environments, public policy is not only a creator of social conditions and contexts; it is also shaped by governments in several ways. Therefore, in order to effectively promote some desired policy, it is also necessary to be aware of the manifold context surrounding it (Milio 2001). For example, a policy to expand anti-smoking education will have very different results depending upon whether other policy initiatives, such as tobacco advertising bans and CPI-indexed tobacco taxation, are in operation. The environment influences policy-makers' judgments about policy direction; thus, it is important to know whose views policy-makers accept about what is important and what is happening in the real world (Milio 2001).

The development of explicit public policy usually follows a sequence that involves:

- **Issue identification**—an awareness of a need that is a legitimate issue for the health care system to be involved in.
- **Policy assessment**—a decision that a policy solution is desirable and a review of all possible policy options.

- **Policy selection**—the process of choosing a preferred policy option, usually achieved by a stakeholder group following an analysis of the strengths, weaknesses and potential impacts of the various policy options.
- **Policy advocacy**—the process of implementing strategies to inform and persuade. The stakeholders often do not have the authority to adopt policy, so must 'sell' it to a decision-making body.
- **Policy adoption**—the process of adopting the policy.
- **Policy implementation**—the process of policy implementation.
- **Policy evaluation**—the process of monitoring the success of a policy related to specific criteria. This is a critical step in the policy-making cycle, necessary to ongoing knowledge development in the policy field.
- **Policy reformulation**—the process of policy review and revision based on the results of evaluation, environmental changes or new evidence (Calgary Health Region 2005).

Often, the greater the conflict of interests in the issue at hand, the longer the time-lag between stages in the process. Any particular policy is also influenced by what happens during the entire policy-making procedure, from establishment to adoption, implementation, evaluation and redevelopment (Palmer & Short 2000). Lloyd was critical of the development of Australia's national health policy, arguing that the protracted process of release of the draft document, *Towards a National Health Policy* (Health Ministers Forum 1994), the media report heralding the release of the final document, and its unavailability to the public health community several months later revealed 'the tortuous and vexatious quality of political decision making' (Health Ministers Forum 1994, p. 357). Lloyd further contended that the process 'highlighted the complex nature of health policy development in Australia, particularly when this involved negotiation between different tiers of government' (Health Ministers Forum 1994, p. 357). The policy process is a 'multi-person drama' which is continuous, sometimes conflict-ridden and more political than rational. It is a political activity that involves bargaining and negotiation between conflicting interests (Milio 1985).

Lloyd (1994) supported the public health 'vision' articulated in the draft *Towards a National Health Policy*, which noted that health status is dependent, in part, upon social and environmental factors outside the health system. However, he claimed that the rest of the draft document focused on the role of health services in maintaining, promoting and protecting the health status of Australians. Lloyd argued that the paper ignored the fact that 'health is not determined by service intervention alone', and that the consultation process had little impact on what should be the key principles underpinning national health policy (1994, p. 357).

A number of other national policy and strategy documents promoting the health of particular sub-populations exist. These include *A national Aboriginal health strategy* (NAHS Working Party 1989); *National Strategic Framework for Aboriginal and Torres Strait Islander Health* (NATSIHC 2003), see Chapter 8; *Improving Australia's Health: The role of primary health care* (National Centre for Epidemiology and Population Health 1992); *Enhanced Primary Care Program* (Commonwealth Department of Health and Ageing 2005a); *National Non-English Speaking Background Women's Health Strategy* (Alcorso & Schofield 1991); *Healthy Horizons* (National Rural Health Alliance 1999, 2002b), see Chapter 11; *National Drug Strategy* (Ministerial Council on Drug Strategy 2004); *National Alcohol Strategy* (Ministerial Council on Drug Strategy 2001); *National HIV/ AIDS Strategy 2005–2008* (Commonwealth Department of Health and Ageing 2005b); *National Strategy for an Ageing Australia: An older Australia, challenges and opportunities for all* (Commonwealth of Australia 2002).

Many of these policies and strategic initiatives are addressed in later chapters. The list highlights the proliferation of health policy at the national level in Australia and raises the question of the extent to which these policies support or compete with each other for time, money and resources. The fate of any given policy, quite apart from its merit, depends upon the competition among old and new policies for attention—the top of the agenda—and for the funds available to policy-makers (Milio 1999).

More than a decade ago, the Green Paper on child and youth health was produced (AHMAC 1994). Lloyd (1994) argued that the Green Paper artic-ulated a comprehensive process of policy consultation and development because it differed in three significant ways from the national health strategy paper, *Towards a National Health Policy* (Health Ministers Forum 1994). First, its depth of detail allowed for 'ample attention to be given to the identification and development of underlying principles and points for intervention, as well as a clear sense of direction, by linking sets of proposed outcomes with seven nominated key action areas' (Lloyd 1994, p. 358). Second, the Green Paper was linked to other relevant reports such as *National Aboriginal Health Strategy* and *National Child Protection Strategy*.

The Green Paper considered how a national policy might be articulated with other relevant national initiatives. Third, the paper's 'vigorous pursuit and consolidation of a social and environmental view of health' emphasised the need for broad-ranging government approaches to meet the health needs of children and young people (Lloyd 1994, p. 358).

The Health of Young Australians (1995) was endorsed by the Australian Health Ministers' Conference in June 1995 as a national health policy for children and young people. In 1997, *The National Health Plan for Young Australians* was published as an action plan to protect and promote the health of children and young people. In 2005, the National Public Health Partnership published *Healthy Children—Strengthening promotion and prevention across Australia.* This document aims to improve Australia's ability to prevent disease and injury, and promote good health in children up to twelve years of age.

As a number of authors have reminded us (Lloyd 1994; Gardner & Barraclough 2004), policy-making often involves competing interests and demands. There is always the danger that a particular document or statement will be regarded as representing the sum of all knowledge, debate and planning on a particular matter. In fact, any health policy should be reviewed critically and examined in its wider context (Gardner & Barraclough 2004).

A great deal of public health policy and strategic development has taken place over the past two decades at the national level, much of which promotes the use of health promotion principles and practices. What are the implications for health promotion? The final section of this chapter sets out what we believe to be some (though not all) of the most important issues for health promotion over the next decade.

The three broad areas that are likely to impact on health promotion practice are research, health promotion's role in implementing national health strategies, and sustainable partnerships for health.

RESEARCH AND HEALTH PROMOTION

A perspective of health which recognises that individuals are part of a social, cultural and physical world is the best foundation for health promotion. Kickbusch (1999) claimed that, in an **ecological** understanding of health, socioeconomic factors and social class differences constitute only the beginning of an in-depth understanding of people's way of life. This understanding extends to include components of their social environment such as cultural dynamics and social change, social support and social relationships. A challenge is posed to develop new types of research on health behaviour that sees the individual as an integral part of a social group and that acknowledges the biological, as well as the non-biological, components of health.

By these statements, Kickbusch extended the health promotion **research framework** to consider the cultural, political and social dimensions of individuals' lives. Traditionally in health promotion, the concept of risk behaviour has been the dominant conceptual lens through which research issues have been perceived. It has usually been understood in a narrow sense as behaviours that may negatively impact on health (Kickbusch 1999). Much health education epidemiological research gained prominence as it focused on such risk factors as smoking and alcohol consumption. Kickbusch claimed that this approach was strongly criticised as it separates behaviours (1999). She urged researchers to understand the context in which behaviour patterns occur and to augment their knowledge base to incorporate evaluations of the social and psychological outcomes of such contexts. Furthermore, she suggested researchers investigate contexts of coping in people's everyday life, as well as researching methodically the outcomes of nurturing and caring on wellbeing in addition to morbidity and mortality patterns (Kickbusch 1999).

Kickbusch also challenged us to consider a 'new epidemiology of everyday health actions suggesting new priorities for allocating resources for preventive care and supportive services'. She argued the 'need to focus on definitions of significant health actions and health potential as people define their needs and researchers concentrate on those factors people see as a threat to their everyday wellbeing' (1988, p. 242).

In summary, it is acknowledged that if health promotion emphasises the complex interrelations between the immediate and the underlying social and environmental causes of ill health, a wider range of issues should be examined. This process would greatly expand the theoretical base for practical action.

Utilising a **program development cycle**, Girgis et al. (1993) defined a five-stage process in researching a health problem. The stages include: determination of health indicators; descriptive research—for example prevalence and description of target groups; determination of the efficacy of an intervention; dissemination of an effective intervention; and adoption and implementation.

Citing Nutbeam et al. (1990), the *Pathways to Better Health* (National Health Strategy 1993b) authors recommended a model to relate **basic research inputs** to health promotion:

- analysis of causality, primarily through epidemiological and sociological studies of health and ill health in populations;
- understanding the scope of desirable content of interventions through the study of the personal, social and environmental characteristics that influence health;
- understanding community needs through demographic profiles and community consultation;
- establishing an appropriate theoretical base to guide the development of an intervention—this includes individual, organisational and community change theories and management practices.

The gap between research and health promotion practice has been noted in both Australia (National Health Strategy 1993b) and internationally (Beaglehole et al. 2004).

Mechanisms to **build partnerships** between researchers, most often academics and practitioners, were proposed by Kok and Green (1990). The authors suggested the following: that programs incorporate planned, small-scale research and development projects prior to larger scale implementation; that researchers need greater sensitivity to implementation and feasibility issues; and that researchers and practitioners should work cooperatively to develop reliable and feasible research designs in light of the practicalities of implementation.

ESTABLISHING INTERSECTORAL PARTNERSHIPS FOR HEALTH

The process of advancing the health of the population over the past twenty years has shifted from behavioural and lifestyle change towards structural and environmental change. This has resulted from increasingly sophisticated analyses of determinants of health, from research demonstrating the improved effectiveness of such change in terms of improved health status, and from the experience of many people working to promote health in a range of settings. Some of the most influential models, such as the Ottawa Charter (WHO 1986a), incorporate this framework.

One of the major challenges for health promotion in the future will be the development and sustainment of intersectoral partnerships for health (WHO 1997b). Any discussion of establishing sustainable partnerships forms part of a broader discussion about intersectoral collaboration. Harris et al. (1994) used an organisational perspective to analyse the process of working intersectorally. The authors identified four sets of factors that influence the success of intersectoral action: the context within which organisations are operating; the characteristics of each organisation independently; the characteristics of the partnership between organisations; and the knowledge and skills of the individuals involved (Harris et al. 1994).

In their review of intersectoral action in health promotion, the authors identified many different kinds of partnerships working at many different levels. Harris et al. (1994) argued that taking an organisational perspective moves one away from viewing partnerships almost solely in terms of the individuals who develop and maintain them. The authors contended that taking an organisational perspective enables one to focus on the organisational conditions that influence, significantly, individuals' capacity to perform this function successfully.

While the early literature defined intersectoral action as being decidedly informal and short-term in nature (Warren 1967), more contemporary standards characterise intersectoral action as involving formal, multipurpose and long-term alliances (Wandersman et al. 2005). Wandersman et al. (2005, p. 293) defined coalitions as 'inter-organisational, cooperative and synergistic working alliances'. Similarly, Harris et al. (1994) characterised intersectoral action as a range of activities that involve a relationship or collaboration with other sectors and involve united planning or action on a health-related concern.

While there is little research that has assessed the effectiveness of intersectoral collaboration, several researchers have discussed factors that contribute to its effectiveness. Specifically, intersectoral collaboration should be issue-oriented, structured, focused to act on specific goals, committed to recruit member organisations with diverse talents and resources, and durable (Norton et al. 2002). Intersectoral action allows for the exchange of mutually beneficial resources and directs the interventions at multiple levels—for example, policy change, resource development and ecological change (Wandersman et al. 2005). McLeroy (1994) identified three factors that contribute to the generation of collaborative working alliances:

- **Demographic appeal**—provides an opportunity to involve the broader community in solving local problems and changing community needs, as well as a framework for tailoring programs to local conditions.
- **Empowerment**—the process can strengthen inter-organisational relationships, providing a mechanism for addressing local problems and demonstrating the effectiveness of working together.
- **Effective resource management**—better coordination of services and improved working relationships among organisations reduces overlap of services, possibly reduces costs, and may provide more efficient use of local resources.

We might well ask ourselves: why work intersectorally? Tones and Green offered a comprehensive list of reasons for working intersectorally, namely to:

- achieve organisational objectives, enhance efficiency and effectiveness
- improve coordination of policy, programs and service delivery
- broaden the scope of influence to include other services and activities
- greater economic benefits
- lessen bureaucracy and regulation
- offer more business and commercial opportunities
- provide access to data and information
- offer access to a range of skills and competencies
- provide opportunity for innovation and learning
- encourage more involvement of local communities (2004, p. 139).

Major challenges for health promotion will be to establish intersectoral partnerships and to sustain those partnerships by, for example, taking good account of the organisational factors that support or restrict them and by using consultative and collaborative approaches as fully as possible. Further effort is essential to help government, non-government and community groups recognise that each contributes, directly or indirectly, to advancing the health of the population, and that working collaboratively enhances that contribution.

CHRONIC DISEASE

In Australia, much of the burden of disease is attributable to chronic diseases, including coronary heart disease (CHD), chronic obstructive pulmonary disease (COPD) and stroke. While 'chronic disease' is often used to refer to both non-communicable diseases and to communicable diseases which have become chronic, for the purposes of this chapter 'chronic disease' refers to non-communicable diseases only. Chronic diseases are conditions that are persistent, usually not curable, and of complex aetiology (AIHW 2002a). Chronic diseases, while not immediately life-threatening, are the most common cause of premature mortality, as well as indirectly contributing to mortality resulting from other causes of death (AIHW 2002a).

A variety of perspectives, chronic disease targets and reviews have transpired in proposals by a range of organisations, including the National Health Priority Action Council, the NPHP, the Australian government's Rural Chronic Disease Initiative and the NHMRC (Gross et al. 2003). While there has been a great deal of discussion regarding the need for more cost-effective and coordinated policies for the prevention and management of chronic disease, according to Gross et al. (2003) various Australian governments continue to debate the issues when they should be demonstrating strong leadership and initiating changes in health care funding systems.

While there is considerable variation in the nature and extent of their impact, chronic diseases are important because of their considerable burden on individuals, communities and health services. Some conditions contribute significantly to premature mortality, whereas others impact more on morbidity (AIHW 2004a). A large number of these chronic diseases are partly or wholly preventable—various factors that impact on their progression are modifiable and, consequently, effective prevention strategies are essential (NPHP 2001; AIHW 2004a). The paper *Preventing Chronic Disease: A strategic framework* (NPHP 2001) outlines a framework for comprehensive action that utilises data in relation to the determinants of ill health, understanding risk factors, and a life course perspective on predisposing factors. Founded on public health philosophies and methodologies, the model focuses on health promotion and illustrates how health promotion practice can be employed within a continuum of care.

Research demonstrates that health services can be developed to manage chronic disease more successfully. Nevertheless, it is crucial that such change is complemented by, and supportive of, people's autonomy and active involvement (NPHP 2001). Increasingly, it is accepted that a more comprehensive approach to chronic disease prevention is essential. There are diverse national, State and community initiatives directed at developing guidelines and initiatives to generate action to enhance the early diagnosis and management of chronic disease as well as addressing risk and protective factors. For example, the federal government increased spending from July 2005, through Medicare, on new chronic disease management services for people with chronic diseases or complex care needs. This is aimed at augmenting care planning options for GPs, expanding patient eligibility and enhancing the assistance that practice nurses and other allied health workers can provide. The NPHP (2001) advocates an approach that extends contemporary developments, acknowledging that a systematic, comprehensive and cooperative preventative effort may considerably improve health outcomes.

CONTEMPORARY ISSUES

There are many issues that currently impact on decisions regarding health priorities, and which are expected to increase in significance in the future. These include population ageing, transformations in service delivery models, and coordinated care.

Population ageing

Like most other industrialised countries, Australia's population is ageing, with increasing numbers aged 65 and over. This is due to decreases in fertility rates and a decline in mortality. In 1997, 12 per cent (2.2 million) of the population were aged 65 and over; this is projected to rise to between 24 and 26 per cent (6 to 6.3 million) by 2051 (ABS 1998a). The older age group (85 and over), constituting 1.2 per cent (216 000) of the population in 1997, is expected to increase to between 4.4 per cent and 4.8 per cent (1.1 to 1.2 million) in 2051 (ABS 1998a).

The future cost of health services will be determined by supply and demand, both of which are hard to predict. The ageing of the population adds only 0.6 per cent to expenditure per year, so does not have a significant influence on cost. In contrast, changes in medical practice due to improvements in technology add significantly to health costs each year. Furthermore, the decisions made now about health workforce planning will influence the future supply of the health workforce (AIHW 2000).

Shift to community care

A shift from institutional-based care has happened in the disability, mental health and aged care sectors, and new models have been introduced to replace some traditional hospital-based systems, for example, day surgery. Average lengths of stay in public acute hospitals decreased from 5.1 days in 1993–94 to 4 days in 1997–98, largely due to the increase in the number of day surgery patients, who do not need to stay in hospital overnight. The combination of aged care services has changed considerably since the 1980s, with an expansion in community-based care and no increase in residential places for the population aged 70-plus (AIHW 2000).

Coordinated care

People with complex care needs, those with chronic conditions, for example, are of special concern. Partially due to the ageing of the population, the size of this group is growing. It is problematic for those with complex care needs to access adequate care when various services are provided by diverse and often disconnected providers. In 2000, Commonwealth, state and territory governments collaborated to trial nine coordinated care programs, throughout Australia. They involved the selection of a care coordinator who assumed multidisciplinary care planning and service coordination (AIHW 2000). The interventions were expected to decrease hospitalisations and reduce costs. Generally, however, there was no significant improvement in the participants' health and wellbeing, and only three of the trials demonstrated a significant reduction in hospital admissions compared to the controls (Esterman & Ben-Tovim 2002).

REVIEW

The notion that the health of the Australian population improved in the twentieth century can be supported by analysis of mortality and morbidity patterns. This improvement, though, is qualified by the continued poor health of sub-populations such as Aboriginal and Torres Strait Islander peoples. Furthermore, there is no room for complacency in our society regarding infectious diseases, particularly pandemics such as HIV/AIDS, and developing epidemics such as avian influenza. Effective health promotion is influenced by the extent to which the health promoter understands the determinants of health within a social and environmental framework.

There have been a number of significant international and national developments in public health and health promotion policy that have set up many challenges for public health practitioners. These developments include revision of the national health goals and targets, the implementation of a national health strategy and the production of a national health policy. All have implications for the nature and scope of public health and health promotion practice in Australia in the future. These issues, together with an ecological approach to public health (discussed in Chapter 2), provide us with a conceptual framework to organise practice. The next chapter looks at the application of this framework in practice.

REVISION

Consider the main issues addressed in this chapter. Review each of these points in light of your understanding of national health policy developments and their implications for public health and health promotion practice.

1. *What are the main determinants of health status in Australia, and how do these determinants influence health promotion practice?*
2. *Identify and analyse each of the main stages in Australia's approach to health advancement over the past decade.*
3. *What lessons for the public health practitioner are to be learned from national health policy developments in Australia? Considering the list of national health policies, how integrated are they with each other and with other policies that impact on the health of the population?*

4. *Analyse the three main contemporary implications for health promotion practice in light of your understanding of the role of health promotion in public health in Australia.*
5. *Identify each of the activities that make up the sequence of policy development.*

PART II

PLANNING AND MANAGING HEALTH PROMOTION PROGRAMS

The ability to plan and evaluate health promotion programs, and to manage health promotion programs successfully, are important skills for contemporary health promotion practice. This section of the book contains two chapters that address these issues.

Chapter 4 outlines the principles of program planning and evaluation and their integration in successful practice. A range of program planning models is introduced. The importance of well-articulated programs based on sound theory, with clearly identified evaluation markers, forms the basis of all program development.

Skills are required to manage programs and activities for maximum gain and accountability. The theories of modern management and the implications of good management practice for health promoters form a backdrop against which management checklists are discussed in Chapter 5.

4

Program planning and evaluation

- *Evidence-based health promotion*
- *Integration of program planning and evaluation*
- *Program development*
- *Elements in program planning*
- *Program planning models*
- *Health promotion program evaluation*
- *Contemporary issues*
- *Beginning the evaluation*
- *Evaluation in action*
- *Evaluating community development*

In the first three chapters of this book, we introduced you to a history of public health, the emergence of ecological public health and the nature and scope of health promotion. We noted that health promotion had become integral to public health practice. Health promotion is multidisciplinary, and its interventions or programs and settings or practices are diverse—in schools, hospitals, community health centres, worksites, local government and in the community itself. Because of this diversity, program accountability becomes the responsibility of all health promotion workers. This requires a knowledge of and proficiency in program planning and evaluation to maximise outputs and outcomes, particularly within the current financial competition for health investments.

In this chapter, we discuss a selection of program planning and evaluation models that can be applied to health promotion initiatives. Current debates in evaluation are also identified. It is not our intention to replicate the substantial literature on health promotion program planning and evaluation. Excellent texts are available, for example, see Hawe et al. (1990); Pawson & Tilley (1997); Rossi et al. (1999); Glasgow (2002); Green and Kreuter (2005); Windsor et al. (2004); and McKenzie et al. (2005). Instead, we synthesise the literature in order to highlight the important principles.

Several definitions of 'program' exist. We have selected the following definition, because it is comprehensive in its scope:

> A grouping of resources (including persons, funds, equipment and supplies) performing activities all of which fall within definable boundaries enabling the scope of the program and its activities to be measured, and achieving outputs and outcomes aimed at fulfilling a definable set of objectives. (Health and Welfare Canada 1977)

A program's scope and depth are determined by its organisational setting. Some organisations use the terms 'project', 'program' and 'intervention' interchangeably. Whatever term is used, human and fiscal resources, equipment and supplies are involved; and goals and objectives, timelines and evaluative mechanisms shape the program's output.

EVIDENCE-BASED HEALTH PROMOTION

In 1996, the Health Advancement Committee of the Department of Health and Aged Care commissioned, through the National Health and Medical Research Council (NHMRC), a report entitled *Promoting the Health of Australians: Case studies of achievements in improving the health of the population* (NHMRC 1996). Now rescinded by the NHMRC, this report was one of the first attempts in Australia to demonstrate the evidence that multiple health promotion strategies can have an impact on population health issues, for example, tobacco control and injury.

The initiative coincided with a growing worldwide investigation linking evidence to professional health practice. Beginning with 'evidence-based' medicine and the establishment of the Cochrane Collaboration in 1993, systematic reviews of evidence have influenced all health discipline boundaries. Combined with the growth of the World Wide Web and information at the click of a mouse, practitioners can become adept at sifting evidence from such synthesising and diffusion initiatives as the Cochrane Collaboration for Health Promotion and the Campbell Collaboration (see 'Useful websites').

For health promotion, it is argued and generally accepted that with quality findings from intervention studies, practitioners can make better decisions to achieve effectiveness in their interventions (Tang et al. 2003). The nature of what constitutes 'health promotion' evidence, and its influence on policy and practice, has been debated and discussed (Perkins et al. 1999; Nutbeam 2004; Rychetnik & Wise 2004; de Leeuw 2005). Evidence is an integral component in working within models of health promotion best practice.

What are models of best practice health promotion?

'Best practices in health promotion are those sets of processes and activities that are consistent with health promotion values/goals/ethics, theories/ beliefs, evidence, and understanding of the environment, and that are most likely to achieve health promotion goals in a given situation' (Kahan & Goodstadt 2001).

How do they affect my practice?

'Best practice' for practitioners means that there is an accumulating evidence for what works under what conditions and for what groups and with what theories, program planning and evaluation tools. For example, if you are planning a tobacco control program for adolescents, you would begin by examining the evidence about what interventions have been most effective in the past. You could search the literature in journals, and systematic reviews completed either through the Cochrane Health Promotion and Public Health Field or other review databases. With this evidence, and the distinct values, goals, ethics, theories, beliefs and the context within which your program is planned (Kahan & Goodstadt 2001), you are beginning to work within a 'best practice' model of health promotion. The program planning and evaluation models proposed next will also assist this development.

INTEGRATION OF PROGRAM PLANNING AND EVALUATION

Kok (1993) suggested that inadequate planning and evaluation of programs are the reasons why health promotion is not effective in some cases. He urged health promotion professionals to reflect critically on their practice and to become skilled in planning and evaluation. His exhortations are still relevant today.

Green and Ottoson (1998) said that health promoters need to assume the role of 'sympathetic critic' when developing and evaluating programs. This role requires an open mind to the possibility both that the proposed program has great potential and that it might fail! It requires the ability to maintain an open mind on hopes and doubts even though all the people around you may be either demoralised or blindly enthusiastic.

This role of sympathetic critic is similar to what Schon (1995) called the art of the 'reflective practitioner'. Schon wrote extensively on the merits of reflective practice, arguing for a dual process that he called reflection-in-action and reflection-on-action. Practitioners need opportunities to think critically about puzzling or problematic features of their work, intending to encourage the practitioner as researcher, and researcher as practitioner, to improve the quality of their thinking in action and thereby to become 'reflective practitioners'. Usher et al. reassert this paradigm of reflective practice in revisiting Schon's work and emphasising that reflective practice needs to contain a continual re-scripting and critique of one's own practice (1997, p. 169). The framework of reflection-in-practice is applicable in health promotion program planning where evaluation can be a process of reflection-in-action (how well are our programs being implemented?), as well as a process of reflection-on-action (what impact are our programs having, and what outcomes are they achieving?).

Kok (1993) strongly recommended that health promoters increase and maintain their skills in program planning and evaluation. He offered a series of questions to aid health promoters:

- How serious is the health problem?
- Which health-related behaviour is involved?

- What are the determinants of that behaviour?
- Which combination of health promotion interventions—education, provisions, regulations—might change the determinants and behaviour?
- How can those interventions be implemented?

Kok's particular viewpoint in this discussion focused on a behavioural approach to the redressing of a health problem. Nonetheless, for health promoters working in a community where the health issue identified is not a behavioural risk factor, such as tobacco smoking, but rather an issue such as social isolation, the sequence of steps in program planning remains the same. These include: *mutually agreed-upon health issues;* an *understanding of the determinants of the issue*; and the development of *program plans that are multifaceted* and address the predisposing, enabling and reinforcing factors of the problem. The program components should be based on theoretical foundations to ensure as high a degree of success as possible. Knowledge of theories of behaviour, community and organisational change are recommended, as is a thorough literature search of previous successful interventions in the journals and databases.

It is obvious that programs cannot be evaluated in a vacuum. They are more easily evaluated when specific goals and objectives are articulated. Several authors (Hawe et al. 1990; Green & Kreuter 2005) have claimed that one of the flaws in health promotion practice has been the inability to build an evaluation plan into the planning stages of program design and implementation. Poor definition of anticipated outcomes has long been a stumbling block to progress in health promotion (Green & Lewis 1986; Hawe et al. 1990; Green & Kreuter 2005). Evaluation is crucial in assessing the process, impact, outcome, efficiency and effectiveness of a program.

The **program evaluation framework** (Figure 4.1) shows the successive steps involved in evaluation in a circular format. The six steps are:

- Engage stakeholders.
- Describe the program.
- Focus the evaluation.
- Gather credible evidence.
- Justify conclusions.
- Ensure the use of evaluation findings, and share the lessons learned.

These steps are interrelated and not necessarily linear; each builds on the successful completion of previous steps. Each stage in the framework is also allied with four criteria for 'good' evaluation:

- **Utility.** Does the evaluation have a constructive purpose; and will it satisfy the information needs of the various stakeholders, in a timely manner?
- **Feasibility.** Are the planned activities practical and resources used judiciously? Is the evaluation minimally disruptive to your program?
- **Propriety.** Is the evaluation ethical and does it protect the rights and welfare of those involved?
- **Accuracy.** Will the findings produced be valid and reliable? (Centers for Disease Control and Prevention (CDC) 1999)

Figure 4.1: Framework for program evaluation

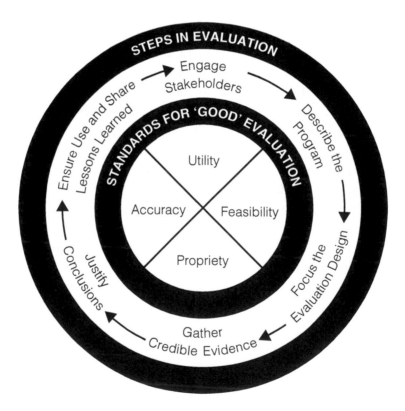

Source: Centers for Disease Control and Prevention (2000, p. 1)

PROGRAM DEVELOPMENT

Involving your community in planning a health promotion program adheres to one of the main principles of such planning—that is, the need to develop a collaborative planning partnership and mutual agreement about the issues with the people for whom the program is planned. This collaboration can take place in various ways. (These are more fully explained in Chapter 7.) With relationships and issues determined, the next stage can begin.

Establishing a program

- **Finding the right entry point.** It is important to find a common understanding with your community, not only about the issues, but also about the action that can be taken to address them. The 'community' could be a local residents' group, a group of workers or a school community. Working collaboratively with your community, using appropriate needs-assessment techniques, draws everyone together in the process. From this entry point, programs can be developed.
- **Developing a constituency and providing leadership.** McKenzie and Smeltzer (2001) suggested the need for a commitment to the proposed action from the leaders in the group you are working with, so that the program is seen as legitimate and, therefore, its chances of success are improved.
- **Creating an identity.** The use of the media and/or logos or symbols (stickers, T-shirts and so on) can be important, not only to enhance program participants' commitment and energy to the program, but also to provide outside support and interest in the program. For example, the local newspaper might provide free space for an article on the program, or a local service club might provide extra person power for tree planting in a school-based initiative.

ELEMENTS IN PROGRAM PLANNING

The steps to be taken in program planning are similar in a variety of health promotion settings, including workplaces, communities and schools, although the labels may vary. In the school health area (see Chapter 6), the elements of curriculum development have been extensively documented (Booth & Samdal 1997). They include:

- stating objectives
- selecting content
- selecting strategies or methods
- selecting organisational location
- selecting evaluation procedures.

Hawe et al. (1990) used a schema of goals, objectives, sub-objectives and strategy objectives as their preferred stages in developing a program, arguing that these stages easily relate to evaluation questions. Goals correspond to the health problem; objectives correspond to risk factors; sub-objectives relate to contributing risk factors; and strategy objectives correspond to program activities. Kok (1993) identified the sequence of steps in program planning as: **needs assessment; goals and objectives setting; selection of program components; implementation;** and **evaluation.** These steps are still appropriate today. Additional processes required to support planning and evaluation activities may include: assessing, having a vision, planning/revising, evaluating/reflecting, relationship building, skill sharing/capacity building, coordinating/cooperating, decision-making, communicating, documenting, and managing resources (adapted from Kahan & Goodstadt 2005).

The selection of strategies and activities in any health promotion program should be based on theory. Kurt Lewin, the famous social psychologist upon whose work much health education theory has been based, is reported to have said, 'There is nothing as practical as a good theory' (1951, p. 169). Yet few health promoters use theory as a guide to establish explanations and predictions of human behaviour, or to establish program strategies and methods that bring about the desired change. This comment is substantiated by Kok (1993) and Bartholomew et al. (1998), who argued that the lack of theory might also be the reason a particular choice of strategies and methods often does not work. Models of individual health behaviour, such as the health belief model, the theory of reasoned action, or its more recent variant, the theory of planned behaviour, as well as models of interpersonal behaviour such as social cognitive theory, have been used widely and are reviewed in various publications (for example, Glanz et al. 2002; Nutbeam & Harris 2004; Kerr et al. 2005). Staging models, such as the transtheoretical model (for example, Prochaska et al. 2005), have often been used in combination with social cognitive theory (for example, Baranowski et al. 1997) to improve the potency of a health promotion program; and ecological planning approaches (for example, Sorensen et al. 1998; Sallis & Owen 2002) are commonly used in public health and health promotion. A combination of models or theories can often assist in the development of more individually tailored and targeted strategies (Oldenburg et al. 1999). The lesson for all health promoters is to understand theories of behaviour change, community organisation and organisation development, as these theories can more accurately inform strategy and activity selection.

So much attention may be devoted to the objectives, content, strategies and methods of a program that the 'process' of implementation may often be overlooked. Parkinson (1982) considered three approaches to overcome this. These fundamental approaches have been expanded on by McKenzie et al. (2005):

- **The pilot approach.** This is an important first step in implementing a health promotion program. Green (1986) calls this the *site response*; that is, obtaining feedback from participants involved in the program, as well as from staff planners, on the *quality* of the program in all its dimensions—from educational materials (for example, pamphlets or displays) to the appropriateness of the staff chosen to deliver the program. This valuable feedback from the pilot phase is also known as *process evaluation*, an evaluation of the processes involved in implementation.
- **The phased-in approach.** This occurs when programs are implemented at different sites, areas or regions. A pilot program may have yielded a positive process evaluation, and/or the evaluation may have yielded adjustments to the program. The decision is then made to phase the program into various settings over time because of resource constraints.
- **Immediate implementation of the total program.** Programs that have been effective in the past, or programs that have a standard approach, are often implemented in their totality.

Our view is that a pilot approach to any newly developed program is imperative. This approach serves to engage your community in the design, process evaluation and execution, thereby ensuring commitment from the community itself.

PROGRAM PLANNING MODELS

Numerous books and articles have been written on health promotion program planning (Nutbeam 1998; Bartholomew et al. 1998, 2001; Goodstadt et al. 2001; Ewles & Simnett 2003; Green & Kreuter 2005). These and other program planning models have been used in the past twenty years in a variety of health promotion settings—in schools, workplaces, communities and health care settings.

Table 4.1: Program planning models for health promotion

Planning model	Key elements in each model
Ewles and Simnett (2003) Seven-stage model	Seven stages: identify needs and priorities; set aims and objectives; decide the best way of achieving aims; identify resources; plan evaluation methods; set an action plan; take action.
Green and Kreuter (2005) PRECEDE/PROCEED	Eight phases that build on one another: phase 1 identifies goals and problems of concern to the target population; phase 2 identifies specific health goals and problems; phase 3 diagnoses predisposing, enabling and reinforcing factors; phase 4 assesses organisational and administrative capabilities and resources; phase 5 develops program components and implementation; phases 6 to 8 cover evaluation.
Goodstadt et al. (2001) A generic model for planning and evaluating health promotion	Eight steps: describe program; identify issues and questions; design data collection process; collect data; analyse and interpret data; make recommendations; dissemination; take action.
Nutbeam (1998) Staged model for planning, implementation and evaluation of health promotion programs	Adds capacity-building through staff development, social mobilisation, advocacy and dissemination of results.
Bartholomew, Parcel, Kok and Gottlieb (1998, 2001) Intervention mapping	Five steps: developing matrices for creating 'proximal' program objectives/matrices; method selection; strategies and program design; planning and adoption; implementing and evaluation.

Each of the models presented in Table 4.1 uses a step-by-step approach to program planning—Ewles and Simnett (2003) propose a seven-stage linear model focused on writing objectives which encompass cognitive, affective and skill domains in behaviour change programs. Green and Kreuter (2005) expand their diagnostic planning model, PRECEDE (Predisposing, Reinforcing and Enabling Constructs in Educational/Environmental Diagnosis and Evaluation) to PROCEED (Policy, Regulatory and Organisational Constructs in Educational and Environmental Development). This model includes additional environmental and genetic dimensions and has been applied successfully worldwide in schools, worksites and communities. Nutbeam (1998) integrates many of the elements from the above models into a comprehensive planning and evaluation model with an additional important element that considers the dissemination of results. Table 4.1 highlights each model's key stages, phases or elements.

Five models of planning

A summary of each of the models in Table 4.1 is given below, and a selection of brief examples illustrates the models in practice.

Ewles and Simnett's (2003) Seven-stage model
This can be used as a template for program planning action. It offers a broad guideline for the steps taken in program planning and is useful in its simplicity.

A shortcoming of this model is the placement of the evaluation planning phase at stage 5; evaluation questions should in fact be discussed and planned at the same time as the objectives are formulated at stage 2 in this particular model (O'Connor-Fleming et al. 2006). However, this model does identify a logical, step-by-step framework for planning health promotion programs. The steps can be applied to a variety of settings—to a school-based program, to a workplace and in a community. Ewles and Simnett also provide guidance on writing objectives. The importance of specificity in program objectives cannot be overemphasised, as a successful evaluation is dependent on their clarity. Educational objectives can be classified into three categories: cognitive objectives; affective objectives; and behavioural or skill objectives.

Cognitive objectives are those that are related to giving information, explaining it and ensuring students or clients understand it—thereby increasing their knowledge. **Affective objectives** are concerned with attitudes, beliefs, values and opinions. Attitudes are a combination of concepts, information and emotion. For example, if a person has a particular attitude, it means that he or she is likely to respond in a particular way. Educational objectives in this affective area are concerned with clarifying, forming or changing a client's attitudes, beliefs, values or opinions. **Behavioural or skill objectives** relate to learning how to master certain skills and actions.

In health promotion programs, it is rare that only one set of objectives, such as cognitive objectives, will be used. Most often, a combination of affective or behavioural/skill objectives is required. For example, persuading a smoker to stop smoking is primarily concerned with the objective of changing the smoker's feeling of 'determination to continue' into a feeling of 'wanting to stop'. This then could lead into the behavioural/skill objective of acquiring the skills necessary to stop smoking, for example, being able to refuse the offer of a cigarette. Cognitive objectives may also be included and may involve giving the smoker information about the effects of smoking and various approaches to stopping smoking. Again, remember the previous exhortation that, as far as possible, programs be theory based!

It is worthwhile pausing here to consider the process of writing objectives. Health promoters often confuse objectives with activities or strategies—the latter refer to the list of actions that you intend to carry out, for example, developing and printing brochures for a target group would be an activity. Objectives, on the other hand, are precise statements that map out the tasks necessary to reach a goal. An objective is a defined commitment to a predetermined specific outcome that contributes to the goal. Realise that the emphasis is on the outcomes, rather than the activities, of the program.

Objectives should be stated clearly in terms of the timeframe within which an activity will take place, the direction of change to be facilitated in the target population, the magnitude of change anticipated, and a precise definition of the way change will be measured. For example, an objective might read as follows: 'By the end of 2007 (timeframe) there will be a 30 per cent increase (direction and magnitude of change) in correct dental flossing behaviour of Year 8 children, noted through (measured by) direct observation and parental reporting.' Activities undertaken to achieve this objective could be to conduct an oral health promotion program demonstrating correct flossing procedures to Year 8 students, or to produce easy-to-read instruction pamphlets for parents and students.

Ewles and Simnett's (2003) approach to writing objectives that include cognitive, affective and behavioural/skill domains is based on the belief that the combination in education programs of these three domains is linked to behaviour change. Whether a health promoter is working in a community to reduce isolation among the elderly or to improve traffic calming near a primary school, writing objectives as specifically as possible is an important principle to follow. It provides program clarity and is significant for evaluation purposes.

Green and Kreuter's (2005) PRECEDE/PROCEED model
The expansion of PRECEDE (Predisposing, Reinforcing and Enabling Constructs in Educational/Environmental Diagnosis and Evaluation) to include Policy, Regulatory and Organisational Constructs in Educational and Environmental Development (PROCEED) offers health promoters a comprehensive program planning model. First developed in 1980 as a diagnostic planning tool, the recent expansion includes a developmental stage of health promotion planning that involves an implementation and evaluation process. The richness of this model and its proven efficacy in program development in school, community and worksite settings makes it a 'must know' for health promoters.

The strength of the model includes the recognition of various starting points for health promotion. Typically, most risk factor intervention programs address a health problem, such as heart disease. While recognising this approach, the authors give legitimacy to analysing social conditions which often inform any analysis of community needs. For example, these 'conditions' or 'environmental issues' can be as broad as social isolation in the workplace, lack of public transport in neighbourhoods, or student alienation and loneliness in large schools. These 'quality of life' concerns are the starting points in this model. The elements of the model are set out in Figure 4.2.

PRECEDE/PROCEED directs the health promoter's initial attention to outcomes rather than inputs. This accent on outcomes—'quality of life' issues—pushes the health promoter not to focus on program inputs (for example, what resources to develop) but to begin at the end, with the output of the total programming enterprise.

Phase 1   Consider quality of life issues of concern to people in the population in question (patients, school students, community

Figure 4.2: PRECEDE/PROCEED model

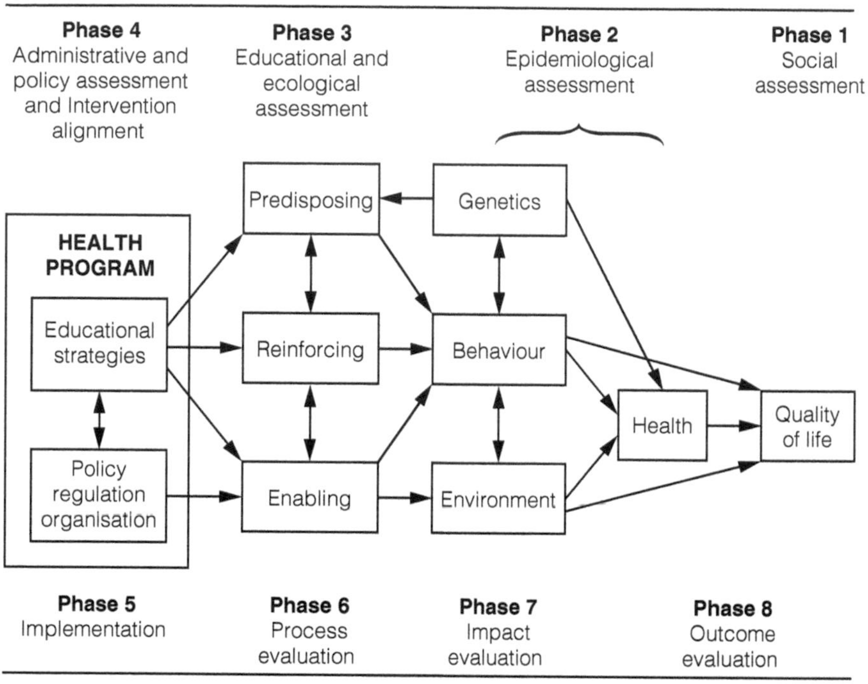

Source: L.W. Green and M.W. Kreuter 2005, *Health Promotion Planning: An Educational and Ecological Approach*, 4th edn, McGraw-Hill, New York, p. 10.

groups). Many methods exist to ascertain these quality of life issues—for example, community surveys, meetings with student bodies and focus groups.

Phase 2   Identify specific health problems that appear to be contributing to the social problems noted in phase 1. This is your epidemiological diagnosis. These are then ranked, and a selection is made to identify to which of these problems resources can be assigned. (Often resources are scarce, and care should be taken that both fiscal and human resources can be assigned to the program—and not just in the short term.)

The reality of much health promotion practice is that often these phases have been attended to or are assumed. Health promoters, including those working as school health educators, typically develop programs after phases 1 and 2 have been completed by someone else; for example, a drug and alcohol program is to be implemented in a school by the school physical education teacher. This program has been developed statewide and is to be implemented irrespective of whether the local school community has identified it as a priority.

Phase 2   (continued) Identify specific health-related behaviours and environmental and genetic factors that appear to be linked to the health problem chosen. Note that in Figure 4.2 Green and Kreuter (2005) link all three factors to the health problem and/or quality of life issues to be addressed. This recognises that any, or a combination, of the factors can impinge on health and/or quality of life issues. This gives you an opportunity to work with your community in deciding which factors have priority.

For example, suppose you work with a group of elderly people and the issue of access to transport to a community health centre is identified as affecting their quality of life. Of equal importance is their desire for more information about arthritis pain relief. The group identifies the transport issue as a priority and you plan to address that issue first; and arthritis information is offered at the community health centre anyway.

Phase 3   From the vast array of potential influences on behavioural and environmental change, Green and Kreuter (2005) identified three broad categories of factors that have a direct impact on the selection done in phase 2. These are:

- Predisposing factors—attitudes, values, beliefs, and perceptions that affect personal motivation.
- Enabling factors—barriers created by societal forces or systems. Limited facilities, forces, resources, laws and statutes, skills and knowledge. These factors include those that make the desired change in the environment or behaviour possible.
- Reinforcing factors—feedback from others may assist, hinder or prohibit either a change in behaviour or a change in the environmental factors impinging on a particular social condition. (For example, the mayor and local council might give positive feedback to a group of elderly citizens

who have approached them for help with a change in bus routes and timetables.)

Phase 4   Decide about organisational and administrative capabilities and resources. Often, at this phase, it is realised that human and fiscal resources are either not forthcoming or not as substantial as first promised—staff may have been reassigned or budgets spent! It is important when embarking on any systematic planning process that this phase is thought about at the outset. It is, of course, difficult to gauge budget requirements when engaged in a planning process, but informing managers of projected requirements early on alleviates the potential for stress. This is a worst-case scenario but one which occurs often. Green and Kreuter (2005) provide guidelines for the development of timelines and budgets.

This phase is critical because of the abovementioned 'politics' of program planning—those organisational and administrative arrangements that can promote or impede planning.

Phase 5   Develop and implement the program, keeping in mind the resource limitations, time constraints and abilities of the staff who are implementing the program. It might be necessary to build in a training program for such staff. Decisions about whether this is a pilot project, a phase-in or a full implementation program should have been made. Check that the right combination of intervention strategies, assessment of administration problems and resource allocation has been achieved.

Phases 6–8 Evaluate each phase. The evaluation should be developed as a part of continuously working through the entire model.

There are several features inherent in Green and Kreuter's (2005) model that make it comprehensive. First, health and health behaviour are influenced by multiple factors; therefore, health promotion efforts to effect behaviour change must be multidimensional, multisectoral, and participatory—that is, they must address the predisposing, enabling and reinforcing factors that impact on behaviour. Second, social conditions which impact on health are included in the diagnosis and given full recognition. Health promoters can plan simultaneous integrated activities to address social conditions. Most program planning models adopt a disease-prevention framework as their *modus operandi*; for instance, if we address risk factors that are linked to particular diseases, there is less likelihood of early onset of that health problem. This is indeed true, but health promotion research has shown that this approach, taken alone, has only marginal utility for some population groups. Health promotion that focuses solely on behaviour does not take into account or recognise the importance of the social context of people's day-to-day lives, which can influence the uptake of risk behaviours. The strength of PRECEDE/PROCEED is that it provides the scope and depth needed to address multiple factors that impact on health.

Goodstadt et al.'s Generic model for planning and evaluating health promotion
The WHO European Working Group on Health Promotion Evaluation was instituted in 1995, with participants from the Centers for Disease Control and Prevention (US), Health Canada and the Health Development Agency (UK). The group's objectives were to: examine the current range of quantitative and qualitative evaluation methods; and provide guidance to policy-makers and practitioners to facilitate the use of appropriate methods for health promotion evaluation and to increase the quality of evaluations.

The working group did not set out to provide a specific evaluation model; instead their aim was to clarify what it means to evaluate, what knowledge means regarding health promotion and how this knowledge may be acquired through evaluation (Goodstadt et al. 2001). Nine key principles regarding evaluation in health promotion were outlined. Evaluation:

- is an evolving discipline;
- can make a major contribution to practice;
- suffers a shortage of evidence on effectiveness;
- comprises a range of models;
- offers a legitimate role for quantitative and qualitative methodologies;
- employs a wide range of social science disciplines and approaches;
- builds on a range of planning models;
- requires theory to be effective; and
- offers many potential roles to evaluators.

The group outlined a generic model for planning and evaluating health promotion consistent with the Ottawa Charter (WHO 1986a).

Nutbeam's Staged model for planning, implementation and evaluation of health promotion programs

In Figure 4.3, Nutbeam (1998) builds on the increasing evidence base of health promotion, and addresses the gaps between research and practice, particularly with respect to the dissemination of research results. The gap between research and practice, due to the lack of dissemination of results to the broader promotion community, has been documented (Oldenburg et al. 1999). Nutbeam attempts to close this gap in his integrated planning and evaluation model, first presented at a national health promotion conference in 1998. The starting points of problem definition and solution generation are also the basis of other models (Green & Kreuter 2005).

Nutbeam makes explicit the notion of capacity building through staff training. This is often overlooked in the reality of everyday planning for programs. Additionally, social mobilisation/advocacy are built into the model, so that the criticism that is sometimes levelled at health promoters—that their programs are 'top down'—is responded to. A vast literature and practice base has developed in health promotion over the past 25 years. However, communicating the outcomes and failures of programs is also a significant responsibility—this adds to the body of evidence about what does and does not work and under what circumstances. Nutbeam's (1998) 'Dissemination of Results' guide reminds us to include a communication strategy in our plans.

Bartholomew, Parcel, Kok and Gottlieb's Intervention mapping

The basis of intervention mapping is Green and Kreuter's (1999) PRECEDE/PROCEED model. The steps and procedures included in intervention mapping provide a system for the integration of theory, empirical findings from the literature, and information collected from the target population (Bartholomew et al. 1998, p. 546). The authors argue that their 'map' is explicit enough to demystify the process for collaborative planning. The map contains a comprehensive needs assessment and capacity framework as a starting point.

There are five detailed steps in developing matrices for creating 'proximal' program objectives/matrices: selecting methods; specifying practical strategies and designing the program; planning for adoption; implementing the program plan; and planning the evaluation (see Figure 4.4). The strength of 'mapping' is that 'proximal' program objectives are specified in step 1. These are designed as matrices, which create the

Figure 4.3: Staged model for planning implementation and evaluation of health promotion programs

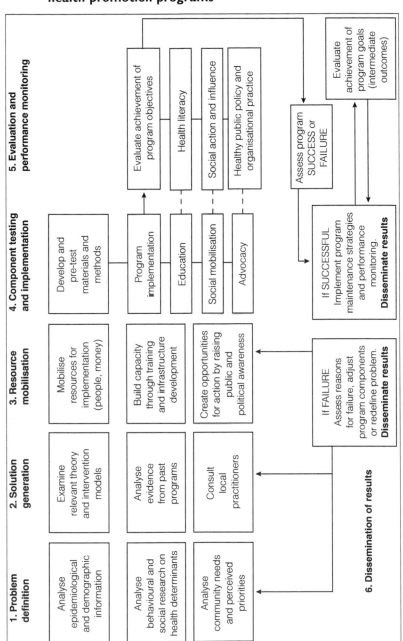

Source: Nutbeam, 10th National Health Promotion Conference, 1998, Adelaide; reprinted with permission of the author

intersection of behavioural and environmental performance objectives—in reality, they contain explicit change objectives which specify what individuals need to learn or what must be changed in the environment as a result of the program. They represent the starting point for change, as well as for examining the determinants of the problem.

Intervention mapping was used successfully in the Cystic Fibrosis Family Education program in the United States. The program has been evaluated thoroughly. It combines social cognitive theory, education and training, and self-management strategies. The uniqueness of intervention mapping is the level of detail, particularly with respect to the application of theories to underpin strategy selection. This builds on Kok's (1993) arguments regarding the need for theoretically robust health promotion program plans.

HEALTH PROMOTION PROGRAM EVALUATION

Program evaluation often raises anxiety among health promotion practitioners. Some feel that the skills required are too difficult, or that resources are not available to allow a 'scientific' evaluation; others believe that programs being scrutinised too thoroughly will lose funding (O'Connor-Fleming et al. 2006). Still others believe that health promotion is about 'enabling and empowerment' and that the concepts are too difficult to evaluate. Despite these sentiments, Nutbeam (1993a) claimed that all aspects of a program can be evaluated, and that evaluation can be flexible enough to respond to each stage of development and implementation. Additionally, King comments that there is generally a lack of information about program effectiveness in health promotion, and there is a need to build an agenda for dissemination about successful program elements, to build practice-relevant research and to investigate successful dissemination approaches that can enrich practice (1996, p. 7).

What is evaluation?

Various definitions of evaluation exist. Green and Kreuter define evaluation as the 'comparison of an object of interest with a standard of acceptability' (1999, p. 220). This definition identifies the three essential components of

Figure 4.4: Steps of the intervention mapping framework

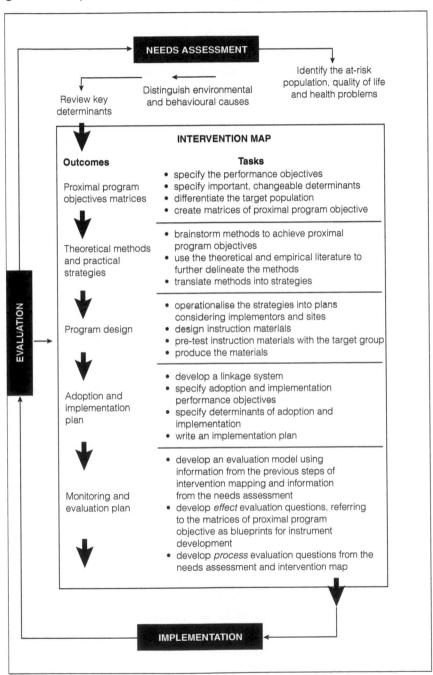

Source: Bartholomew, Parcel and Kok (1998, p. 548)

evaluation: a comparison, an object of interest and a standard. Without a comparison of some kind, even if it is only a comparison with an imaginary ideal or a purely subjective preference, there can be no evaluation. The definition is broad enough to include both processes and outcomes that can be evaluated; and it presents a range of standards of acceptability, leading us to realise that a variety of assessment procedures may be employed in evaluation.

Hawe et al. define evaluation as 'the process by which we judge the worth or value of something' (1990, p. 6). How you evaluate depends on what you think is important, how the evaluation is conducted, and whose interests the evaluation serves (Hawe et al. 1990). Obviously, evaluation must be relevant to the goals and objectives of program activity, and the measurement of these activities needs to be appropriate (O'Connor-Fleming et al. 2006).

CONTEMPORARY ISSUES

The multiple determinants of health indicate a wide range of areas of action for health promoters—public policy development (economic and legislative strategies), public participation (community development), media advocacy, social action, organisation development, social support and networking, dissemination of results, capacity building and personal skills development for behaviour change. This impressive array can be viewed from various perspectives—changes in a community's capacity to cope, environmental changes, changes in public policies, individual behaviour changes, the strengthening of social supports and networks, and healthier organisations. Health promotion needs a variety of evaluation models to address an expanding repertoire of strategies.

Earlier health education practice focused on individualistic orientations targeted at 'lifestyle modification' and behaviour change. As the concept of health promotion expanded in the 1980s, critics of this singular approach to research and evaluation emerged. Lincoln (1992), and Simpson and Freeman (2004) claimed that, as health promotion is dealing with the complexity of human understandings, beliefs, fears, attitudes and prejudices, the research and evaluation repertoire needed to be expanded to include models for inquiry that are more 'resonant with human, social, behavioural and cultural phenomena', as the human, cultural and social side of health promotion is not well understood using the classical scientific method. Lincoln asserted that the repertoire be expanded with the legitimacy given to action research and ethnographic methods to be matched to the complexity and context of life. She labelled her particular paradigm the 'constructivist' paradigm, and argued that grounded theories of human aspiration for health needed to be developed which utilise qualitative methods and constructivist philosophies. The breadth of health-enhancing strategies in the Ottawa Charter (WHO 1986a) raised questions about appropriate evaluation models and measurement. The social view of health promulgated within the 'new public health' demand a holistic method of analysis that is sufficiently powerful to advance understanding of the dynamics of social change (Baum 1992a). In addition, the social and policy approaches generally accepted as important instruments for having an impact on health have not traditionally been considered in program evaluation.

With respect to these challenges, Thompson (1990, p. 70) proposed that evaluation questions be expanded, and suggested three particular components that reflect a philosophy of health promotion. These combine both social policy and educational and behaviour approaches in tune with 'new public health' philosophies; these questions can frame your evaluation:

- **Program concept**—does the program address the health challenges of reducing inequities, increasing prevention and enhancing coping skills?
- **Program processes**—do the program interventions both strengthen factors that sustain health and reduce factors that cause vulnerability to health?
- **Program impact**—what health improvement targets have been achieved?

These layers focus our questions and assist in making the evaluation relevant to its overall aim and purpose. The Integrated Domain Model (Kahan & Goodstadt 2005; see 'Useful websites') provides an elaboration on these core foci and assists with ensuring the evaluation is relevant for the program context.

In their Heartbeat Wales study, Nutbeam et al. (1993a) pointed out the difficulties in maintaining evaluation designs in long-term, community-based health promotion programs. As success in any such program rests on the ability to influence a range of predisposing factors, these 'new intervention approaches pose special challenges for developing appropriate and manageable evaluation designs that can be maintained throughout the life of a program' (1993a, p. 127). From the Heartbeat Wales experience, Nutbeam et al. (1993a) formulated three substantive areas in which to monitor program inputs and reach. These were: supportive environments; creation of new resources; and coordination, monitoring and communication. By quantifying the inputs, Nutbeam et al. (1993a) asserted the importance of comprehensive process evaluation in both the intervention and, in their study, reference areas. They emphasised the need for alternative experimental designs in assessing the effectiveness of long-term intervention programs. Judd et al. (2001) argued also that effective long-term evaluations will be achieved when standards are agreed upon between funders, evaluators and communities, particularly considering community realities.

Smith and Glass (1987) offer four paradigms that can guide decisions about how, when and what to evaluate. These paradigms are still relevant and are useful starting points for evaluation decisions.

The first paradigm is evaluation as **applied research**. Field experiments, quasi-experiments, and randomised clinical trials are examples of methods used. Rigour and validity are central; methods are primarily quantitative, objectives clearly specified and program goals limited. Evidence from the evaluation is presented to policy-makers for decisions based on the material. An example of this approach is an evaluation of a lifestyle modification program utilising pre- and post-tests and control groups.

The second paradigm is evaluation as part of **systems management**. A setting such as a school is a system with inputs, processes and outputs. The role of the evaluator is to relate to each of these components within the evaluation design; the manager of the 'system' makes decisions to modify particular aspects of the components. The evaluation is formative and provides feedback to improve levels of performance. Stufflebeam's (2003) Context, Input, Process and Product (CIPP) model is useful for evaluating policy implementation and activities within organisation systems.

The third evaluation paradigm is that of **professional judgment**. Models that employ direct observation and interviews with clients enable professionals to make judgments about programs against established standards. An example of this paradigm is the accreditation or critical review by outside experts, of a health care setting such as a hospital.

The fourth evaluation paradigm is **evaluation-as-politics**, which focuses on the link between evaluation and organisational politics, as occasionally policy-makers may ignore the results of evaluations. Thus, it is necessary at the outset to engage all stakeholders in the outcome of a program evaluation. Qualitative case studies can be combined with quasi-experimental studies, in order to provide as comprehensive an approach to the evaluation questions as possible (Smith & Glass 1987). Each of the four paradigms can guide the evaluator in becoming aware of the context in which an evaluation takes place.

BEGINNING THE EVALUATION

Obviously, it is important to understand the purpose of the evaluation. Owen (2004) provides us with a helpful list of issues: Is the evaluation for the purpose of determining the way a program is to be implemented? synthesising information to aid program development? clarifying a program? improving the implementation of a program? monitoring program outcomes? determining program worth? Owen stresses the importance of determining the audience for the evaluation prior to developing an evaluation plan.

The context in which decisions about the results of an evaluation are going to be made cannot be overlooked. Program evaluation does not occur in an organisational vacuum, so it is important to *analyse* the evaluation audience and the scope of the evaluation, to ensure that adequate resources are available. This includes identifying at the beginning *key* decision-makers and their concerns to ensure the credibility and use of the findings. The agenda of these people, and the values they hold about the program, provide an evaluation context for your efforts. Such decision-makers can be the staff sponsoring the evaluation and/or making decisions based on the results, the staff running the program or the target group participants. Furthermore, if the program is publicly funded, the public also has a right to the results. If you clearly understand the evaluation context, you can be hopeful that key decision-makers will not be adversely surprised by the results of your evaluation. Once you have completed this process, you will have set the background for your evaluation efforts.

Two processes are involved in evaluation. The first is observation and measurement—the collecting of some form of data through interviews, survey questionnaires or direct observation. The second process is the comparison of what you observe with some criterion or standard of good performance—a standard of acceptability. Specifying the standard against which you are going to measure program efforts is essential. Otherwise, once the data are collected, it will be tempting to call any level of improvement or change a success! Setting out clearly the process by which the program is to be judged does not eliminate values that influence how the judgment is made, but at least it holds them up to public scrutiny (Hawe et al. 1990). Evaluation can occur at various levels:

- **effort**—resources available and used by the program; activities planned and carried out, and the relationship between activities and resources
- **effectiveness**—attainment of program outcomes
- **efficacy**—benefits of the program to the clients
- **efficiency**—achievements relative to costs
- **execution**—adequacy of delivery, accessibility, quality, side effects, client satisfaction.

The choice of the aspect to study will depend on the questions you need to answer and the stage of development of the program. A program can be assessed in different ways at different times.

EVALUATION IN ACTION

In this section, we examine two evaluation models.

Model 1: Program evaluation using applied research methods

This is the traditional model of evaluation used by most health promoters. Program goals and objectives are written as specifically as possible to enable an effective evaluation to be made. Hawe et al. (1990) present an extensive step-by-step approach to the writing of specific program goals and objectives, as well as the methods employed in evaluating program goals and objectives in terms of program processes, impacts and outcomes. The book is highly recommended for students and practitioners because of its comprehensive approach and its extensive detail on evaluation levels.

Levels of evaluation
There are three commonly agreed-upon levels of evaluation—process, impact and outcome. *Process evaluation* measures the activities of the

Figure 4.5: Evaluation methods checklist

Type of evaluation	Quest.-comm. participants	Focus groups	Document review/Minutes	Face-to-face interviews	Journal	Group interviews	Observations	Other
Project reach—key questions								
Participant satisfaction—key questions								
Project implementation—key questions								
Project quality—key questions								
Impact evaluation—key questions								
Outcome evaluation—key questions								

Source: Parker and Steele (1993), adapted from Hawe et al. (1990)

program, its quality and who it is reaching. *Impact evaluation* measures the immediate effect of the program (does it meet its objectives?). *Outcome evaluation* measures the long-term effect of the program (does it meet its goals?) (Hawe et al. 1990, p. 60).

These evaluations are conducted in sequence. Health promoters often begin by trying to evaluate the impact of programs, without having focused enough attention on 'ironing out the bugs' by examining whether or not the program has been implemented correctly. Hawe et al. suggest four questions that need to be asked about a program during a process evaluation. Attention needs to be given first to these questions (below). Doing so helps to ensure a thorough process evaluation. (See Figure 4.5 for a checklist of methods that can be used to gather data on each of these questions in a process evaluation, and on evaluation questions in impact and outcome evaluation.)

- Is the program **reaching** the target group? Are all parts of the program reaching all parts of the target group?
- Are participants **satisfied** with the program?
- Are all the activities of the program being **implemented**?
- Are all the materials and components of the program of good **quality**? (1990, p. 61)

In assessing **reach**, program planners want to know whether the intended audience for program activities is being accessed. If people are not attending program activities, what are the reasons? The time may not be suitable, transport may be a difficulty, or publicity may be inadequate. The contributing factors to poor program reach need to be examined.

In assessing participant **satisfaction**, we are interested in gathering feedback on what aspects the participants are satisfied with or not satisfied with. In a health education program involving group work, questions could be asked about the venue, the program content, and the expertise and attitude of the facilitators. Again, we are interested in measures that can be adopted to enhance participants' satisfaction and the impact of a program.

In assessing **implementation**, we are concerned with understanding the suitability and effectiveness of program activities. For example, is the program being conducted the way that it should in terms of agreed content?

Assessing **quality** is a critical stage. We are interested in knowing whether the content, readability and the cultural perspective of program materials are appropriate. Conducting focus groups prior to the final development of materials such as pamphlets and videos is one method suggested for determining this aspect.

Process evaluation should not be overlooked in any health promotion intervention. Most, if not all, health promotion programs are expected to show an effective impact on participants; some fail because the above process evaluation questions have not been asked.

With respect to measuring program effects, both qualitative and quantitative methods of investigation are available. Hawe et al. (1990) are helpful in their recommendation that one conduct an evaluability assessment— that is, make sure that a program is ready for evaluation prior to embarking on the impact and outcome evaluation. They provide useful tips for planning impact and outcome evaluations, along with helpful guidelines for gathering data on knowledge, attitude and behaviour change, and a discussion on measuring health status. A range of evaluation designs, with their strengths, limitations and applications, is also presented (Hawe et al. 1990, pp. 118–23).

Another version of this approach is the widely accepted and adopted RE-AIM model proposed by Glasgow et al. (1999) that assesses five dimensions of initiatives:

- Reach—the degree to which an initiative reaches those in need.
- Efficacy—the assessment of the positive and negative consequences of an initiative, incorporating behavioural, quality of life and participant satisfaction indicators in addition to physiologic outcomes.
- Adoption by target setting or institutions—this assesses the proportion and representativeness of settings that adopt a change, as well as barriers to adoption.
- Implementation—measures the consistency of the delivery of an intervention, that is, the extent to which a program is delivered as intended. At the individual level, it determines adherence.
- Maintenance—the evaluation of the intended effects in individuals and populations over time, that is, the extent to which a program becomes institutionalised or part of the everyday culture.

Model 2: Health promotion as systems and policy management

Stufflebeam's (2003) CIPP model of evaluation is presented, as it is particularly appropriate for school-based curriculum evaluation and the analysis of policy initiatives. Four elements are proposed in this evaluation model: context, input, process and product.

Context evaluation defines the environment in which change is to occur. Input evaluation determines how one can utilise resources to meet program goals by identifying capabilities of the agency or organisation in implementing a program. Strategies that may be appropriate for meeting the goals are assessed; this might involve an analysis of the human and fiscal resources required and the commitments of staff and/or clients to the particular policy or program goal. Process evaluation is an ongoing evaluation of the implementation of the plan, with a record of how the intentions are being implemented in day-to-day practice. Product evaluation measures, interprets and judges the effectiveness of a program or policy—for example, student learning outcomes in a curriculum evaluation. Each of these levels also assists program or curriculum managers with decisions they need to make.

Context evaluation informs planning decisions by examining and adjusting existing goals and priorities and targeting needed changes. The environment or context of programs and policies can affect their strategic directions. Input evaluation can assist decisions by examining barriers and constraints that are taken into account in the development and implementation of programs. Process evaluation can guide decisions about program improvements and modifications. Product evaluation serves decisions about future policy and program directions.

Both Stufflebeam's (2003) CIPP model and Stake's (1983) 'responsive evaluation' are important additions in the assessment of policy, school and professional curriculum areas. The Australian federal government accepted the CIPP model to evaluate the Diabetes Prevention Pilot Initiative in 2006.

EVALUATING COMMUNITY DEVELOPMENT

Community development is an accepted health promotion approach as it coincides with the 'new public health' conceptual framework that emphasises the critical role of social, political and psychological factors in both the development of ill health and its prevention. An evaluation of strategies that aim to increase levels of participation in health matters provides valuable input for both program managers and communities engaged in the community development process. The task of evaluating community development strategies can seem daunting, as the goals and objectives are often imprecise—because the community development process itself is dynamic. An evaluation of community development can make use of indicators of the impact of such psychosocial factors influencing health potential as community participation, social support, alienation and empowerment.

Attempts have been made to measure community participation in primary health care (Potvin et al. 2003) through work in Canada, and social support measures are available (Gottlieb 1983); and, with the increasing prominence of the concepts of alienation and empowerment in the social science and health literature, the task of refining the measurement of these variables is ongoing (Perkins & Zimmerman 1995).

Hawe teases out concepts of community development, empowerment and community organisation. She proposes, as part of an evaluability assessment process, that 'workers, community partners, and other key parties consider what changes they would like to see as a result of the program and what would make them think the project was successful' (1994, p. 199). Drawing on community psychology, Hawe (1994) redefines the term 'empowerment' into manageable components—for example, attitudinal, consciousness, skill and structural dimensions. This breakdown creates a framework through which appropriate evaluation questions can be asked.

Baum (1992a, 1998) suggested that multiple methods of evaluating community development should be used, including:

- interviews (usually semi-structured or unstructured), questionnaires and focus groups to obtain opinions and data; during this stage, key informants should be involved;
- participant observation to provide another perspective on topics under consideration;
- diaries kept by staff to document field work and day-to-day records of activities; and
- minutes, attendances at meetings, and official documentation to provide quantitative indicators of programs.

In addition, analysis of media coverage during an initiative can be relevant for community-based campaigns and can be compared with the coverage prior to the project commencing.

In summary, 'strengthening community action' is consistent with the philosophy of health promotion and one of the action areas of the *Ottawa Charter for Health Promotion* (WHO 1986a). Community development is one of the strategies employed in this process. Many people participate in community development, and often have competing agendas. Gaining agreement on the goals and indicators of success and clearly articulated objectives is a critical ingredient in an evaluation, but is not an easy task. Community-driven projects are often without stable funding or have only short-term funding. Project staff often have limited time, so documentation of ongoing activities by the methods cited is invaluable for process evaluation. Ideally, objectives that are clearly written—setting out place, person, time and amount of change—will provide benchmarks that assist at the impact level of an evaluation. The models presented here should assist you in beginning your evaluations.

REVIEW

There is evidence that health promotion has an effect on population health. Health promotion program plans and evaluation methods need to reside within robust evidence and utilise proven methods and theories for effectiveness. This practice embraces the core values, ethics and goals of communities or clients. A collaborative approach for evaluation design can be agreed upon. Health promotion practitioners are able to use a variety of program planning and evaluation models in their work. Our repertoire of program planning and evaluation models has to reflect the wider understanding of the impact of social and environmental determinants of health. In this chapter a variety of models were outlined, in an effort to address current health promotion possibilities.

REVISION

Consider the main issues addressed in this chapter. Review each of these points in light of your understanding of program planning and evaluation.

1. *What do you understand by evidence-based health promotion practice?*
2. *How do you understand the principles of program planning and evaluation against the backdrop of changing health promotion practice?*
3. *What are the traditions of program planning and evaluation in public health and health promotion?*
4. *What are the main models of program planning and their application in health promotion programs?*
5. *What is the scope of evaluation in health promotion, and what models are appropriate to your practice?*

5

Managing health promotion programs

- *The changing management role*
- *Health promotion practice*
- *Core competencies in health promotion*
- *Workforce development*
- *Managing health promotion activity*
- *Strategic management*
- *Program/project management*
- *The manager's checklist for success*

This chapter discusses the health promoter's role as a manager of an organisation or agency and the more specific responsibility of the management of projects and programs. In contemporary practice it has become evident that the health promotion practitioner needs a wide set of management skills. There is clear recognition that there is a role for the health promoter in the management of programs, from their development and implementation through to their conclusion and evaluation.

The chapter does not include an exhaustive analysis of current management literature. Rather, it introduces the reader to general issues of health promotion management and to the range of skills needed to manage projects effectively and efficiently.

THE CHANGING MANAGEMENT ROLE

When we discuss the modern organisation and the role of management, we often think of large Australian organisations in the public and private sectors. While there are a number of common issues about management in organisations that we will address in this section of the chapter, the management of health promotion activity is a major task for health workers. For that matter, management in a range of health-related settings is becoming an important consideration for practitioners as the sphere of their work and areas of responsibility extend beyond the traditional settings for health promotion practice. The regionalisation of health and education departments throughout Australia, coupled with the devolution of management and budgetary responsibilities, has meant that management skills have become a necessary and important element of professional competency.

Stace and Dunphy commented on the challenges that face organisations in the successful management of change associated with the adaptation to new environments. They suggest that 'in organisations that are large and small, commercial and not-for-profit, the boundaries of our knowledge are being stretched to breaking point' (2001, p. 4). They feel that 'most successful managers realise that they have to experiment, take risks and move beyond the boundaries if they are to create a sustainable future for their organisations' (Stace & Dunphy 2001, p. 4). This general comment about organisational change is relevant to health promotion practice as well as to practitioners working in a range of organisations, be they for-profit or not-for-profit.

Why is **adaptive management** becoming so important in Australian organisations? The increasing rate of technological, social and economic development has created a climate in the modern organisation of constant change (Breckon 1997). Several authors (Dunphy & Griffiths 1998; Stace & Dunphy 2001) have referred to the direct influence of world economic and social structures on the transition taking place in Australian organisations today. While changes in the world economic environment were taking place in the 1970s and early 1980s, the impact of those changes on Australian organisations came almost a decade later in the late 1980s and that impact is still gaining momentum. Technology and increasing access to improved information transfer systems are transcending geographical and other barriers.

Swayne et al. (2006) suggested that organisational and management structures have changed over the last decade. The structural changes have necessitated changes in the ways in which managers go about their work. Traditionally, organisational structure was based on two forms of specialisation: hierarchical and functional. *Hierarchical specialisation* meant that managers managed workers who did the task. *Functional specialisation* ensured that workers doing similar things in similar ways were grouped together. In responding to changes in the technological, economic and social environment, the emerging Australian organisation is typified by a flatter organisational structure, where more responsibility is devolved to the worker and where the supervisor provides the necessary help to do the task and manage the changes (Breckon 1997; Dunphy & Griffiths 1998). In some organisations, the structure and style of management have evolved even further, with workers organised into semi-autonomous work groups comprising the appropriate mix of skills and experience to achieve a particular outcome (Mendoza 1994; Stace & Dunphy 2001). In many health departments and not-for-profit organisations throughout Australia, health advancement units and health promotion teams operate much like semi-autonomous work groups, where teams of staff with a wide range of expertise work on specific projects managed by a project manager, or health promotion director in the case of non-government organisations.

It is important to note that no matter how the organisation is structured, nor how many managerial skills an individual might possess, the mere possession of those skills does not automatically guarantee managerial efficiency and effectiveness. What factors can you think of, within an organisation and outside, from your own experience and the experience of others, which have supported a person's endeavours to manage? What factors have acted as barriers to successful management of projects? A range of factors influencing the ability of a person to manage can be identified. These include the people who make up the workforce; the nature of the organisation, in terms of both its structure and its culture; the policies and plans guiding the organisation, in terms of both the extent to which they exist and how they shape the organisation's activities; political imperatives, both outside and within the organisation; and, most importantly, the material resources and financial support available on an ongoing basis to enable strategic planning to take place (Simnett 1995; Ewles & Simnett 2003).

Stacey and Griffin (2006) and many other authors (e.g. Mendoza 1994) have referred to the process of effective and efficient management as 'being able to walk the talk'. That is, a good manager is more than theoretically competent; a good manager is someone who is able to effectively and efficiently apply management processes, not always according to the rules. 'Knowing about' management does not always translate into effectiveness and efficiency, because effectiveness and efficiency are defined by the dynamic interaction between knowledge, skill, experience and organisational context (Mendoza 1994; Stacey & Griffin 2006). Figure 5.1 demonstrates the interaction between the factors conducive to effective management.

Figure 5.1: Factors conducive to effective management

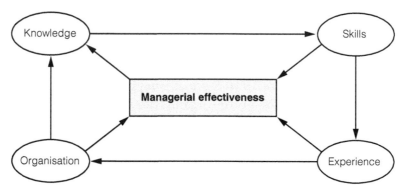

Source: Mendoza (1994)

What is management?

Its common usage notwithstanding, the term 'management' has many connotations; consequently, there are many contemporary definitions of its meaning. The *Macquarie Dictionary* defines management as 'the act or manner of managing; handling, direction or control; skill in managing; executive ability'. Management denotes both a function and the people who discharge it. It denotes social position and authority, and a discipline and field of study (Stace & Dunphy 1994). Simnett suggested that, in general terms, management is about being effective and efficient in your work, effectiveness being the extent to which the results you set out to achieve are actually achieved, and efficiency being about how you achieve those results compared with other ways of achieving them (1995, p. 9). Management not only involves tasks and discipline, but also people. Management style is about the extent to which individuals have a vision, integrity and a dedication to the task at hand (Child 2005).

This definition is a useful one for the health promotion student and practitioner. Several authors have suggested that we should be talking about a 'management group'. Within the management group, there will be people whose functions include the traditional managerial function, that is, responsibility for the work of others. There will be others who do not carry this responsibility within their specific roles and functions. There will also be a third group of people whose job is that of team leader or project manager, for example.

Accordingly, the first criterion in identifying those people within the organisation who have management responsibility is not command over people, it is **responsibility for contribution**. 'Function rather than power has to be the distinctive criterion and the organising principle' (Drucker 1990, p. 18). This is a useful way for us to consider management in the health promotion context, as health promoters are likely to have as much allegiance to their professional skills as to their organisation. For example, the health promoter within a workplace setting might prefer to be thought of as a member of a particular academic speciality, such as psychology, rather than as a manager of a project or a unit. This has implications for the various relationships that exist within an organisation.

Regardless of the diversity of functions and roles that health promoters perform in their day-to-day practice, it is possible to categorise some of the main stages in the management process. The management process is traditionally defined as the process of planning, organising, leading and controlling the utilisation of resources, both human and material, to accomplish the agency's purposes. Success in implementing the management process requires a **capacity to make decisions, solve problems** and **take action to use resources effectively and efficiently**. Where hierarchical and functional specialisation in the organisational structure has been reduced, and there is a flatter organisational structure, the management process changes to: **planning**, in conjunction with other relevant managers and their own staff; **leading**—that is, giving leadership, and training and developing staff; and **monitoring**—that is, focusing on performance results (Mendoza 1994).

In fact, when we consider the management process we might realistically conceive of it in a number of different ways depending upon whether the management role is seen to be traditional, transitional, or new and emerging. We noted these changing management roles earlier in the chapter when we examined structural changes in contemporary Australian organisations and the consequent changes in managerial responsibilities.

Out of all this, we can identify five basic elements of the work of a manager. The first stages involve ascertaining from the **stakeholders** what their **expectations** are and then **setting objectives** that align with this process. The latter step involves determining what the objectives will be, deciding how they can be reached, and communicating them to all staff. Managers must also **organise**. In this stage of the process, a manager needs to be able to analyse the activities and decisions required to achieve the objectives. Activities are divided into manageable tasks, and people are selected to run the activities and do the tasks. Another important stage involves **motivation and communication**. This entails making a team from the people responsible for various tasks. This is the manager's integrating function. Managers are also responsible for **establishing measurable targets**, both for the organisation as a whole and for every person in it. Therefore, managers must work with, and develop, their team members (Drucker 1991, pp. 20–1; Breckon 1997; Swayne et al. 2006).

A health promoter's experience with the management process could occur at various levels. For example, he or she may be involved in setting priorities for health promotion action in a region; in strategic, operational and action planning for an organisation or school; or in managing one or several health promotion projects. What skills does the health promoter use to manage these tasks? How effective and efficient is he or she in this management process? Later sections of this chapter address these issues. However, before we come to them we need to consider both the range of skills that define health promotion practice and the core competencies of the profession.

HEALTH PROMOTION PRACTICE

The role of the health promoter has been an evolutionary one. Traditionally, health educators used knowledge and skills related to behaviour change, educational approaches for the transmission of information, and program planning and evaluation, among other tools. The role of the health educator has expanded to embrace socio-political understanding, including advocacy, lobbying and networking; knowledge about organisations and organisational change processes; and the politics of coalitions and community power. With the regionalisation of health departments in various states throughout Australia, and the subsequent devolution of responsibility, the health promoter has had to take on a range of managerial skills, in terms of both unit or agency management and program or project management.

Ewles and Simnett (2003) identified six clusters of competencies necessary for health promotion practice, as follows:

- managing, planning and evaluating
- communicating
- educating
- marketing and publicising
- facilitating and networking
- influencing policy and practice.

Parker (1993) undertook a pilot study to determine what health promotion practitioners identified as the most frequently utilised areas of knowledge and skill in their day-to-day practice. She surveyed 250 graduates of a Graduate Diploma in Health Promotion, the majority of whom lived in Queensland (80 per cent); 44 per cent were between the ages of 31 and 40 years. Thirty-one per cent were teachers, and 64 per cent worked in hospitals or other health areas. Respondents were asked to comment on sixteen aspects of health promotion knowledge and skills in terms of their perceived 'confidence with' and 'frequency of use' in practice. Program planning, group education, networking with organisations, coordinating programs and health advocacy were the aspects most used. Respondents indicated least confidence in epidemiology, community development, curriculum design (school health), managing budgets, grant writing, submission writing and word processing. Areas that the study participants considered important were management issues, and health promotion training and education.

In terms of the nature of health promotion practice, Catford (1994) suggested ten **vital signs** of quality:

- understanding and responding to people's needs
- building on sound theoretical principles
- demonstrating a sense of direction and coherence

- collecting, analysing and using information
- reorienting key decision-makers
- connecting with all sectors and settings
- using complementary approaches at both individual and environmental levels
- encouraging participation and ownership
- providing technical and managerial training and support
- undertaking specific actions and programs.

If we look back at Ewles and Simnett's (2003) categories of health promotion practice, Parker's (1993) survey of health promotion practitioners and Catford's (1994) list of health promotion practice, we can see some commonality emerging in the nature of health promotion practice and the skills required by the practitioner to effectively manage the multifaceted nature of that practice. We can also see that almost everything a health promoter does, from an individual perspective right through to large-scale management activities, requires at least some management skills—if only in the sense that those skills help to make day-to-day practice more effective and efficient.

CORE COMPETENCIES IN HEALTH PROMOTION

Considerable activity has taken place in recent years in Australia on the development of core competencies for public health, and specifically for health promotion practitioners. On the one hand, this process has involved the identification of the health promotion workforce; on the other hand, the development of competency standards for health promoters to foster effective practice is being further discussed. It could be argued that this activity mirrors the much broader agenda of developing competency standards and competency-based curricula in all areas of the Australian workforce.

The document *Pathways to Better Health* (National Health Strategy 1993b, pp. 53–4) contained a comprehensive list of knowledge, skills and attitudes (or core attributes) required, for best practice in health promotion, by all members of the health promotion workforce. The document's authors argued for the development of standards and criteria to enable more appropriate preparation and continuing education. The five **core attributes** were listed as:

- a knowledge of: population health issues in Australia and their determinants; national goals, targets and priorities for health promotion; and scientific and theoretical bases for health promotion; social change and advocacy processes and methods;
- assessing needs by using both quantitative and qualitative research methods;
- planning programs, which involves planning goals, objectives, strategies, evaluation, performance indicators, and the application of strategies;
- initiating and maintaining programs in organisations and bureaucracies, and understanding funding sources and criteria;
- putting programs in place; managing the implementation process (National Health Strategy 1993b, pp. 54–5).

As to the **generic skills** needed by all health promotion practitioners in Australia, the Public Health Association (1990) offered the following list: writing skills; interpersonal skills; teaching skills; group process skills; advocacy and public presentation skills; research skills; and critical appraisal skills.

In 2000, the National Public Health Partnership (NPHP) and the Australian Health Promotion Association (AHPA) surveyed Australian public health experts in order to revise and review core public health competencies in Australia. The resulting 82 tasks were classified into eight core competencies:

- needs assessment
- planning
- implementation
- communication
- knowledge
- organisation and management
- evaluation and research
- technology (Shilton et al. 2003).

The authors of the study recommended the competencies should be re-evaluated every five years (Shilton et al. 2003). Thus, a revision of the competencies commenced in late 2005. The project comprised three stages:

- Stage 1 entails consultation with health promotion experts from around Australia who will recommend amendments to the earlier competencies.
- In the second stage a questionnaire was emailed to the Australian health promotion workforce. Participants were asked to rate each competency as 'essential', 'desirable' or 'not relevant', and to propose modifications and additions to the list.
- Workshops will be held in the third stage to refine, and promote the uses of, the competencies (In Touch 2005).

When completed, the results will be presented to the International Union for Health Promotion and Education's (IUHPE) Workforce Development and Training Committee to facilitate global discourse on health promotion competencies (In Touch 2005).

Ewles and Simnett (2003) claim that it is impractical to expect all health promoters to be highly proficient in all spheres of health promotion. We would extend this argument by claiming that competencies are also organisationally determined—for example, a hospital setting may not provide much scope for health professionals wanting to work with communities. A health promoter in a non-government organisation, such as the National Heart Foundation, may need particular skills in media work, advocacy, networking, policy development and group education, but may not have a great deal of opportunity to undertake patient education.

Essentially, the culture, politics and dynamics of the setting in which a health promoter works influence, to varying degrees, the emphasis placed on core knowledge and skills for effective health promotion practice (Ewles & Simnett 2003).

It could be argued that the drive to establish competencies in professions was based on a federal government program to influence the way in which the workforce was educated and trained. This agenda was seen as a part of a wider national program of microeconomic reform which sought to make Australia more internationally competitive. One of the key features of these changes was the development of a national competency-based training system (CBT), administered by the National Training Board (NTB), and the establishment of an Australian National Training Authority (ANTA) and state and territory training authorities (Mendoza 1994).

Problems have been identified in the process of developing nationalised generic standards that would relate to all workers and professional occupations. For example, the lists produced are often so broad they are merely statements of the obvious, and the competencies are meaningless because they lack a specific context (Garrison 1992; Mumford 1992). An alternative suggestion, designed to avoid the rigidity of the National Training Board's approach of segmenting all professions into competency categories, is the development of organisation-specific models to enhance skills and to bring about changes in the efficiency and effectiveness of the workforce.

It is important that health promoters be skilled and knowledgeable in their practice, and that the foundations of their practice be based on sound theoretical and ethical principles. There are many areas of knowledge and skills that health promoters employ, as discussed above. Nonetheless, the complex tapestry of human action in health promotion challenges the validity of any institutionalised attempt to provide a highly prescriptive set of generic measures impacting on university curriculum development, professional training and practice.

Mendoza (1993) suggested the use of a **set of principles** as a model to accommodate and encourage the development of competencies within a broad range of concepts, strategies, solutions and settings. The four principles are as follows:

- Competence should include the '**transparent**' **aspects of practice**, the attributes, qualities, motivations, values and attitudes—the artistry as well as the science.
- Any model of competence must **remain a 'working model'**, as health promotion is ever expanding; this is evident in the process of advocating for healthy public policy.
- **Organisational characteristics define competence** as much as an individual's skills and attributes do.
- **Competency models are a basis for reflection**, critical thinking and development for individuals, groups and organisations; rigid institutionalisation of generic competencies (career progression, remuneration) can lead to job rigidity, inflexibility and bureaucratic responses.

A number of activities have characterised the development of the health promotion and public health fields. The public health workforce education and training study conducted in 1994 defined the public health workforce as: 'people who are involved in protecting, promoting and/or restoring the collective health of whole or special populations (as distinct from activities directed to the care of individuals)' (Rotem et al. 1995). Health promoters and educators were one subset of the public health workforce, which included a wide range of professional and occupational backgrounds. The most commonly listed needs for additional training reported by coordinators of surveyed public health agencies were in the area of **management**, including health services management, general management and personnel management (Rotem et al. 1995, p. 438).

WORKFORCE DEVELOPMENT

Swerissen and Tilgner (2000) reported on a workforce survey of health promotion education and training needs in Victoria. The study concluded that effective training must be tailored to suit the specific needs of different professionals involved in health promotion and consider how factors such as time release and financial incentives influence participation across different settings and locations. Implications of the study included that the health promotion workforce requires recognition of its professional diversity and a more responsive and organised approach to education and training programs (Swerissen & Tilgner 2000).

In the United States, in response to serious gaps in the training of public health managers and administrators, the CDC established three workforce training programs aimed at developing management and leadership capacity (Setleff et al. 2003). These were the Sustainable Management Development Program (initiated in 1992), the Management Academy for Public Health (1998), and the CDC Leadership and Management Institute (1999). Although the programs were designed independently and have distinct target audiences, they encompass comparable principles:

- **Emphasis on adult learning.** The programs are structured on adult learning-interaction, application and reflection philosophies, and impart a base of theoretical knowledge which students need to apply to concrete situations.
- **Use of tools which reinforce evidence-based decision-making.** Although the three programs have different target audiences, each is based on the application of appropriate general management tools to decision-making within the public health milieu.

- **Individual feedback.** The central tenet of the three programs is that individual feedback on expertise and behaviour is a major part of personal development.
- **Continuous improvement of the learning process.** Another key guiding principle is continuous improvement. The exact implementation practices vary across the three programs; nonetheless, they all evaluate both content and process.
- **Post-training support for networking and lifelong learning.** All three programs afford post-training opportunities to encourage involvement, continual learning and strengthening networks. An assortment of methods is used to realise this goal, including the Internet and seminars.
- **A focus on teamwork.** In all three programs, learners participate in the course as a member of a team rather than as an individual, increasing the likelihood of achieving and maintaining the development process through shared knowledge and skills (Setleff et al. 2003).

These programs can serve as best practice examples for other public health management programs, although there is a need for more evaluation on long-term outcomes (Setleff et al. 2003).

An important point to make is that health promoters, as change agents, have recognised the need for flexibility. Many health-related agencies and organisations have also recognised the need for less bureaucratic structures—for example, the devolution of responsibility for planning and budgeting to regional health authorities, and closer consultation ties with communities in primary health care policies. There is a need for a competent, yet flexible, workforce of health promoters capable of working in a range of different settings.

MANAGING HEALTH PROMOTION ACTIVITY

It is possible to identify a range of important management skills that appear consistently throughout the management literature. White (2004) identified **critical management skills** that included: developing self-awareness and managing personal stress; creative problem-solving; establishing supportive communication; gaining power and influence; improving employee performance through motivation; delegating and decision-making; managing conflict; and conducting effective group meetings.

While the scope of this chapter does not permit us to address in any depth the multifaceted nature of management, we must note that health promotion practitioners are at times involved in implementing strategies for organisational change. Hence, they need to understand the functions and activities associated with human resource management. Mullins (2005), and earlier Beer et al. (1990), examined the relationship between organisational change and subsequent behavioural change within the organisation, concluding that for change to occur it is more productive to concentrate on the actual work, rather than intangible concepts such as 'participation' or 'culture'. Beer et al. (1990) argued that managers could achieve 'task alignment' through a series of six overlapping yet distinctive steps. These steps are outlined below.

SIX STEPS TO EFFECTIVE CHANGE

1. Mobilise commitment to change through helping people to develop a shared diagnosis of what is wrong in an organisation and what can and must be improved.
2. Develop a shared vision of how to organise and manage for success through a task-aligned vision of the organisation that defines new roles and responsibilities.
3. Foster consensus for the new vision, competence to enact it, and cohesion to move it along.
4. Spread revitalisation to all departments without pushing it from the top.
5. Institutionalise revitalisation through formal policies, systems and structures.
6. Monitor and adjust strategies in response to problems in the revitalisation process.

Source: Adapted from Beer et al. (1990)

Stace and Dunphy (2001) suggest a model for the management of organisational change that contains four main factors. These are the **changing demands of the organisational environment**, both internal and external, on management practice; and, in consequence, the **impact of the business strategies** the organisation chooses in order to succeed in that environment;

the **organisational change strategies** needed to implement the business strategies; and the **human resource strategies and practices** designed to make it all happen.

Whatever strategies you use to accomplish change in the health promotion organisation in which you work, you should keep in mind that *successful change programs focus on results, not activities.* Schaffer and Thomson (1992) and Kakabadse (2004) argued that a manager who sets about translating potential into results is able to achieve measurable change in the organisation. Schaffer and Thomson (1992) discussed four ways in which management can get started along this path:

- Ask each unit or section to set and achieve some **ambitious short-term performance goals.** In the health promotion context, this may mean the development of self-directed teams to undertake program development based on established priorities—for example, for cardiovascular disease.
- Periodically **review progress**, capture the essential learning and reformulate strategies. As a manager, you should review and evaluate progress with your team and learn what is and isn't working. For example, how rapidly is the project team making gains? What sort of support do they need? What changes in work methods can they implement quickly? What obstacles need to be addressed at higher levels in the organisation?
- **Institutionalise the changes that work** and discard the rest. As a manager in a health-related non-government organisation, you might establish a policy and set of practices for the formation and operation of project teams. This policy and set of strategies could form part of a handbook of program development used by staff in the organisation to plan and implement projects.
- **Identify the crucial challenges** for the organisation. Your role as a manager in this context is to guide the development of both strategic directions for your organisation or unit and a 'vision' of how it will operate now and in the future.

Schaffer and Thomson's (1992), and Kakabadse's (2004), suggestions are appropriate for health promotion units and organisations because for many health promoters working in management roles the political imperative of short-term success is as important as the achievement of long-term objectives. In addition, you need to be able to look into the future to ensure that the management of the organisation remains a dynamic and effective process.

A large part of a manager's time is devoted to execution—that is, detailed programming, motivating, coordinating and controlling. What should be kept in mind is that, in practice, these phases do not always occur in a logical sequence, nor do they operate in quite the same way on all occasions (Stace & Dunphy 2001). For example, putting a change strategy into effect may involve policy changes, organisational issues and procedures for controlling the entire process. Nevertheless, for the purposes of understanding management it is important to be able to observe the management process in its various phases and to put these various parts into a logical perspective.

Establishing policy and priorities, developing strategies, building organisational structures and developing managers are all vital to the management of any endeavour. If the organisation is to achieve its goals, then steps must be taken to 'get things done'. This is the **execution phase** of the management process and can be seen to have three broad elements (Stace & Dunphy 2001):

- **short- and long-range program planning**—what actions are to be taken and when;
- **activating**—concerned with direction and motivation;
- **controlling**—seeks to ensure that the results correspond with organisational plans.

How do these three broad elements translate into management tasks and responsibilities for the health promoter? As we discussed earlier, the roles and responsibilities of a health promoter can be both diverse and demanding, requiring the practitioner to be able to shift between a client-centred focus and an organisational focus. Ewles and Simnett (1995, 2003) identified four key aspects of managing health promotion, as follows:

- **working with other people**, including coordination and teamwork, participating in meetings, and effective committee work;
- **communicating with colleagues**, which may involve establishing and maintaining communication channels and report-writing skills;

- **information processing,** through the management of information systems such as paperwork and by giving, receiving and analysing information;
- **time management,** including the use of time logs and diaries for scheduling work.

STRATEGIC MANAGEMENT

Many public health practitioners, particularly health promoters, are involved in strategic management in private or public organisations. Strategic management is rarely an easy task. Ensuring that all the parties involved agree on the **mission of an organisation** can be a real challenge. For example, a private hospital may define its central mission as 'providing quality health care to the public', but each member of the board and staff may interpret that mission a little differently. One person may believe that the emphasis should be on quality care, while another may believe that service to the public mandates health care for a very broad group of clients. It is only when some consensus among the executive over the organisation's mission has been achieved that agreement can be reached about strategies to accomplish the mission (Dunphy & Griffiths 1998). Another underlying problem in any organisation is **determining success criteria** and evaluating alternative strategies. In particular, 'success' for non-profit organisations and service organisations is not only difficult to measure, but is often difficult to define.

What are the strategic issues for health promotion? *Goals and Targets for Australia's Health in the Year 2000 and Beyond* (Nutbeam et al. 1993b) highlighted many of the strategic questions health promoters need to ask in order to successfully plan and manage health promotion activity. For example, what are the health needs of the population, where are the challenges and opportunities, how can progress be made, who should participate, what are the priorities and how fast should we go (Catford 1994)?

Catford (1994) argued that the implementation of strategic management processes in health promotion is often hampered because the organisation does not have a clear strategic intent or a clear idea of its underlying mission. He suggested that strategic intent involves focusing the organisation's attention on: winning; motivating people by communicating the value of targets; leaving room for individual and team contributions; sustaining enthusiasm through new operational definitions; and using strategic intent to guide resource allocation.

The following **five key elements of strategic management**, outlined by Catford (1994), highlight the importance of strategic decision-making for the health promoter involved in management at this level:

- purpose—vision and direction
- participation—joint ownership
- priorities—achieving results
- performance—measures and targets
- partnerships—intersectoral action.

Strategic management in the context of health promotion requires the *ability to make decisions* about the scale of the task and the expectations of all stakeholders involved. Further, it requires an *ability to judge the effectiveness of action and the opportunities for action*, to *understand and deal with changes* in the external environment, and to be *able to demonstrate a return on the investment* (Catford 1994).

We now turn our attention to the process of **strategic planning** (Dunphy & Griffiths 1998). This involves two levels: strategic planning approaches and the planning process.

Strategic planning approaches

While there are a number of approaches to strategic planning, we have focused on the two we consider to be of greatest value to the health promoter—linear planning and integrated planning.

Linear planning follows a logical sequence from broad processes (developing the vision and mission) to more narrow and specific processes (writing action plans). It is done periodically in an organisation's history and has a beginning point and an end point. The main advantage of this process is its comprehensiveness, but this can also be a disadvantage in that the process is slow and often inflexible.

Integrated planning uses the concept of 'strategic fit', in that the various components of planning fit together to make a coherent whole. For example, all the components of the planning process must take place concurrently so that information generated in one area can influence choices and decisions made in another. The advantages of integrated planning are that:

it emphasises the process of planning; it encourages participants to remain involved in the process; and it tends to move more quickly towards action. Its disadvantages are: its lack of comprehensiveness can lead to uninformed decisions; its very flexibility can negatively influence people's confidence in the organisation's long-term plans; and its emphasis on process means that written plans often have lower priority.

No single approach fits every situation or every organisation. One organisation may use both types of planning at different times in its development. For example, an organisation may find that integrated planning helps it to deal with changes in the external environment—such as a change of government—but that linear planning is more useful when the organisation is progressing through a period of consolidation. Whichever approach is used, one of the most important things is to ensure that the process moves from generating ideas and recommendations to the stage of making choices and final decisions.

There are several ways of discussing **levels of strategic planning**. For example, Barney and Hesterly (2006) and Stacey and Griffin (2006) discuss seven elements of strategic planning. These elements are:

* organisational learning
* promoting innovation and experimentation
* using inevitable tensions within the organisation to foster a strong and constructive level of debate
* tapping the creative and intellectual energy of everyone in the organisation
* maximising the benefits of available resources
* building a sustainable organisation
* thinking laterally about what business one is really in.

Mendoza (1990), on the other hand, identified a four-phase strategic planning model that involves situational analysis, goal analysis, strategy analysis and implementation analysis. Because this planning model is easy to implement and because it contains the important steps in strategic planning, it is reproduced in Figure 5.2.

In practice, the process of strategic management is not always clear-cut. In fact, several planning steps may be taking place at the same time. Several common levels of planning can be identified, with the proviso that they are considered as flexible steps which engage the staff at all levels of the process.

Figure 5.2: Four-phase strategic planning model

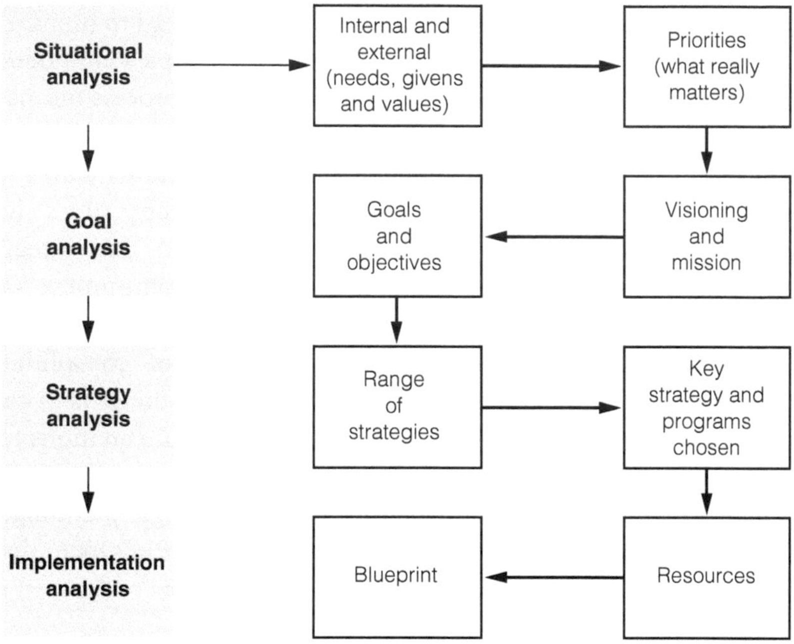

Source: © Mendoza (1990)

Furthermore, many authors (Dunphy & Griffiths 1998) have recommended a clearly articulated strategic intent rather than inflexibly applied top-down plans.

The planning process

Important questions for an organisation to consider are: what planning approaches have been used, and how have staff been involved? how can the whole process be improved? what aspects should be continued on the basis that they have worked well for the organisation and for the staff? and how do you know how well the planning has worked? Questions such as these can be answered by reference to the planning process.

There are seven important steps in the planning process, as the following box shows. In each of these steps, it is important to involve key organisational stakeholders actively.

SEVEN PLANNING STEPS

Step 1   **Set parameters and boundaries.** Determine what your core 'business' will be and how you will go about defining it.

Step 2   **Identify limiting conditions.** What can you realistically achieve? What resources and staff expertise do you have?

Step 3   **Change limiting conditions where possible.** You may be able to produce a more flexible budget than you first thought possible. Or you may be able to introduce some staff development activities or network with another organisation to achieve the same outcomes without the full resources of your organisation being used alone.

Step 4   **Design a plan of action.** How do you proceed to achieve your objectives? This step relies heavily on the data produced in the first three steps, as well as building in ways of dealing with expected and unexpected changes both within the organisation and outside it.

Step 5   **Carry out the action plan.** Put your strategies into practice.

Step 6   **Evaluate what you have done.** Evaluation is an essential component of good planning, as it helps to highlight critical success factors and strengths as well as weaknesses and problems.

Step 7   **Repeat what you have done** on the basis of your evaluation and careful thought and deliberation.

Of course, there are important elements of organisational success beyond the planning process—for example, financial and human resource management, marketing, fundraising and managing information. The roles and responsibilities of the health promoter, in terms of both management and professional practice, are influenced by how the organisation is managed and marketed; or, in the not-for-profit organisation, by how money is raised. Other important success factors include the working relationship or level of cooperation between various units or departments, and the culture of the organisation, particularly in terms of a clear purpose or mission and good morale and motivation among the staff.

PROGRAM/PROJECT MANAGEMENT

In this section, we focus on the role of the health promotion officer in managing the development and implementation of programs or parts of programs—projects. (Some organisations use the terms 'project' and 'program' interchangeably.) The processes of program planning and evaluation were covered in Chapter 4. The following discussion links with the material on program planning by addressing those aspects that require the application of management skills to support the achievement of program goals and objectives. The management element is often neglected in discussions of program development. We consider each of the stages of program development and implementation from the management perspective.

The first stage in the process is the **planning stage**. There are several arrival points at the planning stage. For example, a needs assessment may have been undertaken by the health promotion team and a set of priorities identified. Alternatively, a project may be indicated because of some political imperative, or it may be a part of a broader regional/organisational planning initiative. The reasons for arriving at the planning stage may well affect how one manages the program. If a team feels that a project has been foisted on them, they may resent, or be disenchanted by, the process. Whatever the circumstances, the manager needs to be able to **manage the flow of information** to all members of the team and to key stakeholders and clients.

Hawe et al. (1990) discussed the need for managers to develop a project timeline and budget and a staff handbook outlining the processes to be followed in the implementation process. This is a good idea, as the expectations of the various tasks are clearly identified for both manager and staff and the team should have a clear idea of where they are going and what they are trying to achieve. At this stage, budget implications and resourcing needs will have been considered, as well as the development of a series of strategies for the planning stages through to evaluation. The manager will need to consider feedback mechanisms for all key participants in the process so that he or she is aware of their needs and any concerns that may arise during implementation.

The second stage of the process involves **managing the implementation**. The skills needed to manage the planning process and the implementation phase are similar. The implementation phase requires that the manager has **problem-solving skills**, is **able to communicate**, both verbally and in writing, and is **able to manage people, money and time**. He or she also needs to be able to use good interpersonal skills, and to communicate with clients and key stakeholders in terms of both advocacy and information provision. Managing at this level means maintaining an ability to be flexible and to adjust and readjust plans according to a range of factors such as budgets, resources, timelines and the needs of clients. Team management is not the only organisational skill required. The manager needs to be able to manage upwards as well as sideways and downwards.

This brings us to the third important element in the process: being able to **initiate and maintain programs in organisations and bureaucracies** and to **understand funding sources and criteria**. At this stage, many of the broad management skills discussed earlier in this chapter become important. Managers need to understand the politics and the culture of the organisation. They must have a 'big picture' view of the organisation, the broader public health arena and the needs of their community. They must also be able to identify appropriate sources of funding, and to develop and implement strategies together with the team to secure adequate funding. Grant writing and producing submissions for funding are also key skills for health promoters.

THE MANAGER'S CHECKLIST FOR SUCCESS

The following checklist for managers summarises the major issues we have discussed in this chapter. This checklist is still relevant for 21st-century managers, as can be seen in the contemporary literature (Stacey & Griffin 2006; Swayne et al. 2006). We hope that it will provide you with valuable guidelines for effective and efficient management of health promotion endeavours. However, there is one thing to remember. A friend and mentor once said: 'Always be wary of consultants selling you the six key steps to management success.' How true those words are! Managing organisations and people in the 21st century is not as simple as that. Although mindful of the advice from a friend and of the inherent dangers of listing six, or even 36, steps, we offer this checklist for developing better management practices. Use it with caution and reflection.

KEY ISSUES: ASPECTS TO CONSIDER

1. **Know who you are, first and foremost**
   - Be critically reflective on your practice as a manager. Develop a clear perception of your own competencies.
   - Know your role. Focus on developing your skill as a manager. Learn to 'walk the talk' of successful management.
   - Know why you are in a management role. Opportunity? Content expertise? Management expertise?
   - Know what motivates you to be a manager.
   - Know your capabilities, limitations and excesses. Recognise that your very strengths are potentially a source of difficulties as a manager.
   - Let the staff know your strengths and limitations. Appropriate public knowledge is fertile material for developing trust.
   - Develop continuous self-improvement plans based on your own self-awareness and the feedback of others. Review these at least twice a year. Advise the staff of your plans.
   - Use mentors, inside and beyond your workplace, in developing your abilities.
   - Live the values you espouse—or change your values. Put your exposed and practised values to the test by seeking feedback.

2. **Know the staff**
   - Recognise that all staff want to know three basic things: What do I have to do? How am I going? What can I do to improve? Get these things right and a lot of good things will happen.
   - Know the capabilities, limitations and aspirations of staff.
   - Assign work on the basis of providing challenges, opportunities and rewards, as well as direct linkage to organisational priorities.
   - Adopt a developmental rather than judgmental approach to staff development. Work collaboratively with staff on performance development agreements that put the onus on staff member, supervisor and organisation—not merely on the staff member.
   - Make sure staff know what you expect of them and what constraints they operate under. In short, define the 'boundaries'.

- Allocate time with each member of staff to get to know them. Use a diary to keep a check of when you last had a chat.

3. **Know your organisation**
   - Recognise that your effectiveness is largely an outcome of the way you 'fit' with and respond to the organisation's internal environment.
   - Learn the shared values of the organisation—the underlying values, philosophy, guiding concepts and aspirations which affirm the more concrete and visible aspects of the organisation.
   - Know the style of the organisation—the way in which aims and objectives are translated into actions and behaviours. In particular, know and understand the style of management.
   - Take time to learn about the history of the organisation.
   - Learn the key organisational systems quickly. These are the policies and procedures for planning, accessing, implementing, monitoring and reporting.
   - Become familiar with the 'real' organisation structure. Develop alliances with those areas important to your area's work.
   - Know the strategies of the organisation and other key sectors. Know the capacity and collective skills of the organisation. Know which skills are valued.

4. **Know your stakeholders**
   - Be very clear about who the stakeholders are and what they expect from your area.
   - Establish stakeholder 'feedback loops' at all levels of your area. Actively seek feedback.
   - Know what the gaps are between what stakeholders expect and what your area provides.
   - Know what constraints exist in meeting stakeholders' expectations. Communicate these to stakeholders.

5. **Focus on the future**
   - Don't just do something—sit there and think about the direction in which the unit is going, where it needs to go and how it can get there.
   - Develop a vision, and communicate it clearly and consistently to staff. Involve them in determining how it can be achieved.

- Maintain a 'big picture' focus. Your role is concerned with strategic positioning of the unit for survival and development and performance improvement.
- Delegate, delegate, delegate. As much as possible, delegate operational tasks.
- Develop with staff critical success factors (based on stake-holders' needs), key performance indicators, measures and formulas for monitoring performance, and targets and time-frames for improvement.
- Review progress towards targets quarterly.

6. **Focus on systems for improvement**
   - Apply the 85/15 rule—that 85 per cent of problems are directly attributable to systems and 15 per cent to people.
   - Maintain continuous improvement of systems—products, procedures and processes—the 'three Ps'.
   - Involve staff at all levels in identifying and implementing continuous improvement projects.
   - Undertake continuous improvement on specific functions and cross-functional issues.
   - Start on those problems recognised by all and that are most easily changed.
   - Put in place systems for monitoring improvement.
   - Communicate, consult, collaborate—the 'three Cs'. Learn the difference between the 'three Cs'. Be flexible. Use the 'C' appropriate to the situation. Adopt a contingency style of leadership. Advise staff which 'C' you intend using and why.
   - Communicate in person with staff rather than via memos, emails and the like.
   - Practise simple, concise, accurate communication.
   - Orient your communication to the needs of the other person.
   - Whenever there is a crisis, tight timeframe or high risk, adopt a directive leadership style with staff. Using one of the 'three Cs' in these situations is usually inappropriate.

Source: Mendoza (1994)

REVIEW

In this chapter we covered two broad issues. We discussed the nature of management, the skills associated with good management, and the management and planning processes. We also examined the core competencies of health promoters as a means of determining the nature and scope of their management role, both in terms of general management skills and more specifically in terms of program/project management.

The changing nature of contemporary health promotion, the changing view of human resource management, the structural changes to health departments, including regionalisation, and the evolving management role for health workers in health-related non-government organisations have all influenced the roles and responsibilities of the health promoter. Further, many health promotion units operate project teams, with project managers responsible for the development, implementation and evaluation of projects of various sizes and budgets. Too often, the importance of developing and using effective project management skills is neglected. In order for the health promoter to be an efficient and effective practitioner, it is essential that he or she use management skills that allow the necessary focus to be maintained on the needs of the clients, the organisation and the staff. Poor management skills mean that time and energy are diverted away from the essential health promotion tasks. Moreover, *good managers are able to adapt to changing circumstances, to plan ahead and to value the contribution of their colleagues.*

REVISION

Consider the main issues addressed in this chapter. Review each of these points in light of your understanding of management issues in health promotion.

1. *What is the theoretical basis of management in general and, more specifically, how does it apply to the needs of the health promoter?*
2. *How can you apply such management concepts to generic health promotion activity and, more specifically, to program/project management tasks?*
3. *Critically analyse the knowledge and skills necessary to manage health promotion programs and projects effectively.*

4. Can you trace contemporary developments in the delineation of core competencies and associated roles and responsibilities for the health promoter, and apply these to the theory and practice of management?
5. How can you apply the information provided in the 'manager's checklist for success' to your own health promotion management practice?
6. Apply some of the practical ideas discussed in this chapter to your own health promotion management practice.

PART III

SETTINGS AND COMMUNITIES FOR HEALTH PROMOTION

In Part III, the theory of health promotion and the skills identified in Parts I and II are illustrated through the discussion and analyses of policies and practice in an array of settings.

Settings provide a strategic approach in realising that health opportunities are determined by the physical, social and cultural traditions of people's lives and work. A setting refers to a social and culturally defined geographical and physical area of social interaction (Wenzel 1997). A 'settings' approach in health promotion can be an important feature for individual and social action in enhancing health opportunities. It has not been possible to describe every setting in which people live and work—for example, health promotion within sporting clubs and venues, or clubs and pubs. We feature some key settings for health promotion.

Each chapter begins with an introduction to health promotion and its particular role in the setting under discussion. Relevant policies and current initiatives in health promotion are amplified through a number of case studies.

Chapter 6 considers the school as a setting for health promotion activity, and looks at a range of approaches, including the health-promoting schools initiative, as well as current national and state initiatives in promoting the health of the school community.

Chapter 7 discusses the local community as a site for health promotion. Models of community organisation and the role of the health promoter working in communities are outlined.

Chapter 8 examines the health status of Australia's Indigenous peoples. It discusses health promotion in Indigenous communities and explores ways Indigenous people can promote the health of their communities and family.

Chapter 9 focuses on workplace health promotion and addresses the changing role of traditional lifestyle programs and the emergence of comprehensive workplace management models which consider the whole organisational culture that promotes or inhibits health. The future of workplace health promotion in the context of 'managing for health' is considered.

Chapter 10 identifies the health care setting as a site for health promotion programs; primary health care and health promotion are discussed, as are patient education and the role of general practitioners and hospitals in promoting health.

Chapter 11 profiles rural, regional and remote communities. The recognition of rural health as a distinct area needing attention is highlighted, and particular policies and practices to promote health and prevent injury are identified.

6

School health promotion

- *The case for school health*
- *Health-promoting schools*
- *Curriculum development*
- *Future direction*
- *Challenges and opportunities*

Educating children at school about health should be given the highest priority, not only for their health per se, but also from the perspective of education, since if they are to learn they need to be in good health (Australian Health Promoting Schools Association (AHPSA) 2000). Education for health is a fundamental right of every child, and is inextricably linked to educational achievement, quality of life and economic productivity. By acquiring health-related knowledge, values, skills and practices, children can be empowered to pursue a healthy life and to work as agents of change for the health of their communities.

Why have health education and health promotion in schools? The answers to this question reflect two points of view among health and education professionals. On the one hand, it is argued that comprehensive health education is as basic a discipline as are reading, writing and mathematics. Courses in health education should be allocated time, funds, materials and facilities equal to those provided for instruction in the other basics. Opponents of this view believe that health instruction is provided most appropriately and effectively in the home by good example and everyday training. Others would argue that a 'back to basics' focus in schools means that in an already overcrowded curriculum, the inclusion of health education is neither feasible nor justifiable. However, the literature demonstrates that health education belongs in schools (WHO 1997a; Lister-Sharp et al. 1999; St Leger 2001; Maes & Lievens 2003).

Over several decades, society and health problems have changed, as have schools and students. Children and young people today grow up in an environment that increasingly encourages risk-taking behaviours (Chen & Kennedy 2001). Such realities as the changing nature of the family unit (AIHW 2003), the pervasive advertising of fast foods through campaigns targeted specifically at the young (Gross & Cinelli 2004), and long hours of television viewing that contribute to obesity and social isolation (Chen & Kennedy 2001) are but a few examples of the factors that make up an environment in which health-enhancing decisions by children and youth are made more difficult (Chen & Kennedy 2001). These health and social problems underscore the importance of collaboration between children, parents, families, schools, agencies, communities and governments in taking a coordinated approach to school-based health education (WHO/Regional Office for Europe 1998).

In the last two decades, public and professional interest in school health curricula has been heightened by the rapid growth of knowledge about health, and by the prominence of certain health issues such as HIV/AIDS, drug abuse, child abuse and mental health (Queensland Health 2002). The development and implementation of the National Health Goals and Targets, which included the school as a setting for the advancement of the health of young people and, more recently, the emphasis on health-promoting schools have influenced the case for school health.

THE CASE FOR SCHOOL HEALTH

Increasingly more organisations and individuals are recognising that educational and health outcomes are closely connected, and that schools have the potential as positive settings through which to influence both of these sectors (Deschesnes et al. 2003; St Leger 2004; Tones & Green 2004). In the past few decades, there have been a number of international initiatives to enhance both learning and wellbeing through schools.

You will recall from our discussions in Chapter 2 (see 'Primary health care phase' and 'Defining the new public health—and beyond') that the

WHO has played a major role in promoting health education and health promotion in the international arena, in addition to advocating access to school-based health education for all children throughout the world. This advocacy has spanned five decades of effort by United Nations agencies in advancing comprehensive school health education (CSHE). Concern for, and action on, school health began in Europe and North America after the First World War. The WHO expert committee on school health services was convened in 1950 to outline policies and principles applicable in different countries. The first report of the WHO Expert Committee on Health Education (WHO 1954) identified a number of opportunities for school-children to learn about health. The role of teachers and the importance of planning were recognised by the WHO in the late 1950s and early 1960s through the publication of the document *Teacher Preparation for Health Education* (WHO 1960) and a source book *Planning for Health Education in Schools* (WHO 1966).

In 1986, the WHO and UNICEF published *Helping a Billion Children Learn about Health*. This document addressed the complexity of health learning among school-age children. It described the current state of health education for this population, and proposed strategies and guidelines for strengthening health education in schools. The WHO also organised a number of working groups in collaboration with UNESCO and the United Nations Family Planning Association on CSHE during 1991. The basis of this activity was the promotion of CSHE 'which recognises the multitude of factors at work in the critical years when children and youth are maturing' (WHO 1992, p. 2). In 1991, the WHO, in collaboration with UNICEF and UNESCO, convened an expert consultation to undertake two major tasks: acquire a common understanding of CSHE; and outline actions for countries to consider supporting the implementation of such programs (WHO 1992).

In the document *Comprehensive School Health Education: Suggested guidelines for action* (WHO/UNESCO/UNICEF 1992), five principles associated with the promotion and implementation of CSHE were outlined.

- Because of the relationship between health and education, trying to enhance one without also considering the other is inefficient (National Commission on the Role of the School and the Community in Improving Adolescent Health 1990, p. 9).
- Improving the education of girls can have a profound (future) benefit for their children's health (Dhillon & Philip 1992–93).

- Schools are important sources of health education for students, and their families and communities.
- There is a need to strengthen the relationship between in-school learning and out-of-school health behaviour.
- Education in life skills guides people to think critically about health and social issues, encourages problem-solving collaboration and full community participation (WHO/UNESCO/UNICEF 1992, pp. 2–3).

Schools can help young people acquire basic skills needed to create health. Sometimes called life skills, these include decision-making, problem-solving, critical thinking, communication, self-assessment and coping strategies. When people have such skills, they are more likely to adopt a healthy lifestyle (Jones et al. 1995). Contemporary research is beginning to provide evidence that well-planned school health promotion initiatives can have a number of positive influences on knowledge; however, changing the health-related behaviours of young people is more problematic (Lister-Sharp 1999). In particular, such initiatives can improve student understanding about the scientific and philosophical principles of individual and societal health, develop the competencies students need to make decisions about behaviours that influence their health, and teach the skills students need to engage in behaviours that are conducive to health. Schools can also improve the skills students need to maintain and promote the health of the families for which they will in time become responsible and the communities in which they will reside (WHO 1997a).

Before we begin to examine the notion of CSHE, it is important to set the context for discussion by considering the nature and scope of health education. Health education is not only concerned with the communication of information, but also with fostering the motivation, skills and confidence (self-efficacy) necessary to take action to improve *health*. Health education includes the communication of information concerning the underlying social, economic and environmental conditions impacting on health, as well as individual *risk factors* and *risk behaviours*, and the use of the health care system. Thus, health education may involve the communication of information, and development of skills to address social, economic and environmental *determinants of health* (WHO/Regional Office for Europe 1998). Any discussion about principles of comprehensive approaches to school health education and promotion must begin by turning our attention to the elements of the *Ottawa Charter for Health Promotion* (WHO 1986a).

As a framework to guide our action in the development of school health education, the charter clearly articulates five major directions. As we saw in Chapters 1 and 3, the charter represents a mediating strategy between people and their environments, combining personal choice with social responsibility for health to create a healthier future. The charter suggested the need for **health promotion action** to take place in five broad ways:

- build public policies which support health
- create supportive environments
- strengthen community action
- develop personal skills
- reorientate health services.

In accordance with the principles of the Ottawa Charter (WHO 1986a), a set of guiding principles for action to foster the development of CSHE programs were identified (WHO 1992). It was seen that the following are needed:

- **political will and commitment** as well as policy, legislative and fiscal support at international, national and local levels;
- **advocacy at all levels** and through all channels, including the media, to reach policy-makers and other influential individuals and groups;
- **integration** into national education and health policies;
- building on **global efforts**—through such movements as *Health For All* and *Education For All* leaders are exploring ways in which education and health professionals can work together to advance the healthy development of children worldwide;
- **championing** of comprehensive school health education by committed professionals, visionaries and citizens;
- **alliances of various sectors** of society, including all relevant ministries and agencies as well as teachers, health workers, parents, youth, the media and others (WHO/UNESCO/UNICEF 1992).

HEALTH-PROMOTING SCHOOLS

How do we translate the above concepts and theoretical frameworks into action in the school context? The international health-promoting schools movement is one such approach. A health-promoting school (HPS) is 'a school that is constantly strengthening its capacity as a healthy setting for living, learning, and working' (WHO 1996a). Health-promoting schools endeavour to support the conditions that enhance both students' and teachers' learning prospects, in cooperation with a range of other service providers. Health-promoting school programs contribute to health and educational outcomes through:

- fostering health and learning using all the measures at its disposal;
- engaging health and education officials, teachers, teachers' unions, students, parents, health providers and community leaders in efforts to make the school a healthy place;
- striving to provide a healthy environment, school health education, and school health services along with school/community projects and outreach, health promotion programs for staff, nutrition and food safety programs, opportunities for physical education and recreation, and programs for counselling, social support and mental health promotion;
- implementing policies and practices that respect an individual's wellbeing and dignity, provide multiple opportunities for success, and acknowledge good efforts and intentions as well as personal achievements;
- striving to improve the health of school personnel, families and community members as well as pupils;
- working with community leaders to help them understand how the community contributes to, or undermines, health and education (WHO 1996a).

Health-promoting schools concentrate on:

- caring for oneself and others;
- making healthy decisions and taking control over life's circumstances;
- creating conditions that are conducive to health (through policies, services, physical/social conditions);
- building capacities for peace, shelter, education, food, income, a stable ecosystem, equity, social justice, sustainable development;
- preventing leading causes of death, disease and disability, including helminths, tobacco use, HIV/AIDS/STDs, sedentary lifestyle, drugs and alcohol, violence and injuries, unhealthy nutrition;
- influencing health-related behaviours, such as knowledge, beliefs, skills, attitudes, values, support (WHO 1996a).

The European Network of Health Promoting Schools Conference (WHO/Regional Office for Europe 1998) recommended that health promotion training for teachers should be compulsory, at both teacher training and in-service stages. Teachers must be provided with original and workable methods for dealing with complicated curriculum and organisational problems, and given the support to reflect on their practice. Active learning should be given prominence, with teachers extending their learning in psychology, sociology and pedagogy. In particular, there must be consistency between the practical and theoretical aspects of training (WHO/Regional Office for Europe 1998). In addition, teachers need to be encouraged to use research to inform their practice (Wyn et al. 2000). While there is still substantial development to take place, there are encouraging signs that curriculum developments in school health education have embraced the 'Health For All' concept and moved school health instruction towards the 'social view' of health espoused by the WHO some 30 years ago.

Health promotion 'is a process of enabling people to increase control over, and to improve, their health' (WHO 1986a). If this concept is to be applied in the school context, what are the implications for the health-promoting school?

The WHO European Network of Health Promoting Schools (ENHPS) complements existing Healthy Cities, Healthy Communities and Healthy Hospital programs. It reflects a practical approach to the implementation of health promotion programs through key community settings or infrastructures (Booth & Samdal 1997; Colquhoun et al. 1997). The notion of the health-promoting school involves several key elements: it is based on a holistic view of health which recognises the different physical, social and mental dimensions of health, and the principles of equity of access to school education among different population groups and genders. In addition, it emphasises empowerment through the development of knowledge and skills among students; and inclusiveness, so that the whole school community, parents and the wider local community are engaged in developing and implementing school activities (Booth & Samdal 1997; Colquhoun et al. 1997).

Health promotion in the school setting is about linking education and health. Features of health promotion such as equity, empowerment and participation can also be found in education (Ackermann 1997). Since the early 1900s, the school health program has been conceived to include three components: school health services, school health education/ instruction, and the school health environment. While the traditional school health trilogy of services, education and environment remains relevant, a new definition of school health is required. It will include the school as one locus of a broad range of health and educational activities, carried out by a diverse group of health and educational personnel based both in the community and in the school (Nader 1990). Furthermore, school health entails the involvement of society as a whole, and all sectors, both public and private (Ippolito-Shepherd 2003).

The WHO Division of Health Education produced recommendations for implementing CSHE in its position paper, *Health in Education For All: Enabling school-age children and adults for healthy living*, including the recommendation that education for health should be an integral part of the school curriculum (WHO 1990).

Traditionally, the health-promoting school has been defined by a number of players according to three key areas: the formal curriculum; the physical and social environments and the policies and practices of the school; and the school–home–community relationship, including school health services (Booth & Samdal 1997). Health-promoting schools are considered within six domains: the formal curriculum; school ethos (the social environment); the physical environment; policies and practices; school health services; and the school–home–community interaction (Booth & Samdal 1997). In contrast, Colquhoun et al. (1997) have deliberately not defined the health-promoting school because of the multiple perspectives implicit within the concept. While there may be arguments about the relative merits of various definitions of health-promoting schools, it seems reasonable to suggest that there are a number of areas within the school and the wider community that, in collaboration, form a part of the health-promoting schools concept. These include:

- the school health curriculum
- the school environment—physical, social and emotional
- school health policies and practices
- the school–home–community interface.

More recently, the ENHPS concluded the following:

- The success of the health-promoting school program across Europe warrants further widespread implementation.
- Education and health ministries should collaborate in an expansion of the health-promoting school scheme.

- Health-promoting schools contribute significantly to the social and economic development of society at large.
- The health-promoting school is not a prescriptive approach. Although operating to a core set of values and principles, each health-promoting school will reflect local cultural, organisational and political considerations.
- The concept of the health-promoting school is holistic in nature and, in addition to curriculum development, strives to promote a health-enhancing social and physical environment within the community.
- Action learning rather than teaching should be the focus of the health-promoting schools' curriculum. The challenge to teachers is to develop and implement new and innovative approaches to learning.
- Success is dependent, at least in part, upon the extent to which there is an investment in both initial and in-service teacher training.
- Schools should be viewed as a resource for the wider community, with their facilities available for use outside of normal school hours.
- Improved equity should be both a goal for and a consequence of the health-promoting school.
- Young people and their parents should play a significant role in determining school priorities.
- Schools should act as a catalyst in bringing together a wide range of local organisations in a coordinated approach to community health.
- Implementation requires an active partnership between parents, teachers, community organisations and young people themselves.
- Wherever possible, health-promoting schools should use existing international networks (e.g. Healthy Cities) to promote inter-school collaboration across national boundaries.
- Although already clearly successful, there is a continuing need for further development to be evidence based (WHO/Regional Office for Europe 1998, p. 9).

United Kingdom and Europe

The HPS project was piloted in Hungary, the Czech and Slovak Republics, and Poland in 1991 (St Leger 1999; Erben 1998–2000). In 1992, the ENHPS was initiated by the WHO Regional Office for Europe, the Council of Europe, and the European Commission; and by 1998, more than 38 countries were involved, with 500 project schools (Erben 1998–2000). Ten principles of the health-promoting school were detailed in the Resolution of the 1997 ENHPS First European Conference. These principles, listed below, form the framework upon which countries can develop their own ideas and philosophies.

- **Democracy.** The health-promoting school is founded on democratic principles conducive to the promotion of learning, personal and social development, and health.
- **Equity.** The health-promoting school ensures that the principle of equity is enshrined within the educational experience. This guarantees that schools are free from oppression, fear and ridicule. The health-promoting school provides equal access for all to the full range of educational opportunities. The aim of the health-promoting school is to foster the emotional and social development of every individual, enabling each to attain his or her full potential free from discrimination.
- **Empowerment and action competence.** The health-promoting school improves young people's abilities to take action and generate change. It provides a setting within which they, working together with their teachers and others, can gain a sense of achievement. Young people's empowerment, linked to their visions and ideas, enables them to influence their lives and living conditions. This is achieved through quality educational policies and practices, which provide opportunities for participation in critical decision-making.
- **School environment.** The health-promoting school places emphasis on the school environment, both physical and social, as a crucial factor in promoting and sustaining health. The environment becomes an invaluable resource for effective health promotion, through the nurturing of policies which promote wellbeing. This includes the formulation and monitoring of health and safety measures, and the introduction of appropriate management structures.
- **Curriculum.** The health-promoting school's curriculum provides opportunities for young people to gain knowledge and insight, and to acquire essential life skills. The curriculum must be relevant to the needs of young people, both now and in the future, as well as stimulating their creativity, encouraging them to learn and providing them with necessary learning skills. The curriculum of a health-promoting school also is an inspiration to teachers and others working in the

school. It also acts as a stimulus for their own personal and professional development.

- **Teacher training.** The training of teachers is an investment in health as well as education. Legislation, together with appropriate incentives, must guide the structures of teacher training, both initial and in-service, using the conceptual framework of the health-promoting school.

- **Measuring success.** Health-promoting schools assess the effectiveness of their actions upon the school and the community. Measuring success is viewed as a means of support and empowerment, and a process through which health-promoting school principles can be applied to their most effective ends.

- **Collaboration.** Shared responsibility and close collaboration between ministries, in particular the Ministry of Education and the Ministry of Health, is a central requirement in the strategic planning for the health-promoting school. The partnership demonstrated at national level is mirrored at regional and local levels. Roles, responsibilities and lines of accountability must be established and clarified for all parties.

- **Communities.** Parents and the school community have a vital role to play in leading, supporting and reinforcing the concept of school health promotion. Working in partnership, schools, parents, NGOs and the local community represent a powerful force for positive change. Similarly, young people themselves are more likely to become active citizens in their local communities. Jointly, the school and its community will have a positive impact in creating a social and physical environment conducive to better health.

- **Sustainability.** All levels of government must commit resources to health promotion in schools. This investment will contribute to the long-term, sustainable development of the wider community. In return, communities will increasingly become a resource for their schools (WHO/Regional Office for Europe 2002, p. 79–81).

The ENHPS does not claim that there is one exemplary model of a health-promoting school; rather, each example of a health-promoting school is a result of its developers' discussion and consensus, based on the above guiding principles. 'The health promoting school is more a *process* of contextual interpretation than an *outcome* of the implementation of global principles' (WHO/Regional Office for Europe 2002, p. 2).

Coordinated school health programs—United States

In the United States school health education and promotion come under the aegis of the Coordinated School Health Programs (CDC 2005a), formerly known as CSHE. The coordinated school health program (CSHP) has eight elements:

- **Health education.** Aims to support students in maintaining and improving their health, preventing disease and reducing risk behaviours. The topics covered include family health, sexuality, mental and emotional health and injury prevention.
- **Physical education.** Aims to provide for each student's physical, mental, emotional and social development through the provision of information and learning experiences in a range of physical activity subjects, such as physical fitness, gymnastics and aquatics.
- **Health services.** Aims to ensure access to other appropriate services, provide emergency care for illness or injury, promote a safe school environment and provide education and counselling.
- **Nutrition services.** Aims to provide a range of appetising meals that provide for students' nutritional requirements, and the opportunity to learn about nutrition and collaboration with nutrition-related community services.
- **Health promotion for staff.** Aims to encourage staff to improve their health status and morale, through health assessments, health education and fitness activities, with the expectation that staff involvement in health-related activities will provide positive role models and a greater personal commitment to student wellbeing.
- **Counselling and psychological services.** Aims to provide assessments, interventions and referrals, in order to improve students' emotional, psychological and social health.
- **Healthy school environment.** Aims to enhance the physical environment, the psychosocial conditions and the culture of the school which impact on the wellbeing of students and staff.
- **Parent/community involvement.** Aims to encourage parental involvement and community engagement to respond more effectively to the health-related needs of students.

Although established in many countries, and advocated by the WHO, the HPS model has not been instituted in the United States (Nader 2000).

Nonetheless, Nader (2000) maintains that the application of this concept could improve school health in the United States. The HPS addresses the philosophies, policies and procedures of the schools, while at the same time recognising the place of the school within the community and the community's responsibility for school health; in addition, it embraces both a top-down and a bottom-up approach (Nader 2000). The HPS model clearly defines the relationship between health and education, and involves students, families, teachers, administrators and community partners as key stakeholders in program development (Nader 2000). The HPS framework may be perceived as a holistic/whole-school approach, which addresses some of the underlying factors that influence health. In contrast to the HPS approach, the CSHP programs in the United States are characterised by limited integration of health themes (St Leger 1999; Nader 2000). In addition, health goals can be seen as secondary to the chief goal of education, and are apt to be disregarded or underrated (Nader 2000).

The Australian context

The Australian Health Promoting Schools Association (AHPSA) was established in 1994 through the Australian Association for Healthy School Communities and the Network for Healthy School Communities. The association's vision statement is that 'All children in Australia will belong to school communities, which are committed to promoting lifelong learning, health and well being' (AHPSA 2005). A fundamental objective of the development of the health-promoting school framework was to model good health-promotion practice, consistent with the advocating, mediating and enabling strategies of the Ottawa Charter (Rissel & Rowling 2000).

In Australia, funding from the National Health Promotion Programme provided the impetus for the establishment of an Australian network for health-promoting schools (Colquhoun et al. 1997). It developed the concept of the healthy school community through consultation across Australia. The concept recognises the complexity of the interrelationship between education and health, and the school as a key social system (Ackermann 1997).

While health education is an important component of the broader discipline of health promotion, effective health promotion in the school setting occurs when there are, in combination with health education, approaches that involve organisational, economic or political activities for better health. School health promotion with this broad focus can be described as the application of policy and structural aspects of health promotion to school health issues. The health-promoting school attempts to balance the health curriculum and classroom teaching with action directed at improving the links between schools, families, caregivers and the wider community (Nutbeam et al. 1993b).

In 1997, the AHPSA was commissioned to develop a national framework for health-promoting schools. The framework contains eight key action areas and priority outcomes; within these eight areas are a number of strategic recommendations and priority outcome indicators (for more detail see AHPSA 2000):

- advocacy, promotion and publicity
- partnerships, collaboration and networking
- policy development
- seeking equity and valuing diversity
- workforce development
- curriculum development, implementation and evaluation
- research
- monitoring and evaluation.

CURRICULUM DEVELOPMENT

The development of a national statement and profile for health and physical education has necessarily involved a broad conceptualisation of the field that includes a range of subjects and courses of study, including health education. As we discussed earlier in this chapter, one of the traditional focuses in school health education was the development and implementation of health education programs or instruction. In our endeavour to promote the concept of CSHE and health-promoting schools, we should not lose sight of the importance of school-based curriculum development and implementation. The growing emphasis on the need to address health holistically across all school components can be seen in the reorganised health curriculum structures in place in Australian schools. These new health education curricula adopt a holistic view of health and promote the importance of supporting equity, healthy active lifestyles, skill development and personal and community actions as fundamental aspects of health.

The key questions to be answered in curriculum development are: what goals, changes and personal developments are of most worth, and what curriculum plans are most likely to achieve them? Some of the particular issues to be addressed are:

- Who are the learners, and what do they need and want to know?
- What are the skills they will need?
- What are the health practices and attitudes expected of them in the society in which they will live and function as citizens?
- What are the implications of our being a multicultural society?
- What are the important generalisations or ideas representative of the discipline?
- How can this subject matter be presented as a means of organising new facts accumulated throughout life?

In many states throughout Australia, schools have begun to focus on an integration of the curriculum component of school health with community health promotion activity and school-based healthy environment projects.

State and territory curriculum initiatives

In Australia, the states and territories are responsible for education and health; however, the federal government provides the finance and strategic direction for nationally significant initiatives (Rowling & Jeffreys 2000). All Australian states and territories have organised their curricula around a key learning area that is described as Health and Physical Education, or Personal Development, Health and Physical Education (PDHPE).

In New South Wales, the PDHPE syllabus for Years 11 and 12 focuses on a social view of health, where the principles of diversity, social justice and supportive environments are fundamental aspects of health. The Ottawa Charter is introduced as an important concept for exploring health issues. This model is applied to specific study of national health priority areas and issues related to equity and health. The preliminary PDHPE course includes 'Meanings of health and physical activity', 'Better health for individuals' and 'The body in motion' (Board of Studies NSW 1999).

In Victoria, the Health and Physical Education key learning domain has two dimensions, 'Movement and physical activity' and 'Health knowledge and promotion'. The curriculum focuses on the importance of a healthy lifestyle and physical activity in the lives of individuals and groups, and develops an understanding of the importance of personal and community actions in promoting the health of individuals and communities. Concepts, skills and strategies are introduced to assist students to develop their critical thinking and problem-solving strategies in order to make informed decisions about their health (Victorian Curriculum and Assessment Authority 2005).

South Australia has a Curriculum Standards and Accountability Framework (SACSA). This framework structures health and physical education around three main learning strands: physical activity and participation; personal and social development; and health of individuals and communities. These strands complement one another and provide different starting points for health and physical education. Learners gain knowledge and understanding, and develop processes and skills that enable them to achieve healthy behaviour and address specific health-related issues (South Australia Department of Education and Children's Services 2004).

The model used in Western Australia utilises what is known as the Curriculum Framework and the Outcomes and Standards Framework. There are five health and physical education learning outcomes, which provide a framework for the kindergarten to Year 12 curriculum. These are: 'knowledge and understanding', which facilitate informed decisions regarding healthy, active lifestyles; 'attitudes and values', which promote personal, family and community health, and participation in physical activity; 'skills for physical activity', which support confident participation in physical activity; 'self-management skills', which enable students to make informed decisions for healthy, active lifestyles; and 'interpersonal skills', which encourage effective relationships and healthy, active lifestyles (Western Australia Government Curriculum Council 1998).

The Tasmanian Health and Physical Education core curriculum for kindergarten to Year 10 consists of seven main ideas: 'understanding the body', 'developing and applying movement skills', 'perceptions of health', 'healthy lifestyle factors', 'health decisions', 'respecting and caring for self and others', and 'interacting and communicating with others'. The curriculum for Years 11 and 12 aims to present students with health-related skills, values, attitudes and knowledge. Individual and community health issues and responsibilities are a major focus, as is developing the students' decision-making skills regarding their lifestyles (Tasmanian Qualifications Authority 2005).

In the Northern Territory, the Curriculum Framework (NTCF) signals a shift towards a more holistic approach to health and physical education. The health and physical education learning area of the curriculum underscores the multifaceted nature of health, and how these factors shape an individual's development. The health and physical education learning area is organised into three strands: 'promoting individual and community health', 'enhancing personal development and relationships', and 'participating in physical activity and movement' (Northern Territory Government 2004).

In Queensland, the health education syllabus is divided into a Years 1 to 10 health and physical education syllabus, and a Board of Secondary School Studies health education syllabus for Years 11 and 12. The Years 1 to 10 program recognises the multifaceted nature of health, and the importance of physical activity in Australian society. The key learning area provides a basis for developing the comprehension, skills and attitudes needed to make decisions about promoting the health of individuals and communities, developing concepts and skills for physical activity, and enhancing personal development. The key learning area highlights the social justice principles of diversity, equity and supportive environments.

The Years 11 to 12 health education syllabus is concerned with the development of knowledge, attitudes, values and skills needed to promote health and includes studies of the health impacts resulting from interactions between individuals and their social and physical environments. In addition, it entails learning about, and through, physical activity, and highlights the associations between motor learning and psychological, biomechanical, physiological and sociological factors, together with the broader societal attitudes to, and comprehensions of, physical activity (Queensland Studies Authority 2004).

One good example of a comprehensive approach to school health education, structured within a health-promoting schools approach, is the Queensland University of Technology Resiliency Project.

THE QUEENSLAND UNIVERSITY OF TECHNOLOGY RESILIENCE PROJECT

The Queensland University of Technology Resilience Project uses a whole-school approach to promote resilience in children of primary school age, their families and communities, in urban and rural/remote locations in Queensland, Australia. The study population comprises students from Years 3, 5 and 7 (aged 8–12 years), their parents/caregivers and staff, in twenty primary schools in Brisbane and two in Charleville.

The health-promoting schools (HPS) framework is being used as the basis for promoting resilience, defined as 'the capacity of individuals, schools, families and communities to cope successfully with everyday challenges including life transitions, times of cumulative stresses and significant adversity or risk' (QUT Resilience Project 2005). The project integrates activity across the entire school culture. Resilience-building activities are not only being tested through curriculum development and teaching and learning strategies but also through the organisation and ethos of the schools, along with the school–community partnership process. The aim of this multi-strategy health promotion initiative is to assess approaches to promoting resilience, wellbeing and quality of life in children and their communities.

Initial evidence confirms that the school environment makes a major contribution to the development of resilience in children. Schools in which students reported more positive adult and peer social networks, feelings of connectedness to adults and peers, and a strong sense of autonomy, were associated with higher student self-ratings of resilience (Stewart, Hardie et al. 2005).

Indications are that school environments that are positively perceived by parents or caregivers tend also to be rated highly by staff in terms of HPS attributes and principles. Such schools tend to demonstrate more collective decision-making and planning, stronger community participation, a supportive physical and social environment, explicit health policies and access to appropriate health services (Stewart, Hardie et al. 2005).

For up-to-date information about the QUT Resilience Project, visit the website: www.resilience.qut.edu.au

The inclusion of mental health initiatives within the HPS approach is still evolving; some of the difficulties with the evaluation of these are related to identifying and quantifying such factors as stress and resilience (St Leger

1999). An example of a multifaceted approach to adolescent mental health is the MindMatters initiative, a national mental health promotion program, which provides a framework for mental health promotion in Australian schools (Wyn et al. 2000).

MINDMATTERS

MindMatters, a mental health promotion program for secondary schools, is an initiative of the Commonwealth Department of Health and Aged Care. Under the National Mental Health Strategy, promotion, prevention and early intervention for mental health is a major theme. Developed by a consortium including the Youth Research Centre, Deakin University, Sydney University and Australian Council for Health, Physical Education and Recreation (ACHPER), the program includes:

- a resource for schools
- a national professional development and training strategy
- a dedicated website
- an evaluation process
- a quarterly newsletter.

The goal of MindMatters is to provide a comprehensive framework within which Australian secondary schools can promote the mental health of members of school communities. MindMatters utilises a whole-school approach to mental health promotion. It aims to support the development of school environments where young people feel safe, respected and able to participate fully, by helping schools and their communities to create a climate of mental and physical health (MindMatters 2005).

For example, the MindMatters Queensland Focus Schools Project, which started in April 2002 with 22 secondary schools, aimed to support schools in their utilisation of MindMatters to trial its future statewide implementation. The majority of schools aimed to have topics of social and emotional wellbeing incorporated into the curriculum. Some of the themes addressed included:

- resilience
- bullying and harassment

- community partnerships
- teacher professional development
- understanding mental illness
- conflict resolution.

The process began with the identification of priorities, usually using MindMatters audits and school surveys, followed by professional development. Some of the findings included the following:

- Many schools reported that both staff and students had gained a greater understanding of issues related to resilience and mental illness.
- Schools reported an increase in teachers using interactive learning, encouraging equitable participation in class and generally teaching for wellbeing.
- There was an improvement in bullying issues (MindMatters 2005).

Health-promoting schools, as all-encompassing school approaches, are fundamental to youth health promotion because they have the potential to develop comprehensive solutions to the problems and challenges faced by children and adolescents.

FUTURE DIRECTION

A healthy, supportive school environment, according to Rowling and Barr (1997), is made up of the physical environment, including the built and natural environment, and the social environment, including the psychological, social, economic, political and cultural influences within families, schools and their wider environment. Supportive environments in schools represent the interdependence of health and education. Rowling and Barr (1997) identify five main elements that contribute to supportive school environments:

- the **places in school settings**—the classroom, the school buildings and environs, the school climate and the wider community;
- the **involvement and empowerment** of all the people—the students, teachers, other staff members, families, and health and community workers;
- the **processes and practices** involved in decision-making and participation;
- **policies** involving guidelines for action, for resource allocation and for priority setting;
- the **programs**—the organised, coordinated learning in classrooms and across the school activities.

The authors indicate that it is not the existence of these elements *per se* that is important but, rather, the interrelationship and the cooperation, compatibility and coherence between these elements that contributes to creating supportive environments.

What do we mean when we talk about policy development to support health-promoting schools? In fact, what *is* policy, and how can the process be used effectively for the advantage of school health promotion? How often do advocates of school health use the policy process to their advantage? These are important questions for us to consider as we explore the range of possible approaches to policy development and implementation in the school health context.

Bridgman and Davis (2000) noted that 'policy' is commonly used in several different contexts. For example, it can be used to describe a particular field of activity, such as economic policy, or it can describe a desired state of affairs, as in the 'Health For All by the Year 2000' slogan. 'Policy' can be used in specific ways—for example, policy decisions by the Queensland government not to legalise prostitution or marijuana. 'Policy' can also represent a program, such as the establishment of a national breast screening program, or it might refer to output—for example, what the government actually delivers. Outcome can also be seen to be 'policy'.

International debate on health policy has seen a shift from the dominant health service and resource orientation towards a broader policy perspective with emphasis on environment and lifestyle as major determinants of health and, consequently, priority areas for policy-making (Coonan et al. 1990). The concept, adopted by the WHO, of healthy public policy expresses this broader vision.

The primary goal of healthy public policy is to engender a supportive environment to allow people to live healthy lives, by making healthier lifestyle choices viable for people and improving the social and physical conditions under which people live (WHO 1988; Milio 1999). **Healthy public policy** is exemplified by an obvious regard for equity and health in all policy arenas and by accountability for health impact (WHO 1988). All government sectors—for example, agriculture, trade, and communications—need to consider health as a crucial issue when creating policy, and must be answerable for the health impacts of their policies (WHO 1988). The healthy public policy concept did not emerge until the 1980s, mainly formalised and circulated through the WHO. The suitability of any policy may be determined by its effect on the health of the population (Milio 1999).

It has been argued at the international level that the creation of political support for a policy on health-promoting schools is a critical step in the process of recognising this approach (WHO/UNESCO/UNICEF 1992). Just how this political support might be achieved requires creative advocacy efforts. It is possible to identify a range of strategies to be used by the committed advocate of school health promotion. These efforts can occur at a local, state or national level, thus targeting the range of policy-making processes and the relevant decision-makers at each level.

The advocate of school health promotion should use the Ottawa Charter (WHO 1986a) framework to develop alliances with key stakeholders, influential groups and interested parties. Of importance is the role of *intersectoral collaboration*, particularly between education and health, but also between education and other sectors such as social welfare, agriculture, housing and transport, as these sectors also impact on the health of young people, families and the community. School health promotion also needs to have the necessary human, financial, material and community resources to undertake the tasks and challenges being set for it as a part of the health-promoting schools philosophy. At a more global level, *advocacy* of school health promotion needs to focus on developing the interest of international organisations, foundations, business and development agencies, and professional groups.

How do we put all these good ideas into practice? In addition, how do we create a framework for policy implementation? Strategic planning can be used in creating a climate within a school conducive to the development and implementation of a health policy. Strategic planning is a process that involves making explicit the goals of the school, the environment in which it operates, the strategies employed to reach these goals, the program/s indicated by the strategies and, finally, the feedback loop that tells the school whether each of these steps has been implemented correctly. The principles of strategic planning are the same whether they are applied to the entire school community, the health education department or to individual teachers. (See Chapter 5 for details of management and strategic planning.) Strategic planning is simply the means by which a school organises its resources and actions to achieve its objectives. The better the strategic planning, the more readily the goals will be realised.

Some authors (Resnicow et al. 1993) have cautioned us to move beyond consensus regarding the need for school health promotion, and to question the effectiveness and feasibility of this approach. While it has been strongly argued that school health promotion is a major part of a consolidated approach to improve and promote the health of young people, in the long term the goal must be to *create supportive educational environments and healthy public policies that reinforce this action.*

The interaction between the school, the home and the community is another dimension to be addressed when considering the health-promoting school. Booth and Samdal (1997) suggest a number of ways in which parents can support school health promotion, including fundraising and other material and practical support, advocacy in support of school health initiatives, reinforcing school health education messages, and assistance in modifying the curriculum to more adequately reflect local cultural needs. In addition, many government and non-government agencies and professional and community organisations can provide assistance and support to schools (Kolbe 2005). School and community are natural partners in health education and health promotion (WHO/UNESCO/UNICEF 1992). The community in which a school is located can provide resources for learning and for students to practise health-enhancing behaviours. For example, businesses, community leaders, religious and social institutions, parents, health workers and other community members can be involved in student projects in the community. Further, health educators should be constantly seeking educational opportunities beyond the classroom for their students. Teaching opportunities are available through such activities as school health services, voluntary health agencies, the school canteen and a wide variety of events that regularly take place in the school and the local community.

CHALLENGES AND OPPORTUNITIES

School health, by history and tradition, has straddled the three most important systems that impact on youth—the family, the education system and the community (including health care). Yet budgetary, administrative, professional and other barriers between these systems have prevented collaboration. These barriers have caused purported comprehensive approaches to school health education to fail (Nader 1990).

According to Pollock and Hamburg (1985), the greatest single barrier to the provision of a strong, effective health instruction program may be the nature of the subject itself. As a goal, health is elusive. Health education as a school subject is complex and cannot be organised, learned and tested in traditional ways. Though facts about it can be taught and learned, application of that information is the important outcome of health instruction. The main successes of health instruction can only be inferred from the fact that certain behaviours or disorders never occurred or their incidence was diminished.

Lack of community or parental support for health teaching in schools is sometimes a barrier to its establishment or improvement. There are also misconceptions about the nature and scope of health education as a discipline. It is important to note that what functions as an enabler in one school may be a barrier in another (Weiler et al. 2003).

Because health is a means necessary to virtually all other educational ends, health education should be considered a central part of the school's activities (WHO/UNESCO/UNICEF 1992). In spite of the barriers, there are also strong supports for school health education that the educator should draw upon in his or her endeavours to press for school health education. At the Australian federal government level, statements about the goals and objectives for the nation emphasise the critical need for a continuation of the public health revolution based on health promotion and disease prevention. Many government initiatives are beginning to integrate holistic school health promotion within policies and programs—for example, see the MindMatters case study featured earlier in this chapter.

Research and evaluation of the health-promoting school approach is still limited, with little evidence of its efficacy (Lister-Sharp et al. 1999; St Leger 1999; Wyn 2000; Mukoma & Flisher 2004); although most interventions increase children's knowledge, it is much more difficult to effect changes in attitudes and behaviours (Lister-Sharp et al. 1999). Nonetheless, the concept of the health-promoting school is still developing and, in general, the research indicates its potential as a positive influence on the health of children (Lister-Sharp et al. 1999; St Leger 1999; Deschesnes et al. 2003; Mukoma & Flisher 2004), and the need for further evaluation to gauge its efficacy (Lister-Sharp et al. 1999; Rowling 2002; Wagner 2002). Additionally, it is essential that the approach does not become a 'one size fits all' methodology or a 'checklist', but that the whole-school approach is maintained, giving schools the capacity to customise the program to their own conditions, and attain ownership (Noble & Robson 2005).

There is a need for indicators acceptable to both the health and education sectors, as notions such as problem-solving and analytical and communication skills have more validity in the education sector, whereas the health sector is more likely to be looking for changes in behaviour and health status (St Leger 1999; St Leger & Nutbeam 2000).

It is difficult to measure community-based and long-term strategies in line with conventional health research standards since they exploit processes that are more akin to community development than the biomedical disciplines. Some epidemiological methods may be constructive for evaluating the outcomes from whole-school approaches; however, they are better used in combination with those of other disciplines, for example, policy analysis (Wyn et al. 2000).

REVIEW

Schools have the potential to do more than any other single agency in society to help young people live healthier, longer and more satisfying and productive lives (Kolbe 2005). School health education and promotion is at last being recognised as an effective way to improve students' health and their ability to learn. Those working in the field of youth health and education have known for some time of the links between learning and health (St Leger 2004); and they acknowledge that the health-related problems of today's youth cannot be resolved through a one-dimensional approach. Rather, an integrated, comprehensive approach to school health is required (Deschesnes et al. 2003).

The health challenges facing school-age children and youth, and to which health education programs must be directed, are complex and challenging. Their complexity arises because health status is largely a product of both the environmental conditions in which children live and the lifestyle they adopt (WHO/UNESCO/UNICEF 1992).

In recent years, a number of school-based efforts have been launched in response to the many and diverse public demands placed on the school to ameliorate the contemporary problems of society. Unfortunately, while important benefits have resulted from these categoric approaches, many of the efforts have had limited yield, in part because they were developed and implemented in a disjointed fashion. Government intervention policies and grants are often targeted at tackling discrete problems, thus initiatives that concentrate on isolated and contemporary issues have been unavoidable (Patton et al. 2000). Clearly, a more coordinated, comprehensive and systematic approach to these significant problems would be more successful and effective (Patton et al. 2000).

Promoting health in and through schools is a major challenge. This challenge can only be met through collaboration between the education sector and a number of other sectors, particularly the health sector (Lawson & Baumann 2001).

REVISION

Consider the main issues addressed in this chapter. Review each of these points in light of your understanding of comprehensive school health education and health-promoting schools.

1. *Identify the scope and sequence of national curriculum documents on health and physical education as a basis for contemporary developments in school health promotion.*
2. *Describe the current state of health promotion and health education in Australian schools.*
3. *Analyse strategies for promoting health in schools.*
4. *Describe the relationship between school health promotion and community health promotion.*
5. *Analyse the nature of comprehensive school health promotion in light of the barriers to a comprehensive approach.*

7

Community health promotion

- *Defining community health*
- *The development of community health and the community health program in Australia*
- *Definitions and descriptions of 'community'*
- *Defining community health promotion*
- *Balancing behavioural and socioeconomic approaches: an ecological model*
- *Models of community organisation, including community development*
- *Empowerment in community health promotion*
- *Social capital and community health promotion*
- *Healthy Cities*
- *Community health promotion and the Internet: virtual communities*

It is at the community level that health promotion action needs to take place, according to one of the leading architects of health promotion. In 1987, Kickbusch (1987, p. 437) claimed that there is a growing individual, social and political concern for what constitutes health. Her comments are still relevant. People themselves are creating the conditions for a changed attitude to health policies and practice, by taking a greater interest in health issues and pressing for new approaches. The key task of health promotion is to capitalise on this awareness. People can act to create healthier conditions for themselves, for others and for future generations. The creation of healthier conditions includes strategies such as:

- *self-care*
- *social support and mutual aid*
- *advocacy and direct action to preserve community health*
- *intersectoral action, particularly at the community level where people have local authority and a sense of competence*
- *support networks in communities that can encourage people to take more control*
- *support for local health interest groups and development of local facilities and services*
- *free access to valid, relevant and intelligible information*
- *development of popular support for change through consolidation of community resources and effort.*

Community health and the emergence of community health centres in Australia form the starting point for this discussion. We introduce the dimensions of community health promotion and its conceptual demarcations. Models of community organisation and community development are featured, with Australian examples. Attention is drawn to health promotion in multicultural communities.

The worldwide Healthy Cities movement recognises that major population centres provide many opportunities for the promotion of health through engaging people in creating healthy urban habitats. The concept of social capital and its place in health promotion is introduced. Finally, the impact of the Internet on community health promotion is introduced as cyberspace creates virtual communities.

DEFINING COMMUNITY HEALTH

The term 'community health' has many different meanings in Australia. Some of the meanings have arisen as a reaction to perceived inadequacies in the current health system. Community health is often defined by what it is not, rather than by what it is—for example, it is not hospitals, treatment, traditional doctors, technology or bureaucracy, and it has little to do with traditional diseases. The most common interpretation is that community health refers to state public health systems where community health nurses work. Yet another interpretation refers to the role and function of 'community health centres', an initiative established over 25 years ago by the Australian federal government.

If we examine community health in terms of services, community health takes responsibility for the health of a defined population. Green (1986) provided a broad understanding of community health and the intersecting dimensions of organisation ecology. He identified four overlapping spheres of community health practice, some of which have their roots in different disciplines. Community health utilising this view is a multidisciplinary practice. Although Green's model is illustrative of the US experience, it demonstrates the breadth of contemporary community health practice. Another view of community health is the 'healthy community'. A healthy community is one where there is a 'visible commitment to achieving the health and wellbeing of individuals, families and various groups of people' (McMurray 2003, p. 13). This view presents an ecological perspective, with the first goal of community health being 'sustainability'; that is, the community must be able to continue indefinitely without causing excessive disturbance or damage (McMichael 2000, cited in McMurray 2003, p. 13). The various interpretations of community health are:

- A local service—delivered close to where people live and work.
- A non-institutional service—provided beyond the walls of institutions such as hospitals.
- A service for disadvantaged population groups—for people who, because of distance, income, language or social barriers, may not be receiving an adequate share of traditional health services.
- A service for 'unattractive' health problems—for example, drug and alcohol problems and mental illness.
- A service for dealing with modern health problems—illnesses related to lifestyle and environment for which conventional medical services may have little to offer.
- A service to better deal with problems of living—where problems of living are the limitations imposed on our personal, social or work lives by illness. Traditional health services focus on the illness and pay little attention to the problems of living caused by it.
- A service that provides alternative therapies—for many problems, there is no 'best remedy' and it is possible to provide a variety of alternative therapies from which clients can select.

- **A service that promotes a diversity of health providers within the health system**—some health centres have been established to provide a salaried general practitioner service as an alternative source of care to conventional medical services.
- **A prevention service**—probably the interpretation most frequently linked with community health services.
- **A caring, respectful, humane service**—a reaction to the impersonal, technological image of scientific medicine.
- **A coordinated and integrated service**—hospitals, private health professionals and many community agencies tend to act as independent agents responsible only to themselves. This results in duplication of services or gaps in services, and for clients it often means conflicting or inappropriate advice. Community health services try to link professionals and services together in the interest of their clients. Wherever multiple providers are involved in clinical problems, they act as a team rather than as competing individuals, each not knowing what the other is doing.
- **A public health type of service**—a service that recognises how the environment and the life of the community can hinder or advance the health of the individual, and that accepts community change and development as an important element in health strategy.

Most of these descriptions represent a reaction to perceived shortcomings of conventional medical services. Alone or together, they fail to convey a distinct image of community health, as some conventional services such as hospitals are moving to become more responsive to their 'communities'.

An analysis of community health services in the United States, Britain and Canada identified one fundamental concept unique to community health, especially community health services: they take responsibility for the health of a defined population, as distinct from treating illness only in individuals who seek care. Accepting responsibility for the health of a defined population fosters the following service qualities.

- **Health and illness.** Community health is concerned with health and illness. It involves a broad definition of health that captures the full personal, social and economic impact of health and illness on a community.

- **Populations.** Community health is concerned with illness as it affects groups or communities, not solely with individuals presenting with illness. Community health monitors the distribution and changing patterns of illness. It measures the needs for health services and identifies unmet needs. It may or may not provide the services to fill identified gaps, but it takes responsibility for promoting such services. A healthy community is thus the focal point and health services one component.
- **Non-users.** Community health is concerned with non-users of services. Do they indicate that there are barriers to visiting health services? Do they indicate new health problems for which no relevant services exist? Responsibility for the whole community means responsibility for users *and* non-users.
- **Prevention.** Community health gives priority to the prevention of illness. Having responsibility for the whole community provides an incentive to take prevention seriously—because it will reduce the amount of future illness.
- **Best use of health resources.** Community health is concerned with seeing that the most effective and efficient use possible is made of the community's health resources—this includes identifying priorities for health expenditure and placing services where they are most needed. It favours efficient delivery arrangements—for example, group treatments where they are as effective as individual therapies, or teamwork where it is more efficient than a group of independent providers. Self-help or voluntary services are also promoted.
- **Integration.** Community health encourages provider collaboration and integration in order to ensure that health needs are met. Many communities are well supplied with health services, and the reason for unsuccessful care is often the failure to involve other skills or to communicate with other providers. Occasionally, it may be appropriate to enhance existing services, integrate with other services and develop team structures, or develop entirely new services.
- **Local focus.** Community health is a local concern. Responsibility for health is more easily assumed in well-defined communities of modest size. Services based on local allegiances, knowledge and resources favour a broader definition of health, a wider assumption of responsibility and a greater penetration of the community than do services with 'distant' allegiances or organisation.

THE DEVELOPMENT OF COMMUNITY HEALTH AND THE COMMUNITY HEALTH PROGRAM IN AUSTRALIA

The history of community health in Australia is a long one. Well-baby clinics, school dental services, food and sanitation services—all these form the basis of community health. Furthermore, the launch in 1973, by the Australian government, of a distinct Community Health program broadened the notion of community health by providing economic and political support. This program increased the range of services and activities provided but, more importantly, it aimed for community participation in the planning and development of services. Funding under the Commonwealth Community Health program was applied differently in different states.

Owen and Lennie (1992) provided overviews of contemporary trends in health development at a community level in Australia. They described the role of the Consumers' Health Forum of Australia, and pointed out that since the Australian government initiative of 1973, many community-based health services have evolved. Aboriginal medical services have also been established nationally.

In Victoria, the Health Issues Centre, a consumer-based advocacy group, was established in the 1980s. Women's health centres have flourished throughout Australia, after a shaky start in some instances. Furthermore, the ideal of community participation in the development and delivery of community health programs has now been recognised in practice as well as rhetoric, although Owen and Lennie (1992) argue that the levels of community participation in health services vary.

The principle of participation in health reflected a wider momentum of social change. Feminists and environmentalists began to clamour for more responsive health care and development policies. The impact on the environment of uncontrolled development and the dumping of wastes, and the subsequent consequences for community health, began to be recognised in the 1970s as health concerns by the communities themselves.

Community consultation and participation in the development and administration of health services appeared as a clear principle in the Australian government's Community Health program of 1973. The same principle was exhibited in the adoption of primary health care policies in South Australia in 1988 and in Queensland in 1993. Such policies reflect the World Health Organization's (1982) statement that 'community participation should be structured to provide significant and purposeful community involvement'. This also supports the empowerment of communities for health development. A more complete discussion of primary health care appears in Chapter 10.

Community participation allows people, both individually and in groups, to exercise their right to play an active and direct role in the development of appropriate health services and in ensuring conditions for sustained better health. Baum (2004, p. 346) argues that a clear analysis of 'participation' in health is warranted, as the concept is problematic. She poses four questions of relevance to practitioners: Is participation pseudo or real? what is the relationship between participation and power? who participates? what is the role of professionals in participation? The answers to these questions should guide practitioners in being genuine and realistic not only about their commitment to the concept, but also in not raising unrealistic expectations from community members about the extent of their involvement in community consultation processes.

DEFINITIONS AND DESCRIPTIONS OF 'COMMUNITY'

Traditionally, the concept of 'community' in health promotion was applied to a neighbourhood or geographic area. The role of the neighbourhood was particularly pivotal in developments in the United States in the 1960s and 1970s, where community work flourished through such neighbourhood social interventions as the War on Poverty.

Notwithstanding the importance of neighbourhoods and other geographic demarcations in community health promotion, 'community' is also recognised as a network of people who share certain characteristics or concerns. This notion of community accords with its Latin derivation— *communitas*, meaning 'common or shared'. An historical overview of definitions demonstrates the concept's various forms.

Hanchett described 'people with relationships to one another as the essential elements of community. In most communities, place is the strongest element holding people together. However, in other communities, a common goal, a common perspective or a common need provide the glue of the relationship' (1979, p. 8). Peck expanded this notion, claiming that a community is a place where people feel secure enough to share their 'weaknesses, incompleteness, imperfections, inadequacies', and know they will still be accepted (1987, p. 57).

The WHO incorporates and builds on these themes. A specific group of people, often living in a defined geographical area, who share a common culture, values and norms, are arranged in a social structure according to relationships which the community has developed over a period of time. 'Members of a community gain their personal and social identity by sharing common beliefs, values and norms which have been developed by the community in the past and may be modified in the future. They exhibit some awareness of their identity as a group, and share common needs and a commitment to meeting them' (WHO 1998, p. 5).

Each of these beliefs about the term 'community' is relevant for community health promotion practice. First, the concept of community as a 'place' has been central in community health promotion. Such programs as the Minnesota Heart Health Program and the Stanford Three Community Study in the United States, and the North Karelia Project in Finland, are examples where specific towns have been the focus for heart health interventions. These population-based interventions sprang from the concept of 'population-attributable risk', which measures the amount of disease in the population that can be attributed to a given level of exposure. When risk is widely distributed in the population, small changes in behaviour observed across an entire population are likely to yield greater improvements in the population-attributable risk than larger changes among a smaller number of high-risk individuals (Sorensen et al. 1998). These heart health interventions focused on known risk factors for heart disease. In Queensland, the program Healthier Bowen Shire Partnership was funded by Health Promotion Queensland (2000) as a multi-strategy health promotion intervention in a model community. The project aimed to develop an innovative health promotion intervention where the issues and strategies to address these health issues are generated by the community (see the case study below). Second, the women's movement and the environmental health movement are examples of communities of people who share a common bond, be it gender, ethnicity, age or social class. Third, communities of people who share a common chronic condition, and where they are accepted despite their frailties and vulnerabilities, represent another type of community where community health promotion activities are practised.

HEALTHIER BOWEN SHIRE PARTNERSHIP

This was a two-year cooperative initiative of the Bowen Shire Community (North Queensland) with a consortium of public health researchers and practitioners from the University of Queensland, Queensland University of Technology, the University of the Sunshine Coast, Queensland Health and non-government organisations (including the National Heart Foundation). The Centre of Health Promotion and Cancer Prevention Research at the University of Queensland provided leadership on the project. The consortium provided the health promotion expertise and support for the development, implementation and evaluation of strategies.

Funded in 1999, the partnership aimed to enhance the health of community members through the development of the community's capacity to reduce the risk factors of chronic disease (particularly diabetes, heart disease and cancer) using approaches relevant and appropriate to the particular assets, characteristics and requirements of the Bowen Shire community. The specific objectives were to:

- determine the health concerns and quality of life issues within the community;
- identify strategies for the intervention;
- develop networks and cooperation for community action between people, organisations and agencies, on which future health promotion initiatives may be built;
- increase levels of physical activity and intake of fruit and vegetables, to reduce harmful and hazardous levels of alcohol consumption, to reduce levels of excess weight and obesity and to increase the levels of social and productive activity.

Over the longer term, the aim of the project was stated as follows:

The development of a multi-strategy health promotion intervention in a community setting [which] aims to address the incidence of cardiovascular disease, cancer (particularly colorectal cancer) and Type II diabetes in older people, men and those from lower socioeconomic groups in the community. (p. 7)

The primary mission of the project was to fund community-based projects through the Think Healthy Community Grant Scheme. This scheme was initiated to address the priorities identified by the Bowen community. The Bowen Health Promotion Committee (HPC)—established with an extensive representation of community representatives and individuals—developed guidelines and criteria for assessing submissions for funding from local community groups, which helped ensure the sustainability of the project by enhancing the skills and knowledge of the local community. Among some 30 activities, sponsored by the Healthier Bowen Shire Partnership, were a family fun day (community activities in an outdoor setting), Federation picnic in the park (promotion of exercise, fruit and vegetables), school breakfast project (provision of breakfast from the Bowen State High School canteen), and a sports extravaganza (an open day for 28 Bowen sports and recreation clubs).

The initiative was successful in raising awareness of the Healthier Bowen Shire Partnership. A survey of local media demonstrated an increase in coverage in some health-related areas over the two-year period. Surveys conducted in the Bowen Shire and in a comparison community (Johnstone Shire) at the beginning and end of the period, investigated possible changes in behavioural risk factors and in civic and neighbourhood participation.

- No changes were evident over the period of the Partnership's work either in chronic disease risk factors, or in civic and neighbourhood participation.
- Of those surveyed, 48 per cent were aware of the Healthier Bowen Shire Partnership.
- There were high levels of awareness of the Partnership's Think Healthy Community Grant Scheme.

To ensure the sustainability of the project, the Health Promotion Committee (Bowen Shire) has now become the Healthier Bowen Shire Partnership Incorporated, and has maintained its activities beyond the end of the project.

> The Healthier Bowen Shire Partnership has demonstrated that community members can be involved in developing appropriate methods and decision-making processes to promote, approve and fund local community health promotion initiatives.
>
> *Source:* Final Report from the Healthier Bowen Shire Partnership Evaluation Group, August 2002

The Ottawa Charter's (WHO 1986a) action step, Strengthening Community Action, signals that health promotion works through effective community action. Communities, however defined, need to identify health problems or health issues and direct attention to ownership of solutions, thereby gaining control over their initiatives and activities. This means that professionals must learn new ways of working with individuals and communities—working for and with, rather than 'on', them. The Ottawa Charter's *Strengthening Community Action* legitimised the new directions in community health promotion in which community action is applauded and facilitated by health promotion practitioners. At the same time, it built on the pioneering work of the Community Health Program established in Australia in the 1970s. Regardless of how 'community' is used, its definition must be specified clearly, as its meaning is changeable, depending on context and experience (Baum 2004; Labonte 2005).

DEFINING COMMUNITY HEALTH PROMOTION

As outlined, community participation in health is a principle found in several policies aimed at enhancing the health of Australians. This reflects a new era in health promotion, one that employs the expertise of professionals but also involves people in communities in participating in decisions affecting their health. Green and Raeburn (1990) posed the question: Who will have control over health promotion? For some, health promotion belongs to the community; however, some administrators and professionals might not be willing to cede control (Poland et al. 2000). This poses questions for health promoters working in organisations that have espoused the Ottawa Charter (WHO 1986a) as a framework, yet find the role of the community health promoter a difficult one to define.

We believe that the Ottawa Charter advocates an 'enabling' approach to health promotion. The principle underlying each of the charter's five action steps is the provision of appropriate resources and avenues for people individually and collectively—to have an active role in all aspects of health (Green & Raeburn 1990; Raeburn & Rootman 1998). Wherever possible, people should have significant control over what is undertaken in any health care provision.

Education for health emphasises:

> not just the knowledge and skills to reduce behavioural risks, but also those elements that engage people more actively in their community's affairs, such as participating effectively in making health and social policy, demanding enforcement of regulations on environmental polluters, and organising advocacy for new or revised laws and regulations. (Green & Raeburn 1990, p. xviii)

The challenge for health promoters is not only to understand what health priorities are perceived, but also to advocate community-based solutions to identified problems. This broadens the role of health promoters significantly. Traditionally, the practice of health promoters was to provide information to communities about particular health problems. Health promoters often developed materials (pamphlets and brochures, occasionally videos) and disseminated them throughout a community— often in small group education sessions in hospitals, workplaces and schools, or at community group meetings or through displays in shopping malls.

Evidence from major community-based cardiovascular risk reduction education programs in Finland, Wales and the United States that focused on the reduction of behavioural risk factors shows that successful health promotion risk factor reduction programs were based on theory, were well planned and evaluated, and used a variety of strategies (Farquhar et al. 1985; Puska 1992; Weisbrod et al. 1992; Nutbeam et al. 1993a; Sorensen et al. 1998). Health promoters worked with communities in the development, implementation and evaluation phases of these programs to address lifestyle changes within populations. Comparable principles were adopted in Australia in such programs as the Quit for Life smoking campaigns conducted in the 1980s and 1990s. These community-based programs were extremely ambitious and some of their results were modest (Sorensen et al. 1998; Sallis & Owen 2002).

Community health promoters, in their role as change agents, have also worked with communities on changes in living conditions—for example, the removal of toxic industries in Port Adelaide.

Collaborative relationships between health promoters and communities are not new in health promotion. However, the health agenda in such relationships has more often than not been determined by health professionals. What is new is an expansion of the professional/community collaboration to address a community-driven agenda on health matters. The challenge for health promoters is to facilitate a community-driven agenda in a negotiated mutual partnership, rather than in a hierarchical relationship where professionals have 'power' over the community. The dilemma this poses for practitioners is discussed later in the chapter.

There are distinguishing features in the work of community health promoters. Labonte (2005) argued that the tradition of community health promotion has been to present an agenda of identified health problems to a community, whereas asking a community to identify its problems for itself is more in keeping with the principle of empowering communities to plan their own health destinies. Labonte (2005) labelled this form of community health promotion 'community development health promotion'; traditional community health promotion, where agendas are set by professionals in health agencies, is termed 'community-based health promotion'. Labonte (2005) distinguished the two forms by reference to the behavioural and the socio-environmental approaches to health promotion. An explanation of these terms and their application follows. While contemporary health promotion utilises the terms interchangeably, the distinctions shed light on the various approaches and roles that practitioners can play within their own organisation's context.

Community-based health promotion

Community-based health promotion is when health professionals provide information or advice about health problems to a particular community—for example, a nurse discussing the risks of smoking with a group of women. The focus of such programs is on behaviours, such as smoking, which put people 'at risk' of a particular disease. These 'risk factor' reduction programs have been the traditional mainstay of the health promotion programs. For a comprehensive examination of such approaches, see Glanz et al. (2002).

The **behavioural approach** to health promotion predominantly uses community-wide strategies (Labonte 1991b), as listed below.

- **Definition of health problem**—seen as 'behavioural' risk factors for poor health, for example, smoking and inadequate diet.
- **Target populations**—people with 'unhealthy behaviours'.
- **Health promotion strategies**—health education, social marketing, policies that support lifestyle choices, for example, workplace smoking bans.
- **Program development**—negotiated with communities: process of health professionals and/or health agencies defining the health problem and recruiting local members to assist in solving the problem, for example, school-based lifestyle programs and safe driving.
- **Examples of success criteria**—improved lifestyles, behaviour change; enactment of healthy public policies related to health behaviours, for example, restaurant anti-smoking policies.

This reflects the traditional 'health promoter' role in population-based risk factor reduction programs. The health promoter needs to be skilled in data interpretation, behavioural change theory and practice, group work and networking.

The **socio-environmental approach** to health promotion entails a community development approach to health enhancement. It extends the behavioural approach and legitimises the notion of 'strengthening communities' where living conditions or non-behavioural health problems are identified as a matter of concern (Labonte 1991b). This conceptual approach broadens the lens in understanding that health is influenced by cultural, social, economic and political processes. The approach is also called the social ecological model, as it integrates these multiple perspectives and theories.

- **Problem definition**—psychosocial risk factors and risk conditions, for example, lack of social support, isolation, low self-esteem, self-blame; or conditions which increase susceptibility to ill health, for example, poverty, dangerous work or physical environments.
- **Target populations**—people in high-risk environments.
- **Principal strategies**—personal empowerment (direct service providers); small group development (social support); community development to

strengthen actions on health determinants, social marketing; coalition advocacy of healthy public policies.

- **Program development**—process of enabling communities to make decisions necessary to plan and implement strategies, and allowing communities to define their own issues, strengthening community capacity and skills to make changes.
- **Success criteria**—improved social networks, quality of social support; improved community actions for greater access to service provision or resources conducive to sustaining health.

The starting points of the two approaches and the community methods used are not necessarily mutually exclusive. After all, the starting point in the socio-environmental approach is people's experiences of health/wellness in their day-to-day lives. The distinction lies in: who defines the issues, and how the collaborative relationship is negotiated in terms of the role of the health promoter; the expectations of both the health promoter and the community; and the negotiation between the parties of program goals and success criteria. Variations of this approach, and its potential for enhancing quality of life in communities, and the reduction of social inequalities in health, have been illustrated through the work of Dahlgren and Whitehead (1992), Whitehead (1995) and Whitehead et al. (2001). In 1999 in Australia, a review for the Commonwealth Department of Health and Aged Care documented international evidence on social disadvantage in health. It cited international examples and evidence to address socio-economic disadvantage through a framework for a national research, policy program and intervention agenda (Turrell et al. 1999). This work has been broadened to measure, more fully, socioeconomic position in population health (Dutton et al. 2005).

BALANCING BEHAVIOURAL AND SOCIOECONOMIC APPROACHES: AN ECOLOGICAL MODEL

Several authors (Freudenberg et al. 1995; Green et al. 1996; Sorensen et al. 1998; Minkler 1999) argue for a balanced and integrated approach to health promotion. They hold that an essential focus on either the behavioural and/or the socio-environmental approaches is incomplete and that an integrated approach to addressing health problems is needed. It is true that individuals are the only ones who can change their behaviour, yet focusing only on structural and/or policy changes may fail to recognise individual and group differences in people's response to their environment. These authors argue for a socio-ecological approach to health promotion. A socio-ecological approach is the foundation of Green and Kreuter's (2005) PRECEDE/ PROCEED model (see Chapter 4), as it integrates both strategies to address behavioural risk factors, but begins with a diagnosis of the socio-environmental determinants of the health issue/s being addressed. We would extend the argument for an 'ecological approach to health promotion'. Actions can address specific social environments and risk conditions (see above), as well as those physical environments that may militate against health and quality of life in communities. An example might be a health promotion and advocacy effort to address declining water quality in a community. This is in keeping with an ecology of public health (see Chapter 1).

MODELS OF COMMUNITY ORGANISATION, INCLUDING COMMUNITY DEVELOPMENT

The above discussion outlined the dimensions of community health promotion. Here we turn to models of community organisation and highlight community development as an important strategy.

The umbrella term 'community organisation' has become a recognised process in health promotion. Minkler described it as 'the process by which community groups are helped to identify common problems or goals, mobilise resources, and develop and implement strategies for reaching the goals they have collectively set' (2005, p. 26).

The community organisation framework developed in the early 1970s by Rothman in social work practice and further refined by Rothman and Tropman (1987) and Rothman (1995) has been widely accepted by health promoters as a useful one over the past three decades (Minkler 2005; Baum 1998; Egger et al. 2005). Three terms are employed—**locality development**, **social planning** and **social action**. The terms are compatible with 'community development'. For example:

- **Locality development.** Originally conceived to develop the potential of communities within geographic neighbourhoods, the categories of community action rely on a community's capacity to solve its own problems. While the term was originally applied to geographic neighbourhoods and reflects the emphasis on neighbourhood development in the United States in the late 1960s, the definition of community now applies either to a geographic entity or to a group who: share a common health problem (for example, cancer patients); have a mutual interest in a social issue (for example, mothers concerned about playground safety); or share common characteristics (for example, unemployed youths). Minkler (1990) suggests that 'community development' is related to 'locality development', as in both cases community members are engaged in a community problem-solving process.

- **Social planning.** According to Rothman (1995), social planning draws on the 'technical expert' to solve community problems. Social planning is a term with currency in the United Nations and related agencies at work in less developed countries, where 'technical assistance and experts' are provided to solve community problems. This 'technocratic' approach has relied solely on expert advice for solving problems. The basic change strategy is the gathering of facts and epidemiological analyses of community health status. The practitioner is a fact-gatherer and analyst, program implementer and facilitator. Community interests can be reconcilable or be in conflict. Ideally, negotiation of approaches to problem resolution should occur, but often has not.

- **Social action.** Well-known community activist Saul Alinsky (1969, 1972) is credited for much of the early thinking on this method of community organisation. Mobilising community efforts through advocacy and organising to have a voice and be heard is at the base of social action. Classic examples are the civil rights movement in the United States where transformations in legislation and politics proceeded. The women's movement and the environmental movement each demanded more resources and political attention to health and environmental concerns through tactics of persuasion, street marching and political lobbying. The results were profound: women's shelters and health centres were established and legislation examined to eliminate discrimination against women. And 'protecting the environment' became, to some extent, part of public policy. The foundation underlying this strategy is long-term policy and program change. Specific examples from the demonstrations of the anti-tobacco lobby at the Australian Lawn Tennis Association Australian Open are colourfully illustrated by Chapman and Lupton (1994, pp. 164–5).

Well-planned community health promotion interventions have included some, if not all, of Rothman's components. Education about behavioural risk factors and heart disease and the desire to educate communities to reduce these, together with links with existing non-governmental and community organisations, are the cornerstones of many Australian community-based health promotion programs. Classic examples of this approach have also been the major multi-strategy interventions in the United States (Farquhar et al. 1990), where the research team had a clear idea of the heart disease problem it wished to address, and community organisations and members were consulted when objectives were developed.

Although Rothman's model remains a useful backdrop against which the design of community health promotion programs can be organised, it is important to recognise its limitations. A major disadvantage is that it is organiser-centred and problem-based rather than community-centred and asset-based (Walter 2005). Because the notion of community development is an important one in community health promotion, attention is now given to it and Australian examples will be highlighted below in order to demonstrate the processes involved in community programs.

Community development in health promotion

Community development is widely accepted in health promotion practice, and has become an accepted strategy in program development and implementation. Various definitions exist and Butler and Cass provide one:

> Community development is based on an understanding of inequalities [in the health of different groups within our society]. People's health experiences are seen within the context of their social relationships. In this framework, alienation and powerlessness are identified as linked to poorer health outcomes; having a sense of not belonging to the broader society, a sense of not having much control over one's destiny. A developmental approach involves working in ways that facilitate people and communities developing their strength and confidence while at the same time addressing immediate problems. (1993, p. 8)

The question could be asked at this stage whether community development can be employed only with communities who are disenfranchised in some way, as the discussion seems to indicate this. Because the health data indicate disparities in the distribution of ill health between various population groups, innovative strategies that allow communities to identify problems and, importantly, own the process of proposing solutions need to be developed. Community development is the process used here. Furthermore, the process can be used in population groups where the starting point is capturing the reality of the lived experiences of the group, in all their complexity, and where the problem-solving capacity of the group is respected and enhanced. It aims to strengthen local areas or a group's capacity to deal with local problems, and through the process social support and community networks can be strengthened (Dahlgren & Whitehead 1992).

The role of the health promoter employing this 'community development' model is one of coordinator, enabler–catalyst, and teacher of problem-solving skills using ethical values (Rothman & Tropman 1987, pp. 3–26; Legge & Wilson 1996). We would add 'advocate' to this list, as an advocate is one who pleads and/or works on behalf of a client or client group.

Community development in multicultural health promotion

Community health promotion approaches to multicultural communities take various forms. Hiring multicultural workers to work with specific or various ethnic communities is one approach adopted by some agencies (for example, the East Sydney Area Health Service and the Brisbane Southside Public Health Unit). For many multicultural communities the leading health issue is access to information and services, ideally delivered in a cultural context similar to their own. In the following case study, both children and adults from culturally and linguistically diverse communities participated in a project aimed at enhancing mental health literacy.

INCREASING MENTAL HEALTH LITERACY OF CULTURALLY AND LINGUISTICALLY DIVERSE (CALD) COMMUNITIES

The high level of stigma in relation to mental health issues in CALD communities is a barrier to implementing mental health promotion and prevention (MHPP) initiatives. The stigma is linked to various cultural explanations and beliefs about the causes, prevention and management of mental health problems. However, there is evidence that increasing mental health literacy decreases stigma and that an approach involving children is a positive entry point to a CALD community.

In 2001, the Queensland Transcultural Mental Health Centre (QTMHC) invited ethnic schools in southeast Queensland to participate in their Health and Wellbeing Competition. The project aimed to pilot an MHPP strategy with CALD communities that aimed to increase their levels of mental health literacy. The project worked with ethnic school communities, introducing a mental health activity as part of teaching. (Ethnic schools are community schools that teach a language other than English, outside of regular school hours.) The schools are managed, and largely funded, by the communities and taught in community halls or other available facilities. The project also engaged with language-specific radio programs, which are very effective in disseminating messages across CALD communities.

For the project, students interviewed each other and family members using the language they were learning. The two winning interviews (beginner and advanced) from each school were broadcast on community language radio shows. The following year, the schools were invited to participate in the Emotional Health and Wellbeing Poster Competition. Approximately 1350 students (from ten different ethnic schools), aged between seven and seventeen, responded. Teachers guided the discussion of the topic, 'What do we need to do in today's world to keep mentally healthy?' Winning posters were displayed during the awards ceremony and at a Vietnamese Mental Health Day at a local shopping centre. The messages were reflected on the posters, either graphically or in writing, and indicated a good understanding of mental and emotional health and some of the protective factors. The QTMHC supported the schools with multi-lingual resources and ongoing contact.

Indications are that both children and adults involved in the project increased their understanding of mental health, therefore contributing to decreasing the stigma. Some of the lessons learned were that:

- it is fundamental to acknowledge and enhance the capacity of the CALD communities, and encourage ownership;
- it is cost-effective to implement MHPP initiatives where CALD people live, learn and play;
- a gradual, positive approach to mental health enables participation from CALD communities;
- children can be effective in communicating mental health messages to adults in their families and communities.

The project strengthened partnerships with CALD communities. Ethnic schools continue to use QTMHC's resources and QTMHC continues to work with radio program convenors to broadcast mental health messages in community languages. In addition, some have become involved as community leaders in other QTMHC projects aimed at reducing stigma and increasing mental health literacy in multicultural communities.

Source: Elvia Ramirez and Rita Prasad-Ildes, Queensland Transcultural Mental Health Centre

EMPOWERMENT IN COMMUNITY HEALTH PROMOTION

In health promotion, 'empowerment' is a recurring concept. It joins other concepts such as 'enabling' and 'mediating' in much of the discourse. Indeed, health promotion practice itself is considered to be empowering in its use of community organisation processes for the communities themselves. So, what does empowerment mean? Furthermore, who is empowered—health professionals, communities, clients, or all or none of the above? How does a health promoter build an empowering relationship with a community?

McArdle (1993, p. 2) described empowerment as 'the process whereby decisions are made by the people who have to wear the consequences of those decisions'. The WHO defines empowerment as '. . . a process through which people gain greater control over decisions and actions affecting their health' (WHO 1998, p. 6). The role of the professional is clearly, then, one of 'enabler'. Some of the factors that function to 'disempower' people are lack of information about health, lack of access to health services, and unknowing exposure to risk conditions not conducive to health (inadequate food and fresh water, inadequate housing, unemployment). These disempowering socio-environmental conditions are outlined in the Ottawa Charter (WHO 1986a).

Empowerment in health promotion has been the subject of attention (see *Health Education Quarterly*, vol. 21, no. 2, 1994; Booker et al. 1997; Laverack & Wallerstein 2001). The much-quoted definition by Wallerstein and Bernstein states:

> Community empowerment embodies an interactive process of change, where institutions and communities become transformed as people who participate in changing them become transformed. Rather than pitting individuals against community and overall societal needs, the community empowerment construct focuses on both individual and community change. (1994, p. 142)

Given the term's favour in health promotion literature, Labonte (1993) commented that it is surprising how little the concept of 'power' is attended to in discussion. He drew on the work of Foucault (1979) to point out the need to understand the elements of an empowering relationship between professionals and groups of individuals or communities. Foucault's notion of hegemonic power is that form of implicit 'power-over' that is 'invisible and internalised, so that it is structured into our everyday actions and we come to take it for granted'. This internalisation leads to what authors have called 'learned helplessness' or 'surplus powerlessness' (Seligman 1975; Lerner 1986, cited in Labonte 1993).

Lerner claimed that individuals can internalise this powerlessness and create a potent psychological barrier to action, as they do not engage in activities that meet their real needs and they accept aspects of their world that are self-destructive to their own health and wellbeing as unalterable features of their own reality (Lerner 1986, cited in Labonte 1993).

In situations like these, low self-esteem, self-blame and internalised apathy and anger can be evident. These factors are correlated with poorer self-reported health status and increased behavioural risk factor prevalence (Labonte 1993). This internalisation process can also lead to isolation and removing oneself from active participation in day-to-day life activities. Social isolation is recognised more and more as a condition of existence that is detrimental to health, and the theme of social inequality is recognised within the new public health as one that has to be addressed with creative strategies.

Strategies that begin to build social support networks for alienated and isolated individuals can begin to enhance self-esteem (Lerner 1986, cited in Labonte 1993), and recent evidence suggests that social support and control may have both direct and buffering effects on stress and health (Cohen & Syme 1985; Syme 1996; Franks & Cronan 2004; Stewart, Cianfrini & Walker 2005). Some of these measures are embraced within the concept of social capital which is discussed next. Providing support on a one-to-one basis and assisting in small group development with individuals are just two of the health promoter's strategies of empowerment of people proposed in the following empowerment continuum.

Figure 7.1:The empowerment continuum

✗ ——	✗ ——	✗ ——	✗ ——	✗
Personal care	Small group development	Coalition advocacy	Political action	Social movement

The empowerment continuum has been published elsewhere in similar form as a community organisation tool (Jackson et al. 1989; Labonte 1992b; and modified by Baum 1998). We contend that it is a useful starting point for community development work. It offers an opportunity for health promoters engaged in community health promotion to chart their 'empowerment' practice along a continuum of actions, although it does not presuppose that their practice has to begin at the beginning. **Personal care** occurs where nurses or other health professionals are in contact with individuals. Essential to the personal care provided is its developmental aspect, so that the transaction is not a passive one but one that seeks to understand the psychosocial and socio-environmental contexts of the individual's concerns. In **small group development**, the group is central to any process of community change. Without the support of a group, many people will be unable to participate. Mutual support can include strengthening of friendships and neighbourhood networks. In **coalition advocacy**, through issue identification, other natural networks or groups with similar concerns can be brought together for the development and advocacy of healthy policies (for example, HIV/AIDS groups forming umbrella coalitions). **Political action** involves support through political processes for resources, research, funding. Strategies include political lobbying, networking and media advocacy (for example, lobbying for HIV/AIDS activities and resources). **Social movement** refers to a major groundswell of activity, resources and community awareness, and the changing of community consciousness (for example, successes in many spheres of the women's movement and the green movement).

You might be able to relate your own work to one of the points on the continuum and we challenge you to reflect on your practice and whether there is potential for you to develop its scope in terms of this schema.

The very fact that well-intentioned health promoters engage in community development calls for an analysis of the concept of empowerment and the underlying power relationship involved. Labonte (1993) and Petersen (1994) caution that empowerment can assume 'romanticised notions' and that some communities are not always healthy or empowering in their organisation or interaction. In addition, there is a tendency for bureaucracies to make claims about community development such that community expectations with respect to revitalised services and/or resources are raised but often not met.

Hawe (1994) proposed a model for dissecting the notion of empowerment into manageable components. This is a useful framework for practitioners and is reproduced in Figure 7.2.

Much of the health promotion empowerment work rests on the philosophical foundations provided by the Brazilian educator Paulo Freire (1973). He advocated a participatory education process in which people are not objects or recipients of political and educational projects, but collaborators able to name their problems and solutions (Wallerstein & Bernstein 1994). Freire's *contientizacion*, meaning 'creating critical consciousness', is not only a process of community labelling of health problems or issues through a community development process but also a facilitated dialogue in which health promoters/educators help participants to identify root causes of the problems the community identifies. Through ongoing dialogue, participants are challenged to propose solutions and to develop plans for overcoming problems. Freire's techniques have been expanded from his work with illiterate Brazilian communities to other parts of the world.

Figure 7.2: Community empowerment

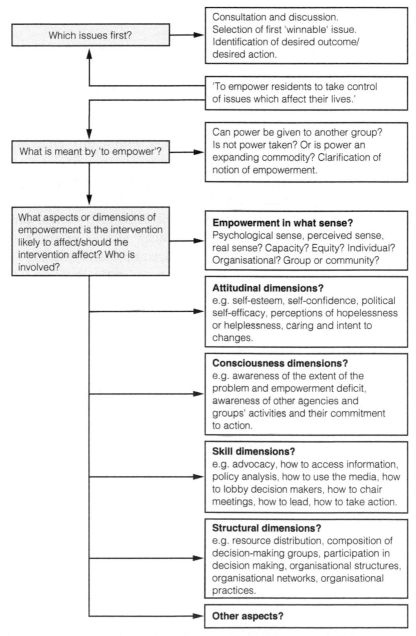

Source: P. Hawe 1994, 'Capturing the meaning of "community" in community intervention evaluation: Some contributions from community psychology', *Health Promotion International,* 9(3), pp. 199–208, p. 206, by permission of Oxford University Press; see original for further explanation.

SOCIAL CAPITAL AND COMMUNITY HEALTH PROMOTION

In the above discussion, the relationship between health professionals and communities has been outlined as a starting point for practice. Recent thinking that emphasises the importance of social support and individual health outcomes, community capacity and citizen engagement has opened another agenda for the socio-environmental approach in health promotion. The concept of social capital resides within this. Drawing on Putnam's (1995) work, social capital focuses on strengthening social cohesion within communities, which is seen as an important future investment for improving population health outcomes (Lomas 1997). People's networks, norms, human connections in the form of trust that can be transferred from one social setting to another, as well as community resources and civic engagement, are all important for strengthening social ties and opportunities and, hence, health (Putnam 1993). Putnam's (1993) arguments stem from his Italian study of regional government and the importance of social capital in economic success.

Putnam's work has been influential in opening discussions on the powerful concepts of classic citizen participation (Arnstein 1969, 1971) and the notion of citizen engagement in building community and increasing social trust (Barber 1996). Another agenda within the social capital 'framework' is that of community economic development. Szreter and Woolcock (2004) claim that social capital creates local economic prosperity through strengthening trust, civic engagement and organisational capability within communities, and is a mechanism for strengthening community economic development, government performance to criminal activity and youth behaviour (Woolcock & Narayan 2000). In Australia, Winter (2000) discusses the potential influence of social capital on public policy. For health promotion, social capital has captured the notion of collaboration, support and building community capital through cooperation across sectors; and Woolcock and Narayan (2000) claim that social connectedness is more consequential in the case of health and wellbeing than in any other sphere. On the other hand, several authors (Baum 1999; Erben et al. 1999; Labonte 1999) remind health promoters that community development activities can build social cohesion and, hence, social capital in communities.

Erben et al., for example, argue that the philosophy of social capital is incompatible with the philosophy of health promotion (1999, p. 173), because maintaining the established social order through these collaborative efforts may in fact mean that social capital becomes 'a resource to exercise power over those who have only limited or even no access to this resource' (1999, p. 180). Essentially, fostering trust, reciprocity and cooperation are laudatory goals. However, one needs to apply the concept cautiously if the spirit of the Ottawa Charter's fundamental philosophy of empowerment remains health promotion's cornerstone. Health promotion activities need to be placed within an empowerment and social change framework to advance health opportunities. Baum identifies 'unhealthy and healthy uses of social capital' (1999, p. 175) from the Adelaide Health Development and Social Capital Study (p. 173). The healthy uses of social capital include many of the elements listed at the beginning of this discussion: trust, cooperation, understanding, empathy, alliance across differences, questioning and openness to new ideas. The unhealthy uses of social capital are: distrust of strangers/differences, 'them' and 'us' mentality, tight-knit but excluding communities, fear of the unknown, dislike of change and new ideas, and racism. Additionally, entrenched norms of behaviour do not necessarily build 'trust and reciprocity' and may mitigate against advancing health—for example, in some groups violence against women is acceptable. An example of both the enhancement of social cohesion as an element of social capital and community 'social change' can be seen in rural communities that have reinvented themselves and their economies through community coalition building, participation and engagement. Unfortunately, it is often in crisis that communities are reshaped. We believe that many of the underlying elements in the discourse on social capital reside already in active engagement, participation and, most importantly, advocacy principles in the healthy communities' literature.

Since Putnam first wrote about social capital (1995), social capital has become 'fashionable' (Pearce & Smith 2003) and a 'cottage industry' (Putnam 2004). The conceptual debates have been extended to examine the role of social inequality in health, in addition to social connectedness and networks, public policy (Shortt 2004) and the government, as Figure 7.3 illustrates.

Putnam refers to the direct effects on health of public policy of 'the State' such as the provision of clean water, and the evidence of inequalities on health, and mechanisms and influences such as social support, communication patterns, social identity and risk behaviour, access to resources and collective actions (Putnam 2004). For health promoters, these concepts

Figure 7.3: Interactions between factors impacting on health

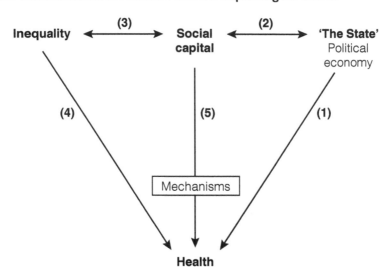

Source: R. Putnam 2004, 'Commentary; "Health by association": some comments', *International Journal of Epidemiology*, 33(4), pp. 667–71, p. 670, by permission of Oxford University Press.

are important. They extend the conceptual understanding of specific influences within the social capital literature on community health. The evidence about the strength of these links is being increasingly investigated by researchers.

There is a conundrum for health promotion practitioners in this presentation of what is seen as a new term for building 'community'. You may be employed on specific health program grants to address a specific health problem, such as diabetes. How does social capital affect your practice? We suggest that awareness of, and being educated about, these developments can assist your program strategy development. Building upon social ties and cohesion ('social capital') within your health promotion program are strong variables in individual and community health as we lean increasingly towards research that focuses on the importance of social contexts for health. Understanding the social capital debate also reminds us of the empowerment continuum (see Figure 7.1) and empowerment as a health promotion fundamental.

Community capacity building

While community organisation and community development have been terms inextricably linked with health promotion and its fundamental core of 'empowerment', these developments converge in community capacity building. What is community capacity building? 'It is not something new, but a refinement of ideas found within the literature and practice of both community development and community empowerment . . . a process that increases the assets and attributes which a community is able to draw upon in order to improve their lives (including but not restricted to their health)' (Gibbon et al. 2002, p. 485).

For health promotion, the scope of practice is extended to not only engage groups and communities in needs assessment and program planning, but also to 'build sustainable skills, resources, and commitment to prolong and multiply health gains many times over' (Labonte et al. 2002). Increasingly, funders of health promotion programs require strategies for the *sustainability* and *transferability* of their funded programs to other sites and communities. Recall the empowerment continuum discussed earlier in the chapter: here, *coalition building and advocacy* and *social movement* implicitly contain mechanisms that communities and health promoters use to sustain ownership of health issues and, importantly, their solutions—although these mechanisms may not originally have been labelled community capacity building.

Community capacity building has been called 'the parallel track for health promotion programs' (Labonte et al. 2002). Essentially, while health promoters are focusing on improving health gains for specific health problems in communities (such as injury, heart disease and cancer prevention), the community development and empowerment processes utilised within these program developments have unintended effects and outcomes through increasing the community's capacity in a number of ways (see Table 7.1). Skills can be developed through rotating community leadership roles, group facilitation, community newsletter and website production, project management and grant writing. These processes can then be measured as 'parallel' health promotion outcomes.

Table 7.1: Examples of a capacity-building approach to physical activity

Operational domain	Description in physical activity program
Participation	Organise events for maximum community involvement by tapping into the community's interests, whether that is better footpaths and lighting, or food security and gardening.
Leadership	Participation and leadership are closely connected. Leadership requires a strong participant base just as participation requires the direction and structure of strong leadership. Work with people's strengths and provide opportunities for shared leadership. Recognise and reward efforts.
Organisation-building	Tap into the organisational structures that already exist, including small groups such as committees, church and youth groups that can tackle the issue within their mandate. Look for opportunities for agencies to collaborate. Work to make the organisations more democratic and empowering for people to come together in order to socialise and to address their concerns and problems.
Problem assessment	Encourage the ongoing identification of problems, solutions to the problems and actions to resolve the problems by the community, both small/personal and large community-wide.
Resource mobilisation	Work together to lever and mobilise resources both from within and negotiated from beyond the community to extend to issues outside the original mandate of physical activity.
'Asking why'	Encourage the community to critically assess the social, political, economic and other causes of inequalities towards developing appropriate personal and social change strategies.
Equitable links with others	Keep the ties open to other organisations, including partnerships, coalitions and voluntary alliances for members to participate as individuals or as a part of the organisation.
Equitable relations with the outside agents	In a program context, outside agents are often an important link between communities and external resources and this is especially important near the beginning of a new program, when the process of building community capacity may be 'triggered' and nurtured.
Stakeholder control	Community members have shared authority in decision-making on all aspects of the program (planning, implementation, evaluation, finances, administration, reporting and conflict resolution).

Source: Labonte et al. (2002, p. 182); reproduced with permission of the Canadian Public Health Association. Originally published in the *Canadian Journal of Public Health*, vol. 93, no. 3, May/June 2002, pp. 181–82.

HEALTHY CITIES

In this section, the intersectoral commitment to the creation of healthy public policies as advocated in the Ottawa Charter (WHO 1986a) is considered by examining cities and communities as sites for this type of action.

The city as a location for broad healthy public policy initiatives was mooted in the late 1980s and, since then, Healthy Cities projects have been established worldwide. It is estimated that by 2007 more than half of the world's population will live in urban areas (Awofeso 2003), and with this prediction the impetus and interest in creating healthier cities from the WHO stemmed from a conference, Healthy Toronto 2000, held in 1984. This and several other initiatives were embraced by the WHO (1986a). However, the concept of a healthy city is a much older concept. Early civilisations had laws and codes to protect the health of residents, and the nineteenth-century public health movement saw the development of sewers, housing codes and improved water supplies. The utopian visions of the garden city movement of the early 1900s flourished and many of us now live in its offshoot, the suburb.

The speed with which the idea of healthy cities has spread across the world is testimony to its timeliness and to the appropriateness of its approach to health promotion. In 1986, the WHO planned five to eight city projects in Europe. By 1997, this exercise had mushroomed to a network of 1000 communities worldwide. Healthy Cities has been variously described as a project, a movement and a vision (Baum 1992b, 1998). Hancock and Duhl (1988) described a healthy city as one 'that is continually creating and improving those community resources which enable people to mutually support each other in performing all the functions of life and in developing to their maximum potential'. A process, and not just an outcome, defines a healthy city—it is conscious of health and striving to improve it. What is required is a commitment to health, and a structure and process to achieve it (Tsouros 1991). The WHO has remained committed to the concept of healthy cities and communities through imaginative networks, funding projects and site visits worldwide.

By 2000, over 4000 communities had joined in and by 2003, 8000 cities were engaged in some healthy cities' actions (Duhl 2003, cited in Tibbetts 2003). In over 1000 cities around the world, better health and quality of life are being addressed with the WHO Healthy Cities Program (WHO/Regional Office for Europe 2005a). The principle underlying the program is that health can be improved by modification of the physical environmental, as well as social and economic factors that affect or 'determine our health'. The program aims to put health on the agenda of decision-makers, build support for local public health action and develop local participatory approaches to health and environmental issues. Moreover, the WHO program has established partnerships for healthy cities through its working group on 'Healthy Cities, Villages, Islands and Communities'. The partnership requires participation from health, environmental, economic, ecological, education and urban planning fields. Key mechanisms of influential partnerships are building on cultural and historical backgrounds, and mutual success, being aware of generating additional financial resources and involving all the important decision-makers within communities.

Awofeso (2003) argues that there have been a number of achievements and cites California's Healthy Cities and Communities program, begun in 1987, which has contributed significantly to improving the state's health profile through a number of intersectoral strategies. The US Department of Health and Human Services asked the National Civic League to assist in launching a nationwide Healthy Cities effort in 1989 (Tibbetts 2003). Numerous toolkits for the development of community partnerships and profiles of successful healthy communities are outlined on its website (www.healthycommunities.org). The breadth of this worldwide activity demonstrates that the actions to promote health through a number of community-based mechanisms in cities, communities, villages and islands are far-reaching and robust.

In Australia, three Healthy Cities projects were funded initially in the late 1980s and were located with the Australian Community Health Association in Sydney. The three were Canberra (ACT), Illawarra (NSW) and Noarlunga (SA). The Australian Healthy Cities project was evaluated and, despite the closure of the national office in 1992, various forms of the projects are continuing.

According to Baum (1992b), within the overall requirement of equity, three sets of criteria can be used to judge the health of a city as mediated through the quality of its environment. They are:

• physical form, including use of land, housing type and standard, communication infrastructure, transport provision and the quality of the built and natural environments;

- interaction, recognising that people come to cities for contact with others—this includes politics, work, caring, education, recreation and home life;
- individual experiences of the city, which include a sense of history and tradition, lifestyle, culture and expressions of creativity and art.

Healthy Cities is a cooperative approach to health planning and urban administration. It is based on the view that improved cooperation between different sectors of government and greater community participation in decision-making can result in an environment more conducive to good health. Each of the Australian projects cited above emphasised the importance of a vision in achieving a healthy community, and each had a different set of sub-projects. (For a useful overview and critique of Healthy Cities worldwide, see Baum 2004, pp. 489–509.)

Healthy cities in a globalised world

The principles upon which the Healthy Cities movement is founded are indeed laudatory: intersectoral collaboration (public health strategists working with urban planners, engineers and the non-government sector), a focus on equity, and collaborations based on a true spirit of social democracy. However, in the past 20 years numerous changes have occurred that confront implementation of Healthy Cities projects worldwide. These include widening social inequalities in some cities, widening income distributions within city populations leading to poverty and violence, and measurement issues to capture the complexities of both process and outcomes of healthy cities approaches. De Leeuw and Skovgaard explore the evidence of Healthy Cities initiatives, and conclude that there is indeed 'fair evidence that Healthy Cities works' (2005, p. 1338), despite the divide between the original intentions of the WHO-led initiative and current drives towards hard 'evidence' of effectiveness. These authors argue that healthy cities are indeed a 'realm to test innovations in public health' (de Leeuw & Skovgaard 2005, p. 1339).

'Healthy communities' was one of the definitions of community health given as an example at the beginning of this chapter. Drawing on the principles of a healthy city and healthy 'settings', numerous initiatives have been implemented in Australia; and federal and state governments have embraced what they term Safe Cities. For example, Toowoomba has the Safer Toowoomba Partnership Inc., an intersectoral, community-based program to enhance the quality of life in Toowoomba through crime prevention and injury prevention. (For more information on this initiative, see the Toowoomba City Council website www.toowoomba.qld.gov.au). Another initiative is the Shoalhaven Aboriginal Safe Community Partnership (SASCP) in New South Wales, which is a collaboration between Indigenous and non-Indigenous people who recognise and encourage the initiatives of the local Indigenous community in promoting a safe and healthy community. The programs include a water-based exercise program for elders to help prevent falls, and swimming lessons for toddlers. In addition, the partnership has produced a Fire Safe poster and an anti-depression toolkit. (For more information on this partnership see the New South Wales government's community builder's website, www.communitybuilders.nsw.gov.au).

Increasingly, individuals and communities are seeking more involvement in the decisions made by governments and organisations that impact on their lives. Many individuals and organisations are concerned about the unproductive relationships with communities that reduce the confidence in public and private institutions, therefore hampering effective decision-making and the accomplishment of social and economic objectives and environmental sustainability. The International Conference on Engaging Communities (ICEC), an initiative of the United Nations and the Queensland government, was held in Brisbane in August 2005 to address some of these issues. The topics covered included 'the development and implementation of public policy and programs, the operation of markets and the activities of corporations, and the achievement of social equity and sustainable resource management' (ICEC 2005). The conference objectives included:

- promoting understanding of the concept of engagement and participative practices and its role in good governance;
- exploring 'what works', showcasing innovation and promoting good practice;
- sharing practice knowledge across the globe at local, regional and state levels; and promoting learning across disciplines and sectors;
- discussing and developing conceptual and theoretical frameworks and directions for the future and the evidence base which underpins this practice;

- building understanding and evidence of leadership, capacity and capability issues for citizens/community and government/institutions;
- creating ongoing national and international networks and collaboration, and creating communities of interest around the issue (ICEC 2005).

A significant outcome of the conference was the Brisbane Declaration on Community Engagement (see the Queensland government's 'Get involved' website, www.getinvolved.qld.gov.au).

COMMUNITY HEALTH PROMOTION AND THE INTERNET: VIRTUAL COMMUNITIES

The technological revolution which has occurred since the mid 1990s presents health promoters with creative opportunities in engaging communities. The capacity to form 'virtual communities' enhances consumer access to health information from international databases. The Internet provides links to interactive chat rooms, computer conferences and bulletin boards. Virtual communities augment face-to-face interactions and will increasingly become a tool for health promoters to link inter-agency and community communication. Technology will break down isolation as like-minded and interested people connect through social networks, across borders and time zones. Some evidence to suggest this is drawn from the United States where Blanchard and Horan (1998) discovered, through a survey of 340 community members, that all respondents indicated an interest in the educational and community potential of the virtual community.

Etzioni and Etzioni (1997) argue that we need to ask the question, what virtues of online communities are absent in offline ones? They suggest that for people who are isolated because of illness, age or handicap, 'virtual health communities' offer online communication potential. Social communities will always offer human contact and a sense of physical place, yet technology provides opportunities for community networking for those who are isolated and/or do not have transport. It also expands our horizons as we examine cyberspace as another exciting 'setting' in health promotion.

With increased access to technology through cybercafes, libraries and 'freenets', health promoters have opportunities to think laterally about harnessing the Internet as another access point for health promotion opportunities.

A number of initiatives have been documented. These build on the work of Milio (1996), who believed that connections through information technology are the way of the future. These information technology opportunities will make a difference to connecting children and older persons to health information. It gives voice also to the isolated and the disabled who may be housebound. In the United States, several authors have demonstrated both the strengths and limitations of health promotion programs focused on behaviour change and the Internet as a vehicle for such change (Evers et al. 2005; Patrick et al. 2005). The former authors argue that there are few studies examining the quality of interactive health-behaviour change programs on the Internet, and that these programs are in the early stages of development (Evers et al. 2005). The latter authors claim that in cancer communication, computer-supported interactive media have been greatly enhanced through 'point-and-click' interfaces to obtain and publish information from the web (Patrick et al. 2005).

In Australia, we need to fund research and programs to discover innovative case studies that can advance our practice in using technology to promote health through a number of means—interactive health promotion and disease management programs, access to quality web-based materials and community health network developments.

REVIEW

Communities, however defined, are central to the promotion of health, and community health promotion is wide in scope and contains many dimensions. Community health promotion embraces planned community-based programs that emphasise the reduction of behavioural risk factors through strategies such as public information and education, legislation, media-based campaigns and economic measures. Community health promotion also includes the collective efforts of communities to enhance their health.

The health promoter who works with communities is a change agent and, as such, needs to be knowledgeable about community and group dynamics and skilled in community organisation theory and practice. In the case studies presented, community development, as a community organisation tool, is an important area of community health promotion.

Increasingly, public health policies have consumer input as part of the policy-making process. Health care policies in practice in several states, and health plans prepared by local governments, include communities within their sphere of influence. Consumer-driven self-help support groups and self-help action groups play an increasingly vital role in promoting the health of community members. Healthy Cities and related initiatives further herald the exciting potential for fostering health in Australian communities. The concept of social capital to foster community cohesion, and the role of the Internet as a potential tool for health promotion, are contemporary issues for community health promotion.

REVISION

Consider the main issues addressed in this chapter. Review each point in light of your understanding of community health promotion.

1. *Describe the concept of community health and its evolution through the introduction of community health centres in Australia.*
2. *Discuss community health promotion in the context of community health.*
3. *Define and describe a community, and identify community organisation strategies in community health promotion, including community development.*
4. *Analyse the case studies of community health promotion in Australia.*
5. *In light of the empowerment continuum, where does your health promotion practice fit?*
6. *Describe Healthy Cities and identify some current Healthy Cities and Healthy Community initiatives.*
7. *Analyse the strengths and limitations of the role of the Internet in the future of health promotion in communities in Australia.*

8

Promoting health in Indigenous communities

- *A note on Australia's Indigenous population*
- *Concepts and perceptions of health*
- *Health status and health service use*
- *The role of Aboriginal and Torres Strait Island health workers*
- *Strategies to improve health*
- *Health promotion in Indigenous communities*
- *A model for health promotion*
- *Ethics in Indigenous health research*
- *Aboriginal and Torres Strait Islander Research Agenda Working Group*

A number of government publications over the past fifteen years have empha-sised the glaring shortcomings in both health status and access to appropriate services of Indigenous Australians (National Aboriginal Health Strategy Working Party 1989; Royal Commission into Aboriginal Deaths in Custody 1988; National Health Survey 1995; Enough to Make You Sick *(National Health Strategy 1992a);* National Aboriginal and Torres Strait Islander Survey 1994 *(ABS 1994);* Australia's Health 1998 *(AIHW 1998);* The Health and Welfare of Australia's Aboriginal and Torres Strait Islander Peoples *(ABS 1999); the National Aboriginal and Torres Strait Islander Health Council (NATSIHC) 2003; the National Health and Medical Research Council (NHMRC) 2003a). Indigenous Australians have the poorest health of all identified sub-populations in Australia. (For the purposes of this chapter, Indigenous Australians refers to Aboriginal and Torres Strait Islander peoples, as this term is used in a range of contemporary publications, including the NATSIHC (2003), the Australian Bureau of Statistics and the Australian Institute of Health and Welfare (ABS & AIHW) (2003), and the Australian Institute of Health and Welfare (AIHW) (2004a).)*

We address Indigenous health status and outline current health promotion initiatives designed to reduce Indigenous health inequalities. Social indicators and health status begin the discussion. Two health problems—child health and circulatory disease—are highlighted. National policies to redress the discrepancies in social conditions and health are profiled through a discussion of the National Aboriginal Health Strategy (NAHS Working Party) (1989). Relevant models of health promotion are presented. The chapter concludes with a presentation of the NHMRC's (2003b) Values and Ethics: Guidelines for ethical conduct in Aboriginal and Torres Strait Islander health research *and the Aboriginal and Torres Strait Islander Research Agenda Working Group (RAWG) 'Road Map' (NHMRC 2003a). The importance of current initiatives in training Aboriginal and Torres Strait Islander primary health care workers is highlighted.*

Because of extremely adverse social and economic conditions in many communities, traditional public health measures—such as ensuring safe drinking water, sanitation and food storage—are fundamental in ameliorating conditions that negatively influence the health of Indigenous people. These public health measures are taken for granted by most Australians. Moreover, let us remember that the Ottawa Charter (WHO 1986a, p. 2) proclaimed that the basic conditions for health are peace, shelter, food, education, income, a stable ecosystem, sustainable resources, social justice and equity. The five action steps set out in the Ottawa Charter (see Chapter 2) are applicable to the promotion of health in Indigenous communities.

A NOTE ON AUSTRALIA'S INDIGENOUS POPULATION

From the 2001 census, the Aboriginal and Torres Strait Islander population of Australia was estimated to be 460 140, which represented 2.4 per cent of the total Australian population. Between 1996 and 2001, the Indigenous population increased by 16 per cent; while three-quarters of this increase can be explained by changes in birth and death rates, one-quarter is attributable to improvements in census collection methods and an increasing willingness to be identified as Indigenous (ABS & AIHW 2003). However, it should be noted that the identification of Indigenous people in data sets is often incomplete (AIHW 2004a). This is due to: doubts regarding estimates of the size and structure of the Indigenous population; the imperfect identification of Indigenous Australians in data collections, such as hospital records; and questions related to the collection of data about Indigenous people living in remote areas and the adequacy of the questions and concepts used (AIHW 2004d, p. 8).

Contrary to popular belief, most Indigenous Australians do not live in rural and/or remote areas of the continent. The majority of Indigenous people live in the southern and eastern parts of Australia. While only 1 per cent of people living in the Sydney and Brisbane Aboriginal and Torres Strait Islander Commission regions were Indigenous, these two regions alone accounted for 18 per cent of Australia's Indigenous population (ABS 1999, p. 15). However, 29 per cent of people in the Northern Territory were estimated to be of Indigenous origin (ABS & AIHW 2005). This corroborates earlier demographic profiles where two-thirds of Indigenous Australians were resident in areas defined as 'urban' by the ABS (centres with over 1000 people or more) compared with 86 per cent of non-Indigenous Australians (National Health Strategy 1992a, p. 87).

The Indigenous population is also comparatively young. In 2001, the median age for the Indigenous population was 21 years of age, while for the non-Indigenous population the corresponding figure was 36 years (ABS & AIHW 2005). This has implications for program and policy initiatives and indicates the importance of schools and communities as settings for health promotion activity (ABS 1999, p. 12).

Indigenous Australians, as a population group, are also heterogeneous. In the traditional living places throughout the continent, and through the early forced removal to other communities and later urban migration, Indigenous people display differences in norms and customs depending on individual circumstance, living place and history. As the NAHS Working Party (1989) proclaimed, any national health strategy needs to consider this diversity.

CONCEPTS AND PERCEPTIONS OF HEALTH

According to the NAHS Working Party, 'health to Aboriginal peoples is a matter of determining all aspects of their life, including control over the physical environment, of dignity, of community self-esteem, and of justice. It is not merely a matter of the provision of doctors, hospitals, medicines or the absence of disease and incapacity' (1989, p. ix).

Traditionally in Indigenous societies there was no word or expression for 'health' as understood by Western society, and it would be difficult for Indigenous Australians to conceptualise 'health' as one aspect of life. The nearest translation in an Indigenous context would probably be a term such as 'life is health is life' (NAHS Working Party 1989, p. ix). The working party defined health as: 'Not just the physical wellbeing of the individual but the social, emotional, and cultural wellbeing of the whole community. This is a whole-of-life view and it includes the cyclical concept of life-death-life' (p. ix); the importance of recognising this definition has been underlined in a number of documents over the last decade and a half, including the Queensland Health discussion paper (2005a).

Health promoters working in Indigenous communities should be aware of this culturally determined perspective of health. The NAHS Working Party also stressed 'quality of life' aspects of health emanating from a social system based on 'interrelationships between people and land, people and creator beings, and between people, which ideally stipulates interdependence within and between each set of relationships' (1989, p. ix). Clearly, an Indigenous concept of health must form a backdrop for any initiative promoting the health of Indigenous Australians.

HEALTH STATUS AND HEALTH SERVICE USE

It is now well recognised that social disadvantage has the potential to compromise individual health (Turrell et al. 1999; Turrell 2002; Thomson 2003). The relationship between social disadvantage and ill health is exemplified in the health status of the Indigenous population. According to the National Health Strategy (1992a, p. 87), and corroborated by the ABS (1999), there have been some gains for Aboriginal and Torres Strait Islanders on broad social indicators, particularly education. However, on indicators of employment status, economic status and housing, this population falls well below the Australian average. Recent research shows that 3.2 per cent of Indigenous males, compared to 0.9 per cent of non-Indigenous males, indicated they have never attended school; for women the respective figures are 3.1 per cent and 1.1 per cent (ABS & AIHW 2003). Furthermore, of

Indigenous people aged fifteen years, 40 per cent said they had left school before age sixteen compared with 34 per cent of non-Indigenous people (ABS & AIHW 2003). Indigenous Australians are less likely than non-Indigenous Australians to own their homes; 32 per cent of households with Indigenous persons were homeowners compared with 69 per cent of other households (ABS & AIHW 2003). At the time of the 2001 census, 42 per cent of Indigenous Australians were in employment, compared to 58 per cent of non-Indigenous Australians; while the mean weekly income for Indigenous persons was $364 compared with $585 for their non-Indigenous counterparts (ABS & AIHW 2003).

On these social indicators, it is evident that health status would be compromised, as health improvements are largely a result of improvements in social conditions and the provision of high quality services of proven efficacy.

The health status of Indigenous Australians is poorer than that of non-Indigenous Australians on various indicators, especially child survival rates, birth weight and the growth and nutrition of babies. With respect to diseases such as diabetes, cardiovascular disease, mental health and mortality, Indigenous health is poorer on all fronts than that of the non-Indigenous population (Thomson 2003; ABS & AIHW 2005), with Indigenous people being twice as likely to be hospitalised as non-Indigenous people (ABS & AIHW 2005). The substantial social and economic disadvantages, cultural dislocation, political oppression and discrimination experienced by Indigenous Australians results in their extreme poor health (Couzos & Murray 2003). A model that acknowledges both the social, environmental and medical dimensions of ill health is needed (Thomson 2003). Where social conditions are worst, the need for effective medical programs is greatest. These debilitating social, environmental and medical conditions prevent improvements in health and need to be addressed at the same time as medical programs are established.

Child health

Indigenous children in rural Australia are particularly vulnerable to infectious diseases, particularly respiratory infection, diarrhoeal disease, and eye and skin infections. Admissions and length of stay in hospital for Indigenous children are higher than for non-Indigenous children (Ruben &

Fisher 1998; ABS & AIHW 2005). A Western Australian study found that respiratory tract infections, diarrhoea, failure to thrive and anaemia were the most common presenting problems (Waddell & Dibley 1986). In a Northern Territory study of admission rates in ten communities, Munoz et al. (1992, p. 531) confirmed that hospitalisation rates were high for children less than two years old. Of the four communities where there was some variation in hospitalisation rates, social, behavioural and environmental variables consistently contributed to a lower hospital admission rate. Housing, electricity and water, internal toilets and showers were the main variables—these four communities had been established as mission stations over 30 years ago. Overcrowding of children in dwelling places was a feature also in admission rates in the Top End.

Indigenous child morbidity, injury and mortality rates are higher than those of the non-Indigenous population. For example, in 2002, Indigenous mortality for children aged 0 to 14 years was 2.7 times that of non-Indigenous children in the same age group (AIHW 2004b). For the period 1999–2001 the Indigenous infant (less than one year of age) mortality rate was more than twice that of non-Indigenous infants (ABS & AIHW 2003; AIHW 2004b). Indigenous perinatal (from at least 20 weeks gestation, or a birth weight of at least 400 grams, to 28 days following birth) mortality is still double the non-Indigenous rate (Johnston & Coory 2005). For the period 1998–2000, the Indigenous perinatal mortality in Western Australia was 21.3 per 1000 births compared with 8.7 for non-Indigenous births; in the Northern Territory, the respective figures were 24.9 per 1000 births compared with 12.1. For all of Australia the figures were 20.1 per 1000 compared with 9.6 (ABS & AIHW 2003). Although still twice the rate of non-Indigenous Australians, the figures for Indigenous Australians in the Northern Territory represent an improvement on the previous two decades, as Indigenous perinatal mortality in 1981 was 47.5 per 1000 (Couzos & Murray 1999).

Although there have been some reductions in infant and maternal mortality among Indigenous Australians, the differential in birth outcomes between the Indigenous population and other Australians has not been eliminated. Indigenous mothers are twice as likely to have babies of low birth weight (less than 2500 grams) than are non-Indigenous mothers (ABS & AIHW 2005). This low birth weight has implications for the health status of the children in later life; specifically, babies who have been exposed to particular adverse conditions in utero may have higher rates of diabetes and hypertension (Hoy et al. 1999; Singh & Hoy 2003). (See section on renal disease later in this chapter.) One of the major reasons Indigenous infants have a higher mortality is because they have a higher rate of low birth weight and pre-term birth; the risk factors for these include maternal smoking, inadequate maternal nutrition and genito-urinary tract infections; accordingly, primary health care initiatives directed at decreasing these risk factors should be a priority (Johnston & Coory 2005). One program showing the potential to reduce the rate of low birth weight of Indigenous infants is the Strong Women, Strong Babies, Strong Culture program in the Northern Territory.

STRONG WOMEN, STRONG BABIES, STRONG CULTURE

The Strong Women, Strong Babies, Strong Culture (SWSBSC) project was developed in collaboration with Indigenous people in the Northern Territory in August 1993, to address concerns regarding the health status of Indigenous mothers and their infants, in particular the incidence of low birth-weight infants (Fejo 1994, 1997; Mackerras 1998).

Senior Indigenous women in three pilot communities (East Arnhem and Darwin Rural) worked with pregnant women in a program that employed both customary Indigenous birth practices and Western medicine (Mackerras 2001). Selected by the Indigenous communities in which they live, these Strong Women workers had relevant cultural knowledge and worked cooperatively with nutritionists, community-based health workers, local schools and other women in the community (Fejo 1994). The interventions were delivered in the local language and were designed to be culturally appropriate (Fejo 1997; Mackerras 1998).

The aim of SWSBSC was for senior women to support young Indigenous women in their preparation for birth, and encourage them to visit clinics for antenatal care early in their pregnancies. In addition, the senior women provided guidance and encouragement regarding healthy pregnancy management in relation to nutrition (including greater use of 'bush' foods), alcohol and smoking, and compliance with medical advice (Fejo 1994; Tursan d'Espaignet et al. 2003).

The specific goals of the program were to increase infant birth weights by earlier attendance for antenatal care, and enhancing maternal weight status (Mackerras 2001). Infants with lower birth weight (less than 2500 grams) have a higher morbidity and mortality than babies weighing around 3500 grams (Mackerras 1998). In addition, lower birth weight may be linked to an increased risk of disease in later life, such as renal disease (Hoy et al. 1999) and hypertension (Singh & Hoy 2003).

Between 1990–91 and 1994–95 the mean birth weight of Indigenous babies in the pilot communities increased by nearly twice as much as that in the control communities. Changes in maternal weight were associated with changes in birth weight; these changes corresponded with the start of the program and were greater than the secular trend in the control communities (Mackerras 2001).

This program, which continues today, utilises the knowledge and skills of both Indigenous people and medical and nutritional professionals, the outcome being an effective program implemented by Indigenous people themselves (Fejo 1994). The SWSBSC program is adaptable to the specific needs and preferences of individuals and communities; furthermore, it is more culturally appropriate as it is delivered by senior Indigenous women (Tursan d'Espaignet et al. 2003). In addition, support for participation in cultural events is a valuable part of the program (Tursan d'Espaignet et al. 2003).

Diseases

Diseases that occur more frequently in the Indigenous population than in the non-Indigenous population include diabetes mellitus, renal disease, circulatory system and respiratory disorders, ear and eye diseases, and specific communicable diseases such as tuberculosis, sexually transmitted diseases, haemophilus influenza type b (Hib) and diarrhoeal disease (ABS & AIHW 2003, 2005). Indigenous adults, while having a higher incidence of infection than non-Indigenous adults, also suffer the complex diseases of 'Westernisation', including diabetes, hyperlipidaemia, cardiovascular disease and obesity.

High diabetes prevalence has been reported in a number of Indigenous populations (Couzos & Murray 2003). These authors compared the prevalence of diabetes in Indigenous and in other populations and noted that the prevalence of diabetic renal complications among Indigenous people is now ten times the national rates, and deaths from endocrine causes had risen dramatically from 1985 to 1994. In fact, Gracey et al. (2000) in a comparative study of Indigenous deaths in Western Australia between 1985–89 and 1990–94 found there was a major increase in deaths from endocrine diseases in both the Indigenous and non-Indigenous population; however, the increase was proportionally much greater among Indigenous Australians. Clearly, diabetes is a major health problem and an escalating one. The authors call for better health promotion, and disease prevention and management, to help achieve acceptable health standards.

Chronic disease

Diseases of the circulatory system (heart, stroke and vascular diseases) are the leading cause of premature and overall death in Australia, and in the period 1999–2001 accounted for nearly 40 per cent of all deaths (AIHW 2004a). The rates of morbidity and mortality from heart, stroke and vascular diseases are higher for Indigenous Australians—mortality rates are 2.6 times, and hospitalisation rates 1.4 times, those of non-Indigenous Australians (AIHW 2004d). Morbidity and mortality rates are likely to be much higher than this, because of the under-identification of Indigenous people in hospital and mortality data. The mortality from acute rheumatic fever and chronic rheumatic heart disease for Indigenous Australians is 19 times that of other Australians (AIHW 2004d).

In general, Indigenous populations throughout the world have poorer health status across a number of indicators than their non-Indigenous counterparts (Voyle & Simmons 1999; Moewaka Barnes 2000; Wilson & Rosenberg 2002; Kirmayer et al. 2003). However, Indigenous Australians experienced the greatest disparity in life expectancy, and the highest mortality rates from cerebrovascular disease, COPD, ischaemic heart disease, pneumonia and influenza and diabetes, compared to their non-Indigenous counterparts, than is the case with indigenous populations in Canada, the United States and New Zealand (Dow & Gardiner-Garden 1998; Paradies & Cunningham 2002; NATSIHC 2003; Bramley et al. 2004).

Researchers have identified an increased prevalence of risk factors for coronary heart disease in rural Indigenous communities. Since the early 1980s a number of studies have been produced. Indigenous Australians living in Inverell, New South Wales, were found to have an increased prevalence of cigarette smoking, hypertriglyceridaemia, hypertension, obesity and diabetes compared with non-Indigenous Australians (Simons et al. 1981; Smith et al. 1992). Subsequent researchers have found the prevalence of obesity in Torres Strait Islander peoples to be three times higher, and diabetes six times higher, than in non-Indigenous Australians (Leonard et al. 2002). In the Australian Diabetes, Obesity and Lifestyle Study 1999–2001 (AUSDIAB) it was found that Indigenous Australians, particularly those in remote areas, have a much higher likelihood of suffering from chronic kidney disease, due in part to the much higher rates of type 2 diabetes, compared with non-Indigenous Australians (Mathew 2004). In addition, Indigenous Australians enter renal replacement therapy at much higher rates than do their non-Indigenous counterparts (Mathew 2004). Furthermore, diabetes prevalence among Indigenous Australians aged over 25 years is similar to that experienced by non-Indigenous Australians who are ten years older (ABS & AIHW 2003).

Although urbanised Indigenous Australians have been shown to develop a high incidence of obesity, diabetes and other risk factors for the development of coronary heart disease, there is no evidence that they suffered from these conditions when they lived as hunter–gatherers (O'Dea et al. 1988). It has been shown that Indigenous Australians who revert to a hunter–gatherer lifestyle for a period of a few weeks demonstrate a reduction in cholesterol levels, body weight and the metabolic abnormalities associated with mature onset diabetes (O'Dea 1984). Changes away from the traditional lifestyle include the replacement of the traditional high fibre, high protein diet, with one principally composed of refined, high fat foods, and the replacement of the 'active' hunter–gatherer lifestyle with a more sedentary one.

The smoking rate for Indigenous Australians is more than twice that of non-Indigenous Australians (AIHW 2002b; ABS 2002b; ABS & AIHW 2005). Forty-five per cent of Indigenous Australians aged fourteen years and over were daily smokers, compared to 19 per cent of non-Indigenous Australians (AIHW 2002b). Of interest is the link between education levels and smoking, where those who had completed at least Year 12 in school were less likely to smoke than those who left school earlier (ABS 1999).

The National Heart, Stroke and Vascular Health Strategies Group has a framework for improving the cardiovascular health of Australians; the specific goals for Indigenous Australians are to eliminate the disparity in health status in the area of heart, stroke and vascular disease by:

- increasing primary health care capacity;
- reducing risk factors for heart, stroke and vascular disease through population-based and consumer-based initiatives;
- reducing disparities in access to primary health care, cardiac rehabilitation and related treatments, end-stage renal services and specialist vascular procedures (Commonwealth Department of Health and Aged Care 2004, p. 8).

Nephropathy (renal disease)

Renal disease has emerged during the last decade as a major health problem for Indigenous Australians. There are four main explanations presented for the excess burden of renal disease in Indigenous people. These are:

- population differences in which renal disease is an outcome of a higher incidence, and greater severity, of various primary diseases;
- genetic differences which determine various patterns of end-stage renal disease (ESRD);
- unfavourable intrauterine environments which affect kidney development, leading to an increased susceptibility to ESRD;
- greater socioeconomic disadvantages which contribute to a higher incidence of ESRD (Cass et al. 2004).

Rates of ESRD among Indigenous Australians are considerably higher than in non-Indigenous Australians; in some areas the incidence rates for Indigenous people entering treatment are 30 to 60 times those of non-Indigenous people (McDonald & Russ 2003).

There is some evidence that foetal exposure to an abnormal uterine environment—specifically vitamin A deficiency, growth retardation and diabetes in the mother—contributes disproportionately to the rising incidence of kidney disease. These anomalous intra-uterine conditions diminish nephron mass by impairing nephrogenesis, thus increasing the vulnerability to kidney damage in later life from diseases such as diabetes and hypertension (Nelson 2003). Singh and Hoy (2003) found a significant association between low birth weight and high blood pressure in Indigenous adults, with larger effects with higher adult weights. This is important because of the high incidence of low birth weight in rural and remote Indigenous people, and the association of high blood pressure with chronic diseases, including diabetes, cardiovascular and renal disease. The following case study illustrates the value of the application of a comprehensive, culturally appropriate approach to the prevention and management of chronic kidney disease.

UMOONA KIDNEY PROJECT

In mid 1997, a collaborative relationship was formed between the Umoona Tjutagku Health Service and the renal units at Flinders Medical Centre and the Women's and Children's Hospital, Adelaide, to undertake a program for the early detection and prevention of renal disease within the Umoona Indigenous community at Coober Pedy (South Australia).

The Umoona Kidney Project is owned by the Umoona community, directed by the board of the Umoona Tjutagku Health Service and run by a project advisory group comprising an Indigenous chairperson, Indigenous majority representation (including members from the Umoona community, the Umoona health worker team and the board of the Umoona Health Service) and two Flinders' team members.

The Umoona Kidney Project uses a family-orientated, holistic approach to renal health. The staff check for early signs of kidney problems in men, women and children (when serious kidney disease is still preventable); and develop community education programs to address the underlying factors (such as smoking and alcohol, and poor nutrition and hygiene) which may predispose people to renal disease. The education program includes:

- healthier ways of preparing and cooking food
- the development of a community vegetable garden
- eating more traditional bush foods

- drinking more water
- reducing infection rates.

Urine was screened using the Bayer DCA 2000 point-of-care analyser machine to measure the albumin:creatinine ratio (protein in the urine, which is indicative of renal disease). The health check-up is free and voluntary, and also provides information about cardiac health, diabetes risk and nutritional status. Participants are examined by doctors of the same gender. Those people without protein in the urine are followed up every one or two years; those with protein in the urine and/or at high risk have more frequent check-ups and are offered treatment, while those with established renal disease are offered immediate treatment.

Early detection of renal disease is crucial because, if identified early enough, progression to ESRD can be considerably reduced or even prevented. Long term, the Umoona Kidney Project is expected to improve the overall health of the Umoona community, help people at risk of developing serious renal and other health problems, and reduce the number of people who have to be separated from their families and community to go to hospital for treatment (Umoona Kidney Project 2005).

So far, the project has identified a significant rate of both early and established renal disease. The Bayer DCA 2000 analyser has been reliable in detecting albuminuria in this remote clinical location, and has been well accepted by Aboriginal health workers and community participants (Shephard et al. 2003).

THE ROLE OF ABORIGINAL AND TORRES STRAIT ISLAND HEALTH WORKERS

The need for specific intervention programs delivered by Aboriginal and Torres Strait Island health workers was documented by the NAHS Working Party (1989).

Content approaches and methods of facilitating education sessions and any accompanying literature must take into account the Indigenous learning styles and environmental and cultural differences (Saunders 2003; Thomson 2003). This is particularly important considering Indigenous Australians' concepts of 'health' (NAHS Working Party 1989; Thompson & Gifford 2000; McLennon & Khavarpour 2004; Murphy et al. 2004). Lifestyle changes and solutions need to be directed by the communities. One approach is to recognise the value of communities envisaging their community as a healthy one. Subsequent actions and solutions can be acted upon through the collective collaboration of health workers and community partners through ownership of both problems and solutions (Golds et al. 1997). The health worker plays an integral role in community health solutions.

In the 2001 census there were 3742 Indigenous people employed in a health occupation—23 per cent of these were Indigenous health workers (AIHW 2004a). Although the numbers of Indigenous health workers has increased by 28 per cent on the 1996 figures (AIHW 2004a), there are still significant numbers of Indigenous people who have limited or no access to Indigenous health workers (Carson & Bailie 2004).

There is a burgeoning of education and training of health workers through a variety of sectors, such as the Aboriginal and Torres Strait Islander Corporations for Health Education and Training and State Departments of Health (Freeman & Rotem 1999; King & Ritchie 1999). Contemporary health worker education and curriculum design ensure that Indigenous learning styles are considered.

A capable workforce is fundamental to ensuring the health system has the ability to address the needs of Indigenous Australians. The Aboriginal and Torres Strait Islander Health Workforce National Strategic Framework (Australian Health Ministers' Advisory Council (AHMAC) 2002), drafted as a guide for workforce development and consolidation, recognises the need for action on methods to enhance the training, recruitment and retention of proficient health workers. The objectives of the framework are to ensure a competent health workforce, which entails the transformation and consolidation of the workforce by:

- increasing the number of Aboriginal and Torres Strait Islander (A&TSI) people working across all the health professions;
- improving the clarity of roles, regulation and recognition of A&TSI health workers as a key component of the health workforce, and improving vocational education and training sector support for training for A&TSI health workers;

- addressing the role and development needs of other health workforce groups contributing to A&TSI health;
- improving the effectiveness of training, recruitment and retention measures targeting both non-Indigenous Australian and Indigenous Australian health staff working within Aboriginal primary health services;
- including clear accountability for government programs to quantify and achieve these objectives and support for A&TSI organisations and people to drive the process (AHMAC 2002, p. 3).

Two examples of successful or promising programs have been initiated in the Northern Territory and Queensland. The Northern Territory has a registration system for Aboriginal health workers to ensure proficiency and support the development of career pathways. In conjunction with on-the-job training, the system enables workers to transfer between A&TSI community controlled health organisations and employment with the Territory government (NATSIHC 2003). Queensland Health has an A&TSI health workforce strategy which includes promoting health careers to schoolchildren, recruitment, retention, professional development and mentoring strategies to support Indigenous staff, and cultural awareness training for non-Indigenous staff (Queensland Health 1999).

STRATEGIES TO IMPROVE HEALTH

Health worker training, even though important, is only one of many policy developments needed to reduce the inequalities in Indigenous health status. The National Aboriginal Health Strategy (NAHS) was an initiative developed in 1989 by the Commonwealth, state and territory ministers responsible for health and for Aboriginal affairs. The Report of the Royal Commission into Aboriginal Deaths in Custody (1988) detailed the living conditions of Aborigines in Australia. The Commission's analysis of these conditions resulted in the developments that led to the NAHS. The strategy has become a blueprint for action to improve Aboriginal health. The overall aim of the strategy was to ensure that by the year 2001 all Aboriginal and Torres Strait Islander people had the same level of access to health services and facilities as all other Australians. This was to be achieved by improving health status, through changes within the health system and through social and environmental changes. The recommendations included:

- reduction of structural problems
- empowerment and self-determination
- improving service and access to services
- information about health
- monitoring of improvements
- health promotion
- education and training support.

Evaluated in 1994, it was found that the NAHS was never effectively implemented, that proposed NAHS initiatives in remote and rural areas with respect to environmental equity targets were under-funded, and that there needed to be substantial increases in access for housing and essential environmental services (*National Aboriginal Health Strategy: An evaluation 1994*). Furthermore, Indigenous health status has remained fundamentally unchanged since 1989, demonstrating the initiative's minimal success (NATSIHC 2003).

Health expenditure in the period 2001–02 revealed that $3900 per person was spent on health services for Indigenous people, compared with $3308 for services to non-Indigenous people (AIHW 2005d). This difference of about 8 per cent expenditure is much smaller than the difference for many of the health status measures (ABS & AIHW 2003; AIHW 2004a). Furthermore, the expenditure for Indigenous Australians has actually declined since 2001 relative to that for non-Indigenous Australians (AIHW 2005d). Patterns of health service use are different for Indigenous Australians, with a greater use of publicly provided services, predominantly public hospital and community health services and a lesser use of privately provided services (AIHW 2005d).

The Australian government instituted the Office for Aboriginal and Torres Strait Islander Health (OATSIH) in 1994 to facilitate an improved delivery of health services to Indigenous Australians. The policy of OATSIH is to improve access to comprehensive primary health care services for Indigenous Australians, with improved coordinated clinical care, population health and health promotion activities to enhance illness prevention, early intervention and disease management. Evidence from Australia and internationally demonstrates that better access to comprehensive primary health care can make a difference to long-term health status. This approach is based on the precept of collaboration with the Indigenous community-controlled health sector. The OATSIH aims to achieve:

- improved access to, and responsiveness of, the mainstream health system;
- complementary action through Aboriginal and Torres Strait Islander-specific health and substance use services;
- collaboration across governments and the health sector to improve service delivery and outcomes (OATSIH 2005).

The major responsibility of OATSIH is to observe health outcomes over time and to develop the evidence base about successful initiatives that enhance outcomes.

The Primary Health Care Access Program (PHCAP) is a significant health policy reform, which provides an opportunity for Indigenous people to gain access to appropriately resourced comprehensive primary health care. Access to primary health care for Indigenous Australians is provided by the Aboriginal Community Controlled Health Service, by GPs, and state and territory health centres. Preventive health checks can occur when a person seeks health care advice for an illness: for example, the doctor can talk with the patient about other problems, or suggest preventative measures such as vaccination, cancer screening or attending a smoking cessation course. Many Indigenous Australians may find it difficult to access medical care, while others do not access available services. Furthermore, some may attend a medical provider only after a disease is entrenched. Many Indigenous Australians are not enrolled in Medicare, consequently limiting their access to health services and subsidised medicines under the Pharmaceutical Benefits Scheme.

The PHCAP provides funding for the expansion of comprehensive primary health care services in Indigenous communities through clinical care and preventative, early intervention and management programs. PHCAP provides for new services in communities identified as having the greatest relative need and the capacity to manage funding and service delivery. Locations for boosting services are identified through consultation in regional health forums, comprised of representatives from Aboriginal

Community Controlled Health Services, state, territory and the Australian government. The forums aid the identification of regional needs, and plan services. In addition, they incorporate both mainstream and Indigenous-specific health services to better satisfy local needs (Commonwealth Department of Health and Ageing 2004).

For significant improvements to occur in the health of Indigenous people, access to primary health care must be enhanced. Thus, the development of the framework agreement that has been signed in every state and territory seeks to address these issues through:

- improved responsiveness of the mainstream health system;
- additional funding where services are currently inadequate in order to provide complementary Indigenous-specific health programs.

The first Aboriginal Primary Health Care Access Program (APHCAP) was launched in 2003 in the northern metropolitan area of Adelaide. The second part of the initiative, which will improve health services for Indigenous people, is to encourage Indigenous Australians to enrol for a Medicare card, thus gaining access to subsidised health services and medication (Commonwealth Department of Health and Ageing 2004).

The issue of Indigenous land rights makes an important contribution to self-determination and, therefore, health and wellbeing. In 1992 the High Court of Australia accepted the argument that customary native title was not extinguished when Queensland annexed the Murray Islands in the Torres Strait in 1879. For the first time since European settlement, Indigenous Australians' land rights were recognised and upheld by law. The common law recognition of native title in the High Court's Mabo decision in 1992 and the Commonwealth *Native Title Act* have transformed the ways in which Indigenous people's rights over land may be formally recognised and incorporated within Australia. In October 2000 the Federal Court's determination on the Wik people's native title claim was an indication of a negotiated settlement between native titleholders, represented by the Cape York Land Council, the state and Commonwealth governments and the commercial fishing industry. It acknowledged the rights and interests of all parties over approximately 6000 square kilometres of land and waters on the western side of Cape York (National Native Title Tribunal 2000). These judgments reinforced the principle of autonomy as an important factor contributing to Indigenous health.

HEALTH PROMOTION IN INDIGENOUS COMMUNITIES

The *Ottawa Charter for Health Promotion* stated that 'the purpose of health promotion is to enable people to gain greater control over the determinants of their own health' (WHO 1986a, p. 1). While this tenet guides much of the work of health promotion, we must recognise that the enhancement of health is very much aided by a variety of strategies: legislative, economic, organisational, motivational and educational.

All health promoters need to be knowledgeable about the socio-political and cultural contexts of their work. This is particularly important in working with Indigenous Australians, whose concept of health, as we have seen, is likely to be different from that of other Australians. Consequently, any health promotion work needs to rest on a thorough understanding of Indigenous people's views of the land, law, family life and community mores.

It is crucial that Aboriginal health workers be the deliverers of programs. For a good example of an appropriately delivered health program, see the Strong Women, Strong Babies, Strong Culture case study earlier in this chapter.

A study of food-purchasing behaviour in a central Australian community was referred to above (Rowse et al. 1994). The outcome of the study was a two-year intervention to change the dietary habits of children under fifteen years of age by working with store managers to improve options for the purchase of healthy foods. Healthy food choices were supplied in the school canteen and supplemented with nutrition education, and family-based workshops were conducted to reinforce the need for a healthy diet. As noted earlier, data were collected over two weeks to check the purchasing patterns of children in the six food outlets in the community (supermarket-style outlets, mission store and takeaway, and council takeaways).

A general improvement in food purchasing was evident in the analysis of the data; this has been attributed to the introduction of a healthy school canteen, to changes in marketing strategies in the council store and to community responsiveness to messages concerning healthy diet (Scrimgeour et al. 1994). These authors contended that there was value in a community-based program that used a number of strategies to deal with an identified health problem. This intervention did so, developing personal skills and knowledge in the children and assisting them to make 'healthy choices, easy choices' by the provision of healthier food at the point of purchase. Indeed, the program presented a model of health promotion in an Indigenous community, where collaborative research and program development and planning were applied successfully.

A MODEL FOR HEALTH PROMOTION

We have adapted the work of Spark et al. (1991) in their work in injury prevention to develop a five-phase conceptual framework to assist health promotion. Importantly, we make explicit a number of principles to guide you. These principles are part of the NHMRC's Research Agenda Working Group (RAWG), which oversaw the formulation of intervention-based criteria. They ensure that there is sufficient Indigenous community consultation and participation, transferability (of the methods to other settings), and sustainability of resulting changes.

Stage one is about joint planning and partnerships between health workers and community members and involves developing strong collaborative relationships and deciding on how the projects are to be managed. In this way, roles can be clarified. Importantly, the principles of community ownership, respect for cultural values and equality of partners can guide this important step. The methods used by Friere inform this process also (Wallerstein & Bernstein 1988). In **stage two** community needs assessments may already be completed; if not, community needs assessments can be undertaken, again according to the principles stated. In **stage three**, sustainability and transferability capacity-building initiatives need to be set. For example, how will the planned education and training initiatives assist with sustainability of the programs? What resources are needed? Is there long-term commitment to the project? Is the health promotion initiative integrated into other long-term programs? **Stage four** is the crux of the implementation process. We have set the principle of Indigenous models of program planning and/or stages of change to guide the implementation progress. The diffusion and uptake of health promotion programs within all communities vary as there are competing demands and different stages of readiness to change. Understanding this can assist also with setting realistic evaluation outputs. In **stage five**, evaluation is implemented but has ideally been integrated in stage two, as have the strategies for sustainability. It is essential that the community be informed about the program's significance and its future.

Figure 8.1: Indigenous health promotion model

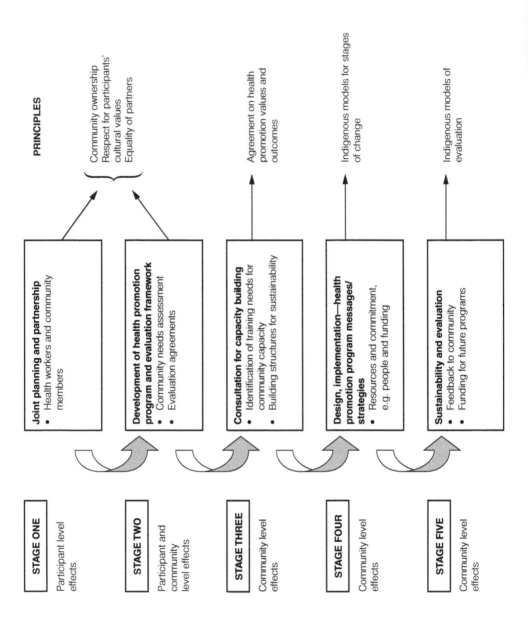

Source: E. Parker and B. Meiklejohn, adapted from Spark et al. (1991), NHMRC (2003a) and Harris and Turner (2005)

Golds (1994) pointed out that one of the priorities of any community health program has to be consultation with the community from the outset—that is, finding out what people see as priorities for their health, rather than what statistics might indicate. When trying to start up community health promotion programs, keep the following points in mind.

- Find out where people meet—sometimes it might be people's houses. Have your meeting in a familiar venue.
- Use culturally appropriate local resources, to which people can relate and respond.
- Invite key community people to your meeting to give testimonials.
- Allow enough time before and after a meeting for people to warm up and wind down.
- Involve local health workers and educators, many of whom are probably already community role models.
- Avoid jargon in your discussions; speak plainly and use lots of visuals.
- Make people aware of risk factors.
- Always return the results of surveys and programs to the community.
- Try to raise awareness, solve problems internally and get to know each other culturally.
- Talk directly to people, not at them.
- Be aware that each Indigenous community is different and adopt a partnership approach to health.

ETHICS IN INDIGENOUS HEALTH RESEARCH

It is important that health promoters practise ethically in all aspects of their work. The NHMRC document *Values and Ethics: Guidelines for ethical conduct in Aboriginal and Torres Strait Islander health research* (2003b) underscores six central values:

- **Reciprocity.** The researcher must demonstrate a benefit (from the research) that is valued by the community, contributes to the community's unity and advances the community's interests, opportunities and outcomes. The guidelines promote an 'equitable and respectful engagement with Aboriginal and Torres Strait Islander Peoples' (NHMRC 2003b, p. 10).

- **Respect.** The relationships between stakeholders need to be respectful and accepting of different peoples' diverse values, norms and hopes, while valuing the contributions of all partners. In addition, researchers need to allow for the potential consequences of research that may initially not be obvious.
- **Equality.** Researchers must acknowledge the value of Aboriginal and Torres Strait Islander peoples' experience and wisdom; otherwise, they may misconstrue information, engender distrust or fail to see a potentially important benefit of research. Notwithstanding peoples' differences, they must all be treated as equals in the research process or there cannot be any trust between stakeholders. The distribution of benefit must be equitable; if one partner in the initiative receives a greater benefit than do others, the allocation of benefit may be seen as unjust.
- **Survival and protection.** Aboriginal and Torres Strait Islander peoples value their cultural uniqueness, do not wish to be assimilated or lose their cultural values. Researchers must ensure they do not threaten this distinctiveness. Furthermore, they must be cognisant of the history and experience of Aboriginal and Torres Strait Islander peoples, and the possibility that research may have negative consequences, for example, on the social cohesion or values of Aboriginal and Torres Strait Islander peoples.
- **Responsibility.** Researchers must ensure they do no damage to Aboriginal and Torres Strait Islander individuals or communities, or to those things that they treasure. In addition, there must be procedures put in place to ensure that researchers are accountable to individuals, families and communities.
- **Spirit and integrity.** Researchers must appreciate the richness and unity of the cultural heritage of past, contemporary and future generations, and the connections which unite them. In addition, researchers need to demonstrate integrity in their intentions, actions and the research process, and may need to demonstrate that the initiative is in keeping with these guidelines (NHMRC 2003b, pp. 10–20).

ABORIGINAL AND TORRES STRAIT ISLANDER RESEARCH AGENDA WORKING GROUP

The NHMRC recognised that a unified and coordinated approach is essential for researching the health of Indigenous Australians, resulting in the establishment of the Aboriginal and Torres Strait Islander Research Agenda Working Group (RAWG). The document known as the Road Map, endorsed in 2002, resulted from the RAWG consulting with Indigenous communities and other stakeholders regarding the responsibilities and priorities for Indigenous health research (NHMRC 2003a). The RAWG delineated six research domains essential to realising substantial health improvements for Aboriginal and Torres Strait Islander people. These are outlined below.

- Descriptive research which outlines patterns of health risk, disease and death. This information should be utilised to inform the development of sound preventive, early diagnosis and treatment-based interventions which are likely to result in meaningful health gains for Aboriginal and Torres Strait Islander peoples.
- A research focus on the factors and process that promote resilience and wellbeing—in particular but not exclusively, during the periods of pregnancy, infancy, childhood and adolescence—and form the basis for good health throughout the lifespan.
- A focus on health services research which describes the optimum means of delivering preventive, diagnostic and treatment-based health services and interventions to Aboriginal and Torres Strait Islander peoples.
- A focus on the association between health status and health gain and policy, and programs that lie outside the direct influence of the health sector.
- A focus on engaging with research and action in previously under-researched Aboriginal and Torres Strait Islander populations and communities.
- Development of the nation's Aboriginal and Torres Strait Islander health research capacity (including training Aboriginal and Torres Strait Islander researchers) and health research practice in relation to Aboriginal and Torres Strait Islander communities (NHMRC 2003a, pp. 3–4).

REVIEW

National attention is now directed at the health of Indigenous Australians through wide-ranging policies and programs. Many of these have stemmed from the NAHS Working Party (1989) recommendations. The solutions need to be community-driven and sponsored with a clear understanding of social and cultural mores. For non-Indigenous health workers a sensitivity to, and respect for, ethical considerations is essential when working with Indigenous health promotion workers as they plan and implement programs aimed at reducing inequalities in health. Thomson (1991) made this still pertinent reminder:

> Unless approaches to Indigenous health are broadened to include greater attention to the health problems of adults, and are matched by broad-ranging strategies aimed at redressing Indigenous social and economic disadvantages, it is likely that the overall mortality will remain high and that the expectation of life of Indigenous Australians will remain comparable with that in countries like India, Haiti, Ghana and Papua New Guinea. (p. 294)

Health promotion professionals working in the field of Indigenous health have claimed to answer the question about how we would know when an Indigenous community is healthy: 'When the environments, cultures, minds and bodies of all members of the community are healthy and conducive to Indigenous people achieving pride, autonomy, longevity and freedom from disease' (Golds et al. 1997, p. 389). The goal can be reached through intersectoral collaboration and action and within a paradigm of health, one that recognises body, land and spirit.

REVISION

Consider the main issues addressed in this chapter. Review each point in light of your understanding of Indigenous health promotion.

1. *What impact does the spatial and demographic location of Aboriginal and Torres Strait Islander communities have on their health?*
2. *Outline the disadvantages faced by Indigenous Australians on a range of broad social indicators.*
3. *Review the dimensions of health status and inequalities within this community, especially in child health, diseases of the circulatory system and renal disease.*

4. *Consider the range of strategies designed to improve Indigenous health, including the training of Indigenous health workers.*
5. *Define health promotion in Indigenous communities by reviewing and critiquing a case study.*
6. *Examine the ethical guidelines for research with Indigenous communities recommended by the NHMRC.*

9

Workplace health promotion

- *History of workplace health promotion*
- *Defining workplace health promotion*
- *The range of interventions*
- *Justifications for health promotion in the workplace*
- *Principles and strategies of workplace health promotion*
- *Comprehensive workplace health promotion*
- *Overcoming barriers to health promotion*
- *Implementing programs*

As a result of the growing awareness of the relationship between conditions in the workplace and the health of workers, health and safety in the workplace has grown in importance as an area of concern for Australian organisations. Formal recognition of the role of health promotion was evidenced in 1988, with the establishment of the National Steering Committee on Health Promotion in the Workplace. Subsequently, various state steering committees were formed to advance the national agenda in the state context.

Interest in health promotion, health education, and self-care and self-help activities has been gaining momentum among industry and union leaders, government officials, health care professionals and the public in general. This interest, together with the costs of accidents and injuries in the workplace, the expansion of medical costs and the imperative of occupational health and safety regulations, has focused industry concern on health promotion programs. However, there is still considerable debate as to what constitutes 'workplace health promotion', why health should be promoted in the work-place, its relationship to occupational health and safety, whose responsibility it is and how best to accomplish its objectives (Chu et al. 1997).

This chapter highlights central issues emerging in contemporary workplace health promotion, particularly in Australia. Like many other developments in public health and health promotion at the international level, various countries have followed different theoretical and practical applications in the different settings relevant to public health and health promotion. For example, as we saw in Chapter 6, in Europe the notion of the health-promoting school has been a dominant theme, while in the United States the concept of compre-hensive school health education has predominated. Although the two concepts are similar, there are differences in their philosophy and application. The history and contemporary practice of workplace health promotion in Australia has both European and American precedents. In many settings in Australia where health promotion and the new public health are practised, a holistic approach to program development and implementation has been advocated. The notion of 'health' advocated by the World Health Organization (WHO 1986a), as 'a product of ways of living (lifestyle) and living conditions (social and economic environment)', reflected a recognition of the dimensions and determinants of health and the complexity of factors influencing the health of populations.

The notion of the health-promoting workplace, like healthy cities and healthy schools, addresses educational, political, economic and environmental impacts on health in the workplace. Participants attending the Symposium on Healthy Workplaces at the 4th International Conference on Health Promotion (WHO 1997b) 'underlined the great importance of work settings for the promotion of health of working populations, their families and friends, the community and society at large. The globalisation of business life, technologi-cal developments and changes in the demographic structure of populations are leading to new types of employment patterns, such as temporary and part-time work, self-employment and telework'. In the face of these challenges, the WHO's global Healthy Work Approach (HWA) 'serves as a catalyst for part-nership between the different stakeholders. This approach is based upon the following four contemporary principles: health promotion; occupational health and safety; human resource management; and sustainable social and environ-mental development' (WHO 1997b). The WHO reiterated the importance of workplace health promotion at the 6th Global Conference on Health Promotion, stating that there is *a requirement for good corporate practice: the private sector has a responsibility to ensure health and safety in the workplace and to promote the health and wellbeing of employees, their families and communities, and to contribute to lessening wider impacts on global health. (WHO 2006b, p. 2)*

This chapter begins with an overview of some of the significant developments in workplace health promotion, both within Australia and internationally. We will analyse contemporary definitions of workplace health promotion and examine theoretical principles for practice and the actual practice of workplace health promotion. Furthermore, we will consider a range of approaches taken in the workplace to protect the health and safety of workers, such as occupational health and safety, workplace health promotion and employee assistance programs. As in many chapters in this book, the theoretical framework guiding the practice of contemporary health promotion, the Ottawa Charter (WHO 1986a), will form the intellectual structure for our discussion and analysis of contemporary workplace health promotion.

HISTORY OF WORKPLACE HEALTH PROMOTION

Possibly the earliest specific occupational syndrome on record in Australia was the illness of Mr H. Parkes, who in 1840 was working in a brass foundry in Sydney. Parkes wrote to his family in Birmingham, England, about his illness: 'I am very unsettled, at present, on account of my health. This brass business does not suit me at all. I think I shall be obliged to go into the country again' (Gandevia 1971, p. 175). It is likely that the small foundry in which Parkes worked had several processes crowded into a poorly ventilated area engulfed by fumes from the heated metals, and consequently he suffered from metal fume fever.

Contemporary workplaces, through legislative initiatives and the advocacy of unions and employers, present a different environment from the one Mr Parkes experienced in Sydney over a century and a half ago. As we saw in Chapter 5, the very nature and scope of work is changing, and roles and responsibilities are shifting and being refined, modified and, in some cases, radically changed or eliminated. Stace and Dunphy (2001) remind us that one of the challenges facing Australian industry in the 21st century will be its ability to cope with rapid rates of economic and technological change and to be proactive in its management style. The changing nature of the workplace poses many challenges. For health promotion, the challenge is to work towards intersectoral collaboration and to engage all of the stakeholders in the decision-making process. Moreover, health promotion activity in the workplace will only achieve success if it addresses structural and organisational issues and recognises the substantial impact of organisational culture (Bensberg 2004).

Workplace health promotion (WHP), as distinct from occupational health and safety, has developed over the last three decades in Australia, even though the worksite is still a relatively underdeveloped setting for health promotion.

In examining the development of worksite programs in the United States, Wilson (1996) referred to four generations of intervention. Programs of the first generation were considered to be initiated for a variety of reasons, most of which were unrelated to health. Smoking policies, for example, were initially imposed for safety and product quality reasons, not for health reasons. The second generation of programs emerged when risk factor identification and intervention technology could be transported to the workplace. These programs were characterised by a narrow focus on one method of delivery, a single illness or risk factor, or programs offered to only one population. Most commonly, this population was upper management, the classic 'executive program' that was often detrimental to worker morale in that workers recognised the company was less interested in their health than in providing executive 'perks'.

Programs that attempted to offer a more comprehensive range of interventions for a variety of risk factors for all employees formed the third generation of programs. In the fourth generation, 'wellness' became both a component of, and the guiding principle for, a corporate health care strategy. A wellness health strategy incorporates all activities, policies and decisions that affect the health of employees, their families, the communities in which the company is located and the consumers whose purchasing decisions determine the company's relative success in the marketplace.

Chu and Forrester (1992), in a report that reviewed workplace health promotion activity in Queensland, produced a succinct summary of major developments in the field. The authors highlighted early workplace interventions that focused on corporate fitness programs and the provision of fitness facilities to meet the needs of executive management, and that were more appropriate for large corporations rather than the full range of workplaces and needs of the workforce. The next set of developments carried on the tradition of a single health issue focus, but offered employees a range of interventions from which to select. These programs included weight control, cardiac risk appraisals, stress management and smoking cessation programs at the worksite. The focus remained on individual behaviour change strategies, usually as a component of screening, education or counselling programs (Chu & Forrester 1992).

As with the early fitness programs, the major critics of these types of approaches were smaller businesses who could not implement many of the programs because they were designed for large corporations. Other critics included government agencies, unions, employees and health promoters, who argued for a more comprehensive approach to workplace health. The major criticisms centred on the narrow applicability of such programs and the restricted focus on individual behaviour change, without recognition of the full range of relevant factors. Some critics pointed to the failure of single-focus programs to meet the needs of the broader workforce and to the lack of consultation with unions and employees. In light of what we know about contemporary models of health promotion, such as the Ottawa Charter (WHO 1986a), it is no wonder that unions were concerned that organisations and management who focused on fitness programs or other 'one-off' interventions were able to shift attention away from issues such as the organisation of work, work hazards and employee participation in decision-making (Chu & Forrester 1992, p. 10).

Despite the criticisms of workplace health promotion, during the 1980s there was a substantial increase in worksite programs, according to a survey of 379 Australian organisations made by Jones (1987). Forty-six per cent of the companies surveyed reported that they were engaged in some form of health promotion activity. Other studies have reported that larger companies are more likely to support and to have introduced WHP initiatives, and these companies tended to feel more positive about their role (Lean 1987; Queensland Health 1990). In a 1992 survey, it was estimated that 34 per cent of all Australian workplaces, and 96 per cent of those with at least 500 employees, provided some health promotion activities (National Coordinating Committee for Health Promotion in the Workplace 1992).

Several writers in the area (Reardon 1998; Chu et al. 1997; Dewe et al. 2000; Chu et al. 2000) have suggested that recent developments in WHP have changed from a singular focus on individual behaviour changes to a recognition of the broader social, environmental and economic determinants of health. While it can be argued that a holistic approach to WHP is occurring in some workplaces in Australia and overseas, we should not be too complacent about the advances. We do know that a range of strategies and methods under the label of WHP are occurring in different workplaces. These strategies and methods include individual behaviour modification, social and environmental changes, and single or multiple interventions designed to achieve short- or longer-term changes. A review of the literature highlights a continuing focus on single interventions that address health-compromising behaviours such as cigarette smoking, poor diet and lack of exercise. One of the substantial difficulties in ascertaining the effectiveness of these programs is that in many cases either they were not evaluated, or the evaluations were not comprehensive.

Few data are available on how programs have been developed and implemented, nor the extent to which the needs of employees were ascertained. One of the criticisms of WHP proffered by employers is that its economic value to the organisation has not been demonstrated. This criticism is accurate in part, as very few contemporary programs reviewed have evaluated their program from the point of view of cost-effectiveness (Pelletier 1997).

In a review of the literature on the economic implications of workplace health promotion programs in the late 1980s, Warner et al. concluded that claims of WHP programs' 'profitability' were based on anecdotal evidence or analyses seriously flawed in terms of assumptions, methodology or data. Furthermore, certain aspects of the economics of WHP programs have been virtually ignored (1988, p. 106). However, the authors did caution that the lack of sound evidence on the economic benefits of workplace health promotion should not be interpreted as a negative assessment of the potential economic benefits of such programs. Rather, they argued for more detailed and extensive research on the economic implications of WHP (Warner et al. 1988, p. 111).

Few systematic studies have provided definitive evidence that health promotion is a cost-effective means of improving long-term health outcomes and decreasing health care costs (Oldenburg & Harris 1996). However, in the European Union at least, there is evidence that quality WHP reduces absenteeism, enhances the working environment and employee motivation, increases the profile of the company and improves perceptions of its value as an employer, and improves productivity (Theuringer & Missler 2003). Several authors assert that improvements in workplace health promotion which promote work–life balance (for example, flexible working hours, family-friendly policies, onsite fitness centres, etc.), can bring about improvements in productivity (Dorrell 2001; Hobson et al. 2001; Chang 2004; Taylor 2005). However, Bloom et al. (2006) found no such relationship with productivity, once good management was allowed for. Their study examined 732 medium-sized manufacturing companies in the United States, France, Germany and the United Kingdom, and found that larger, more globalised and better managed organisations offered a superior work–life balance for their employees and were also more productive (Bloom et al. 2006). However, this higher productivity was found to be a result of good management, not because work–life balance increases productivity. Nor is it the case that globalisation is harmful for employees, and there is no relationship between tougher competition and work–life balance; furthermore, larger workplaces, which are normally more globalised, also have better work–life balance practices. The authors suggest that a good work–life balance is something efficient firms succeed at in any case, as they need to treat their employees well to retain them (Bloom et al. 2006). Improving work–life balance may be appealing, as employees favour it and productivity is not negatively affected; however, it is costly to introduce and maintain and, thus, could reduce profitability (Bloom et al. 2006).

The history of WHP spans several decades and the programs offered in this setting, to date, have relied most heavily on individual behaviour change. Contemporary writing and practice in WHP suggest a broadening of this traditional focus to encompass structural and work culture changes in the organisation, along with behaviour change strategies involving management, unions and government in the formulation of policy and implementation of programs. As the field develops further, research examining the impact of multilayered strategies on the health of workers (both short- and longer-term) and the economic implications of WHP will provide support and direction for health promotion activities in the workplace (Oldenburg & Harris 1996). The requirements of special populations will need to be addressed, and health promotion activity that meets the needs of small- and medium-sized business will require further attention.

DEFINING WORKPLACE HEALTH PROMOTION

Promoting a comprehensive approach to workplace health promotion, the National Steering Committee on Health Promotion in the Workplace defined WHP as: '… those educational, organisational or economic activities in the workplace that are designed to improve the health of workers and therefore the community at large' (1989, p. 8). This type of health promotion involves workers and management participating on a voluntary basis in the implementation of jointly agreed programs using the workplace as a setting for promoting better personal health (Bellingham 1991, p. 5). The Australasian College of Occupational Medicine (1990) issued a position paper on WHP, advocating the creation of supportive environments for health and de-emphasising the individual responsibility of workers.

In the early 1980s, several American textbooks gave illuminating definitions of workplace health promotion. Parkinson (1982, p. 8) defined WHP as 'a combination of educational, organisational, and environmental activities designed to support behaviour conducive to the health of employees and their families'. O'Donnell and Ainsworth (1984) concentrated on the importance of individual behaviour in reducing the risk of illness, and a later work by O'Donnell and Harris (1994) maintained an individual lifestyle focus. The authors defined health promotion programs in the workplace as being 'designed to help employees adopt healthy lifestyles, such as regular exercise, prudent diet, and stress management coping skills. These help reduce the risk for disease and enhance the ability to achieve at work and at home' (p. 453). However, they did recognise three levels of health promotion: awareness, life change programs and supportive environments.

Contemporary workplace health promotion programs follow more closely the tenets of the Ottawa Charter, aiming to produce well-informed participants who attempt to put health-enhancing advice into practice and health-supporting changes achieved largely by the employees themselves (Worksafe Australia 1993; Denner 2001).

Queensland Health developed a set of principles to guide action across a number of health-promoting environments such as hospitals, schools or workplaces in Queensland (Dwyer 1997). These nine principles include:

- management of the program by the organisation;
- participant-based priority setting—setting priorities occurs through participatory needs assessment informed by relevant epidemiological data;
- informed by social justice principles—consider the needs of disadvantaged groups within the setting;

- program design, adaptability, flexibility and organisational relevance—issues that need to be considered at every site;
- use of existing resources in the organisation and the community;
- recognition of policy and legislative requirements—may act to establish the boundaries or constrain program development. The workplace is an example where occupational health and safety legislation has priority over health programs;
- voluntary participation;
- support for a site-based coordinator—can occur through training, resource development and assistance by local health workers;
- evaluation and monitoring—it is important that an organisation monitor the impact of a program on the participants and the organisation (Dwyer 1997, p. 399).

The challenge will be to translate these principles into sustainable programs which meet the needs of a community, through action in different sectors. There are numerous examples of workplace health promotion efforts in the Australian context. Two of these are summarised in the following case studies, illustrating many of the issues discussed in this chapter, such as socio-behavioural, policy and environmental approaches to health in the workplace.

CURTIN HEALTHY LIFESTYLE PROGRAM

Curtin University was the first university in Western Australia to provide an on-site health promotion program to students and staff (Curtin University of Technology 2005). Founded on the principles of the Ottawa Charter (WHO 1986a), the Curtin Healthy Lifestyle (CHL) program was established due to an increasing interest among staff in accessing health and lifestyle information and services on campus (Curtin University of Technology 2005; Woolmer et al. 2005).

The results of a needs assessment in 1989 were used to design a worksite health promotion program to address the needs, interests and concerns of the staff. By 1990, 200 staff had participated in the program, and by 1991 the number had risen to 2000 (Curtin University of Technology 2005). The program's success is a result of both an increase in time and financial support by management, and a policy allowing staff time off for participation (Curtin University of Technology 2005).

A variety of activities are offered at the university, along with environmental and policy changes. These initiatives provide a supportive workplace environment, representing a good example of a health-promoting workplace. They include:

Healthy policies

- healthy lifestyle policy—providing time off work to participate in health enhancing activities
- smoking policy—working towards a smoke-free campus
- alcohol policy—reducing alcohol and other drug-related problems.

Environmental changes

- walk routes and pathways—encouraging staff to walk during breaks
- bike storage facilities and lockers—encouraging cycling to work
- provision of shade—reducing the risk of skin cancer
- removal of all cigarette sales from campus and extensive no-smoking areas—smoking permitted only in two areas on campus
- enhancement of gardens and promotion of the Australia Beautiful campaign to reduce the level of cigarette butt litter on campus
- staff restaurant and student guild catering outlets modified their menus, to provide more healthy food choices.

Behavioural programs

- aerobics, yoga, walking and stair climbing competitions
- participation in the annual City to Surf Fun Run
- stress management, meditation and massage
- formation of groups such as Weight Watchers, local drug action group, bicycle user group, laughter group, juggling group and many other healthy interest groups
- health and fitness risk assessments
- lunchtime seminars
- dietary consults with an accredited practising dietician available for staff and an email newsletter distributed to staff which focuses on healthy lifestyle changes.

The CHL program aims to encourage staff to minimise stress and enjoy healthier and more balanced work and personal lives. The following factors contribute to achieving these aims: staff taking breaks, attending activities during work time, becoming involved with university life, networking with other staff, cultivating hobbies, incorporating physical activity into their day and committing time to attend to their health needs (Curtin University of Technology 2005; Woolmer et al. 2005).

The provision of a safe and healthy work environment contributes to healthier, happier and more creative and productive staff (Curtin University of Technology 2005; Woolmer et al. 2005). This in turn attracts and retains valued staff, reduces workers' compensation claims and assists Curtin University to be recognised as an 'employer of choice' (Curtin University of Technology 2005; Woolmer et al. 2005).

There is no longer a healthy lifestyle coordinator. However, the program is now ongoing, without additional funding or staffing.

WELLNESS AT GREENSLOPES PRIVATE HOSPITAL

Greenslopes Private Hospital (GPH) in Brisbane employs over 1800 staff and has 575 beds, positioning it as Australia's largest private hospital. GPH strives to optimise work–life integration through the provision of support, programs and facilities. The 'WorkLife@GPH' model encompasses all staff benefits including flexible work arrangements, salary packaging, staff development, an on-site child care centre, a social club, and individual and organisational wellness.

The hospital has received numerous accolades, including the ACCI/BCI National Work and Family Award (2005), Australian Private Hospital Association Award for Excellence (2004), Australian National Training Authority Community Services and Health Industry Award (2004) and Queensland Large Employer of the Year (2004), in addition to Health Promoting Hospital accreditation from the WHO (2005a).

In line with the WHO (1999) guiding principles for healthy workplaces, the hospital's staff wellness program adopts a comprehensive, participatory and empowering approach. Moreover, it encourages multisectoral and multidisciplinary cooperation, promotes social justice principles and is sustainable.

The staff wellness program was launched in 2001 and has experienced remarkable growth since its inception, including the launch of a new state-of-the-art wellness centre in 2002 that includes a range of individual and organisational wellness initiatives for staff; these are subsidised or provided at no cost and include:

Club Wellness

- gym
- exercise classes
- personal training
- wellness shop (discounted exercise accessories, such as fitballs and pedometers).

Financial Wellness

- financial planning services
- mortgage brokerage available.

Greenslopes Nutrition at Work (GNAW)

- dietetics
- Mondo Organics Cooking School
- a healthy eating scheme in the hospital bistro

Wellness Assist

- employee assistance program, providing personal support for employees

Wellness2Go (in development)

- modified department-based wellness programs

General

- help with quitting smoking
- wellness clinics, offering services such as massage

- corporate sporting events (e.g. a fun run called Bridge to Brisbane, department volleyball/bocce/lawn bowls)
- an on-site car servicing facility
- wellness walkers (Gone Walking Program)
- health promotion e.g. expos, seminars, 10 000 Steps
- health risk management programs e.g. Lighten Up
- Red Cross blood bank
- WorkLife@GPH initiatives e.g. reward and recognition program for being engaged in the wellness program.

In total, 58 per cent of employees and 87.5 per cent of management have participated in the GPH Wellness Program (Wellness Survey 2005). The impact of the work–life initiatives above can be demonstrated at the individual and organisational level. These impacts are evident in the areas of staff retention and recruitment, health and safety, workplace culture, staff satisfaction and revenue capability. Support from GPH management has been crucial in achieving these outcomes.

Source: GPH Wellness Survey 2005; Katrina Walton, Wellness Coordinator, Greenslopes Private Hospital, Queensland

THE RANGE OF INTERVENTIONS

In defining WHP, we need to be able to discuss its relationship with other well-established processes and interventions in the workplace. One of the main issues is the extent to which health promotion goals and objectives can be integrated with occupational health and safety (OHS) objectives and objectives for microeconomic reform in the workplace. The infrastructure for OHS remains distinct from the health infrastructure in Australia. Occupational health and safety has traditionally been located within the industrial relations sphere, where priority is given to the control of health and safety hazards in the workplace (National Health Strategy 1993b, p. 145).

While health promotion programs that focus on the prevention of 'lifestyle' diseases are distinct and separate from responsibilities employers and employees have in the implementation of proper OHS measures in the workplace, the distinction can sometimes be quite artificial and counter-productive. For example, the implementation of a workplace smoking policy has now become an OHS issue. The onus is on employers to provide healthy and safe working environments. The *Morling* judgment recognised scientific evidence that exposure to cigarette smoke causes lung cancer, respiratory disease and asthma in non-smokers (Everingham & Woodward 1991). This implies that a healthy and safe work environment must be smoke-free. Introducing workplace programs and incentives to help interested smokers to quit, however, is a health promotion activity. Some companies, such as Telstra, provide sunscreen, hats and protective clothing to outdoor workers—OHS measures. The complementary health promotion actions could include on-site skin cancer screenings and educational sessions about self-examination and the importance of protection and early detection. Moreover, structural and organisational culture issues could be addressed to ensure that the working environment for Telstra workers reinforces safety and health as well as job satisfaction and productivity.

New legislation in the 1980s dramatically reshaped OHS in Australia. While the legislation varied from state to state, two of the important features were the duty of care imposed on employers to provide a safe and healthy working environment for their employees, and the training of employees as occupational health and safety representatives (National Health Strategy 1993b).

While the two areas of workplace health activity may appear to be distinct, health promotion interventions are an important complement to OHS action. It is a justifiable concern of unions that employers might seek to improve the productivity and morale of their workers through high-profile health promotion activities at the expense of basic OHS issues. The distinction between OHS and health promotion activities has been made, in part, in order to avoid employers adopting the 'soft' option of benevolent-appearing health promotion actions at the expense of address-ing more difficult, and often expensive, OHS issues. For example, a fitness and dietary education program would be very alienating to employees who continue to be exposed to hazardous gases, chemicals or other substances (Bellingham 1990, 1991, p. 5). While evidence to support the efficacy of health promotion programs in the workplace is scant, there is emerging evidence that OHS interventions prevent workplace injuries and disease, and that some can yield a cost benefit (Oxenburg 1991; Farr 1994).

Shell Australia introduced health promotion to the workplace through its OHS policy in the late 1970s. Three specific topics were originally selected for inclusion in a three-year cycle: heart disease, cancer and a women's program on breast and cervical cancer. Programs for alcohol abuse, smoking and skin cancer have since been added. All programs are available to staff on a voluntary basis. The company's chair reported in 1993 that one of the company's most successful programs was that at the open cut mine at Callide in Queensland. Data suggested there was a decrease in the numbers smoking and a reduction in elevated blood pressure among program participants. The number of employees with cholesterol levels over the recommended limit had dropped by 60 per cent, the level of exercise had increased and, while the quantity of alcohol consumed had not changed, there was a large reduction in blood alcohol content among participants (Charlton 1993, p. 588).

From this discussion, it is evident that workplace health promotion has been variously defined over the past twenty years. A contemporary definition of WHP suggests that multiple strategies which aim to improve the health status of employees and the population at large are now used. Clear recognition is given to people's health and to the fact that the choices they make about their health are influenced by a multiplicity of factors, including type of job, money, housing, education and family circumstances (Worksafe Australia 1993, p. 5). The challenge will be to enhance employee participation in behaviour change by structural and organisational changes in the workplace environment (Zoller 2004). This requires firm commitment by management and participatory involvement of employees (Oldenburg & Harris 1996; Zoller 2004).

This view of contemporary health promotion in the workplace can be contrasted with the nature and scope of employee assistance programs (EAPs). There is substantial literature available on EAPs, as they relate to particular types of interventions and their theoretical and workplace applications, particularly as they occur in the United States. In Australia, EAPs have operated in the workplace using a different model. Traditionally, EAPs were designed to help people solve personal problems that may affect the workplace, such as alcohol and other drug use and abuse, family and interpersonal relationship conflicts, and emotional problems (O'Donnell & Harris 1994).

There has been limited empirical research examining employees' perceptions of EAPs and their willingness to participate in them. Harris and Fennell (1988, p. 423) surveyed 150 employees of a white-collar firm to determine their attitudes, perceptions and willingness to use various resources for help with alcohol abuse and dependence; their beliefs about the causes and the stigma of alcoholism; their reasons for drinking; and their levels of alcohol consumption. Results suggested that willingness to obtain assistance from an EAP was influenced by the individual's familiarity with the program, perceptions of its trustworthiness and opportunities for personal attention, personal level of alcohol consumption, and beliefs about drinking to reduce job-related stress. Men and women were equally willing to use EAPs, but the women's willingness was related mostly to familiarity with the program, while the men's willingness was related mostly to perception of the program's effectiveness, attention to clients and the level of control imposed by the program (Harris & Fennell 1988, p. 434).

In Australia, there continue to be differences in program emphasis between workplace health promotion, OHS and EAPs. It is likely that these emphases will continue into the near future as the three areas continue to have different priorities.

JUSTIFICATIONS FOR HEALTH PROMOTION IN THE WORKPLACE

There is ample research evidence to support the relationship between the work environment and the health of employees (McMichael 1990; National Health Strategy 1992a; AIHW 1994; Oldenburg & Harris 1996). For many people, their day-to-day lives are shaped by their work experiences, in terms of their capacity to earn an income, interpersonal relationships, and the sense of purpose work can provide. The link between unemployment and ill health has long been recognised (Windshuttle 1980; Melhuish 1982; National Health Strategy 1992a; Davis & George 1998). While being unemployed impacts on a person's health and quality of life, those in paid employment also experience illness and injury because of work and the work environment (National Health Strategy 1993b, p. 144).

In 2002–03, Australian data on the total number of new compensable injury and disease cases showed that over 134 000 cases involved one week or more lost from work. This meant that around one in every twenty workers sustained such an injury or disease (National Occupational Health and Safety Commission (NOHSC) 2004). Furthermore, at least 2000 people die as a result of work-related injuries or diseases each year (NOHSC 2004).

In the period 2002–03, the estimated direct and indirect economic costs were \$34.3 billion, or 5 per cent of GDP (NOHSC 2004). Of the compensation cases reported for 2002–03, 68 per cent were males and 32 per cent were females (NOHSC 2004). Injuries accounted for 82.2 per cent of the total new cases reported, while 'other mechanisms' (including diseases) accounted for 17.8 per cent (NOHSC 2004). It is likely that these figures seriously under-report the incidence of occupational injuries and illnesses. Official data collected across Australia are not uniform and do not cover all work-related injuries and diseases, nor do they cover absence from work of less than one week. Moreover, figures are excluded for injuries to the self-employed and outworkers, cases not claimed and cases unsuccessful under workers' compensation legislation (NOHSC 2004). The limited data available on injuries in the workplace for non-English-speaking workers indicate that they appear to sustain more frequent and/or more severe injuries than do Australian-born workers (Lin & Pearse 1990).

Apart from the extensive evidence of the extent of occupational morbidity and mortality, the population of the workplace represents a microcosm of the broader community. The National Health Strategy paper (1992a) highlighted the 'overwhelming inequalities in the health of Australians'. The research suggests that the most disadvantaged groups have the poorest health and that their poorer health largely explains their greater use of primary and secondary health services. In addition, their use of preventive services is less than that of other groups.

Techniques to address this problem should include the development of policy that covers five broad areas (National Health Strategy 1992a, p. 102):

- distribution of economic resources
- education
- living conditions
- access to and conditions of work
- provision of social support.

In terms of access to and conditions of work, clearly unemployment is a central theme to be addressed. But, given that employment exposes people to potential injury, illness or death, and while the need to improve occupational health and safety in the workplace is clearly as essential, 'healthy public policy must go still further and be proactive in planning for healthy workplaces' (National Health Strategy 1992a, p. 104).

The ageing of the Australian population and continuing increases in the cost of health care have combined to increase corporate interest in methods of preventing or reducing disease. The worksite offers specific advantages as a location for risk reduction and health promotion programs. It is a bounded community, one in which there are daily interactions and standardised forms of communication (Oldenburg & Harris 1996). Furthermore, it provides access to sections of the population with poor health or with other special health-related needs (McMichael 1990, p. 16). There is some evidence to support the notion that the workplace provides useful support structures for the successful delivery of health messages to high-priority sections of the community. Moreover, with these high-risk groups the adherence rates for health-promoting behaviours have been shown to be higher in workplace settings than in many other settings (McMichael 1990).

There are other reasons why actions should be taken to improve work-place health, and other factors which make the workplace an ideal site for promoting health. Australians spend approximately one-third of their life at work. We know that a range of occupational hazards endanger worker health and safety. While we must be careful about how we define work-related injuries, they do account for somewhere between 4 and 7 per cent of injury deaths in Australia. In addition, persistent workplace stress erodes individual and organisational efficacy and can lead to illness, accidents and unhealthy lifestyle practices. It can also take a toll on family life. Workplace rules and regulations can affect employee health.

Transformations to the workplace and the recent introduction of new industrial relations regulations mean that much of the Australian work-force must deal with constant change and insecurity. With these changes, and the increasingly globalised marketplace, employees are faced with new and significant challenges (Breucker 2004). These are unavoidable in any industry, and consequently employers need to consider how they can effectively meet their obligations to promote and safeguard their employees' wellbeing (Chu & Dwyer 2002).

In order to manage the complex workplace stresses and the effects on workers' health, Chu and Dwyer (2002) recommend utilising an integrative approach, one that incorporates occupational health and safety, disease prevention, health promotion and organisational development. In addition, both the employer and employees need to contribute to the identification of health priorities and the management of the ecological, organisational and lifestyle influences on employees' health (Chu et al. 2000; Chu & Dwyer 2002).

The workplace provides opportunities to level the 'health playing field' by addressing socioeconomic inequalities in employees' health status. Short- and long-term health benefits can be derived from workplace health programs—for example, lower rates of absenteeism, the reduced cost of workers' compensation, and increased morale (Oldenburg & Harris 1996)—which in turn impact on the productivity of the workforce (Oldenburg & Harris 1996; WHO/Regional Office for the Western Pacific 1999). Workplaces with low turnover lend themselves particularly well to medium- and long-term programs, and many employees consider the workplace to be an appropriate site for the promotion of good health.

Workplace programs tend to have higher participation rates than do health programs offered at other sites. In addition, there are indirect benefits of WHP in the important contributions made to the improved health of the broader community, such as the transfer of health knowledge, attitudes and behaviour skills (McMichael 1990).

One of the main difficulties in arguing for comprehensive WHP is the lack of good-quality longitudinal research. In the late 1980s, Sloan lamented the failure of the literature to examine the entire field of workplace health promotion (1987, p. 181), and concluded that two major types of WHP program were in operation: the single health-habit intervention (most of the interventions), and comprehensive approaches to WHP (primarily an individual behaviour change focus). A paradigm of workplace health promotion does exist: 'it calls for activities, both large- and small-scale, which are designed to induce health-related behaviour change in individuals rather than examining and changing the system of work in which these behaviours may be embedded' (Sloan 1987, p. 186).

PRINCIPLES AND STRATEGIES OF WORKPLACE HEALTH PROMOTION

Achieving a healthy workplace requires a comprehensive strategy—one that provides mutual benefits for the organisation and the employee, on the basis that good health practices on the part of both will lead to individual fulfilment and organisational productivity (Dooner 1990–91, p. 2; Oldenburg & Harris 1996). A healthy workplace is attainable only through the commitment and cooperation of employers, employees and employee representatives, all working together to build creative and supportive social environments.

In advocating health promotion in the workplace, *Pathways to Better Health* (National Health Strategy 1993b, p. 144) recommended the development of a national strategy for workplace health to be coordinated by Worksafe Australia and to build on 'existing occupational health and safety priorities, the potential for workplace health promotion, and continuing workplace reforms'.

According to Dooner (1990–91, p. 2), four key strategies are fundamental to achieving a healthier and more productive organisation. Together they form the foundation that supports a positive work environment. The strategies are:

- shaping collective unity of purpose through clear policy direction
- building organisational and individual efficacy (empowerment)
- eliminating unnecessary organisational stress
- committing to and working towards a healthier organisational culture.

An organisation's overall policy usually sets out what the organisation stands for and what it values, and enunciates the reasons for its existence. It provides the context for organisational objectives, goals, programs and activities. Without an overall policy that articulates clear values and provides clear direction towards the achievement of organisational goals, including a healthier workplace, the organisation may be left with a plethora of programs, each functioning independently of the other and each responding to only a few of the employees' supposed needs.

There are a number of examples in Australian workplaces of programs that represent the breadth of strategies in current WHP practice. For example, in some workplaces regulatory and policy changes have been introduced, while in others there is an emphasis on environmental solutions and behaviour change programs. The more traditional strategies are evidenced by education and information activities and health screening (National Health Strategy 1993b). Sorensen et al. (1990, p. 170) classified worksite and organisational programs into three categories:

- motivation and incentive strategies—screening, health risk appraisal, contests and other incentives;
- educational/skills training activities—written information, lectures, individual counselling;
- environmental and social support activities—restructuring the physical environment, for example, non-smoking policy, canteen changes, building social support by involving family members.

In a study of four cardiovascular health promotion interventions (screening, education, incentives and lifestyle change) conducted in the New South Wales Ambulance Service, Gomel and Oldenburg (1990, p. 137) concluded that more intensive interventions such as use of incentives and cognitive-behavioural strategies produced larger short-term changes in cardiovascular disease risk factors when compared with education and screening alone. Other studies have looked at long-term results of worksite cardiovascular risk factor programs that used individual counselling by occupational health professionals. The conclusions suggested that changes in the level of risk factors favoured the intervention group marginally—varying with the sex, age and occupation of the subject. Nevertheless, the results suggested that individual counselling is generally not effective in long-term modification of mildly elevated cardiovascular risk factors (Edye et al. 1989, p. 574).

When comparisons are made between health promotion interventions in a range of settings, the evidence suggests that workplace interventions concerned with smoking, physical fitness and activity levels have the potential to achieve outcomes at least comparable with those of interventions implemented outside workplaces (National Health Strategy 1993b, p. 148).

If workplace-based health promotion programs can be demonstrated to have a small intervention effect on individual employees, this has the potential to produce an improvement in health outcomes across the whole community, given the size of the population who are employed. In addition, interventions addressing multiple risk factors can be offered repeatedly in worksites, increasing the likelihood of inducing behavioural changes in people who are at various points of readiness for change (Oldenburg & Harris 1996). Most importantly, the workplace offers the opportunity for combining both population-based and early intervention approaches to promoting health (Oldenburg & Harris 1996, p. 227).

COMPREHENSIVE WORKPLACE HEALTH PROMOTION

In order to build a comprehensive approach to workplace health, we need to develop the necessary program framework (O'Donnell 1995). Two principles should guide this exercise: first, not all employees have the same needs and preferences; and second, workplace health programs must be designed to respond to the needs of all employees throughout the organisation (Zoller 2004).

We argued earlier in this chapter that emerging models of WHP incorporate multiple strategies in an effort to modify the work environment and the culture of the organisation, as well as to provide individual behaviour change programs. A number of arguments were presented to support the need for comprehensive approaches.

One of the challenges in the development and implementation of comprehensive WHP is recognition of the differences between workplaces, in terms of both their culture and their size (Breucker 2004). Small businesses are often less enthusiastic and feel less capable about their role in WHP, often feeling they lack the infrastructure to develop large-scale projects like many larger corporations (Breucker 2004).

Although there are national differences in WHP across Europe, a shared understanding of WHP has developed over the past twenty years; it is characterised by a focus on workplace design, psychological issues and an interdisciplinary approach that involves employees (Theuringer & Missler 2003). This is similar to the comprehensive approach advocated in Australia, which directs us to actions aimed not only at changes in the work environment and organisation but also at changes that enable individuals to improve their health. An innovative project targeting industrial workers from a non-English-speaking background in the Auburn area of Sydney, the Industrial Injury Prevention Project, attempted to assist small- and medium-sized industrial sites to establish health-promoting work environments through intersectoral collaboration. The project aimed to reduce the number of injuries occurring at the various industrial sites, to improve access of injured workers to appropriate health care, and to design long-term structures for industrial injury prevention (Berney 1992). Membership of the project committee included representatives of employees, unions and government bodies, together with locally based health care providers. Berney (1992, p. 169) highlighted three main benefits of such intersectoral collaboration: improved project credibility, economic advantage, and ready sources of expert opinion.

Structural changes to the wider worksite environment have the potential to influence individual behaviour, as well as to facilitate the acceptance of health promotion programs by establishing cues supportive of change and building social support. Environmental changes are also likely to support long-term maintenance of change and program diffusion (Oldenburg & Harris 1996, p. 229).

OVERCOMING BARRIERS TO HEALTH PROMOTION

Although the field of workplace health has expanded and developed in a relatively short period, the nature and scope of WHP is not always well understood. While the workplace has many advantages as a setting for the promotion of health among individuals and the wider community, there are also some substantial barriers, not least those deriving from the complexity of the organisational culture and the relationships between key stakeholders such as managers, employees and unions. In view of this, national and state WHP steering committees have tripartite membership, encompassing employers, unions and government representatives.

While these structures have facilitated consultation and broad-based decision-making, there remain a number of other barriers. These include the opinion of some managers that health promotion is outside both the mandate and the capacity of their organisation to implement, and scepticism about the benefits to the organisation, in terms of reduced absenteeism, increased motivation and economic benefits. This is a real issue for employers, and the lack of comprehensive, longitudinal cost–benefit analysis of WHP programs has not served to ease or eliminate their concern. But Sorensen et al. (1990, p. 165) cautioned against using a cost–benefit argument for WHP programs, based on their finding that 'with the possible exception of smoking cessation and hypertension detection and follow-up treatment programs, the potential cost benefits of occupational health programs—especially relatively short-term payoffs—are not clearly established'.

More recently, Oldenburg and Harris identified some US-based programs that had had some success in quantifying issues such as lowered health costs (1996, p. 230). A study by Goetzel et al. (1998) found there was a positive relationship between well-executed, targeted workplace health promotion and health care cost reduction. However, the authors suggested that well-designed economic evaluations of worksite health promotion programs are still somewhat limited and often lack methodological rigour.

Some managers feel spending time and money on activities that occur in work time and that are costly interferes with productivity; and in tough economic times, WHP programs appear less than attractive. Where a range of programs and interventions already operate in the workplace without any coordinated effort—such as EAPs, injury prevention programs and OHS activities—these competing concerns often push WHP off the agenda for managers. Where managers *are* supportive of WHP programs, their support may not extend beyond a narrow focus on lifestyle change programs that produce clear and measurable results.

Pelletier (1997) found that employees who felt that their senior managers, supervisors and co-workers had positive attitudes towards health had improved health status. In addition, feeling valued as an employee, having control over job performance to reduce 'job strain', and being satisfied with work appear to be significant predictors of employee health and health behaviours (Pelleiter 1997, p. 166).

The relationship between WHP and OHS was covered earlier in this chapter. This relationship, in terms of its tensions and its complementary components, serves to heighten the debate between key stakeholders, such as management and unions, as to the overarching framework most likely to advance the health and safety of the workforce.

Unions have expressed concern about the nature and scope of WHP, particularly about the extent to which WHP might divert attention from structural and work practices that both directly and indirectly impact on the health and safety of workers. As Chu and Forrester (1992) pointed out, unions also voice discontent at WHP programs that blame the individual for his or her poor health. Furthermore, unions have expressed concern about the potential discriminatory practice of using WHP programs as a means of selecting workers for promotion or to undertake particular jobs at the expense of 'less healthy' workers (Gun 1990). Unions are more likely to support WHP where initiatives are based on employees' needs and interests (Peltomaki et al. 2003).

Employees, too, are not always supportive of WHP initiatives. Program participation rates and attrition are of crucial importance to the effectiveness of worksite programs. There are obviously a wide range of employee and worksite-related factors which may interact in a complex way to influence recruitment and retention. This lack of support can be due to several factors, not least of which may be the failure of programs to engage workers in the initial decision-making process. On the other hand, some employees may see health behaviours as a matter of personal lifestyle that sits squarely outside management's concern. Where WHP programs involve data collection of one form or another—for example, drug testing, or cholesterol and blood pressure measurements—some workers may be concerned about the confidentiality of this information. Where a workplace does not have the physical facilities to accommodate WHP, the timing and location of programs may influence participation rates. Even when a company's top managers support release time for employees to attend WHP programs, if inadequate development work with all key stakeholders has not been carried out middle managers and an employee's immediate supervisor may be less than enthusiastic.

One of the key tasks for the health promoter in a workplace setting is to understand how the potential benefits and barriers fit with what employers and employees hope to achieve from a program. Without a comprehensive analysis of the attitudes of both management and employees to health promotion, the program developer lacks two essential elements for success.

Oldenburg and Harris (1996, p. 230) state that the use of more organisational and environmental approaches to promote the health of employees in the workplace, in addition to more individually focused approaches, integrated with ongoing occupational health and safety initiatives, will become more the norm than the exception over the next few years. In addition, proficiency in managing organisational change will be a necessity for health promotion and public health practitioners in the future (Baum 2004). Developing into a health-promoting workplace will entail changes in organisations and management, with all stakeholders aware of the objectives of such changes (Baum 2004). The research on organisational change demonstrates the importance of planning, and the ability of organisations to learn and respond appropriately (Baum 2004).

IMPLEMENTING PROGRAMS

According to Dooner (1990–91, p. 5), there are four basic components to a program framework: carrying out a needs assessment; developing a long-range plan; implementing and running the program; and evaluation. An analysis of the concerns and culture of a workplace can be used to identify factors that might affect program adoption.

Sorensen et al. (1990) argued that successful interventions result from a twofold effort. The first component is capitalising on opportunities and resources that can assist program and policy adoption; the second is identifying existing and potential barriers and eliminating or diminishing them where possible.

Worksafe Australia (1993, p. 8) produced guidelines comprising eight steps for workplaces wishing to introduce WHP:

- deciding who will start organising the program—for example, committee, OHS staff, manager, external consultant;
- determining program prerequisites—commitment, workplace leaders, resources;
- liaising with OHS staff;
- selecting health topics—assessing health concerns and needs of employees;
- selecting program format—awareness, healthy environments, group activity;
- resourcing the program and deciding about coordination;
- monitoring;
- concluding.

A similar set of phases is included in a position paper prepared by the Queensland State Steering Committee for Health Promotion in the Workplace (1993, p. 17). In the Queensland approach, the process involves action planning, implementation, evaluation and program reassessment and redesign, with a suggestion that there be training for the worksite coordinator in basic WHP principles.

There is growing evidence in the United States (O'Donnell 1995), and emerging evidence in Australia, that to be successful WHP programs require the following core elements:

- ongoing commitment from management for the idea;
- the establishment or use of existing committee structures to ensure worker participation during all stages of the process;
- a comprehensive needs assessment to ensure that programs are designed to meet the needs of workers;
- links between health promotion activities in the workplace and activities in the community;
- a range of strategies that include behaviour change;
- the creation of supportive social and physical environments;
- the use of company facilities and the program run in company time, wherever possible;
- voluntary employee participation (National Health Strategy 1993b; Bellingham 1990).

In addition, support of unions and informal leaders of workplace groups is essential, as are appropriate resources, involvement of the workplace's OHS staff and, most importantly, development of a comprehensive WHP program with a philosophy that places individual health concerns within broader social and economic contexts (Worksafe Australia 1993; Oldenburg & Harris 1996).

REVIEW

Many authors have argued for WHP to exist within a broader, multifaceted OHS approach (Dooner 1990–91; Anderson 1990–91; Oldenburg & Harris 1996). Throughout the evolution of workplace health promotion, two main approaches have clearly emerged: first, the behavioural approach which focuses on the individual and involves the application of lifestyle interventions in areas such as fitness, diet and smoking cessation; second, a more comprehensive approach which acknowledges that factors influencing the health of the individual worker often lie outside his or her control. Comprehensive programs that incorporate structural changes to the workplace and an understanding of the culture of the organisation are advocated.

Workplace health promotion has not been without its critics. Unions have expressed concern about the potential shift in focus from the health and safety issues impacting on workers to more general issues of exercise or diet. Employers have been sceptical of the benefits of WHP. Small business has been particularly difficult to convince of the need for WHP, seeing the activities as more suited to the structure and needs of larger organisations. Employees have not always embraced the need for health promotion in their workplace. Despite these criticisms and the paucity of data about the benefits of WHP, contemporary programs have continued to expand and develop.

Several common principles in WHP have emerged in the literature over the last twenty years. One is the need to build commitment among all the key stakeholders in the process. Intersectoral collaboration encourages the view that workplaces, like other settings for health promotion, do not exist in isolation. Engaging the wider community in the process of WHP can foster the use of shared resources and activities and, particularly for small businesses, can create a network for participation in existing health promotion activity.

Emerging research evidence suggests that efficient and effective WHP programs are those directed towards the needs of the whole person and the organisation. They require a comprehensive approach to health that is built on sound business principles: careful planning, clear policies and goal-directed action (Dooner 1990–91). Creating a healthy working environment means addressing three broad areas that affect the way people feel: the environment, including physical, work and social environments; personal resources, including the degree of influence people have over their work and their health, the support they receive, and the opportunity they get for active participation in decision-making; and personal health practices.

REVISION

Review each of the following issues, in light of your understanding of occupational health and safety issues, and the nature and extent of health promotion in the workplace.

1. *Discuss the evolution of workplace health promotion and contemporary approaches.*
2. *Define workplace health promotion and the relationship between WHP and OHS approaches to health and safety.*
3. *What reasons are given in support of the implementation of WHP programs and the possible barriers to implementation?*
4. *Describe the main principles and strategies of WHP in light of broader developments in public health and health promotion.*
5. *What is comprehensive WHP, and how can it be developed, implemented and evaluated?*

10

Health promotion in health care settings

- *Socio-historical developments in health care in Australia*
- *Primary health care—its place in Australian health care*
- *Strategies for primary health care in action*
- *Patient education—a focus for health promotion*
- *Health promotion in general practice*
- *Changes in general practice*
- *Health-promoting hospitals*

In 1990, the National Health Strategy examined the range of institutional, community and personal health services primarily concerned with treating and caring for the ill. The common features of each of these aspects of the health system were not the only areas to be examined. Activities that fostered good health, including health education, promotion and public health, also received attention (National Health Strategy 1990). Essentially, rather than health promotion activity being seen as separate from health care services, attention was drawn in the National Health Strategy to the role health care services play in initiating and integrating health promotion activity to improve the health of the population.

As we have seen throughout this book, some of the fundamental conditions determining health lie outside the health care delivery system (Turrell et al. 1999; Turrell 2002; Wilson & Rosenberg 2002). Nevertheless, health promotion—in our sense of the term—can, should and does take place in hospitals, community health centres and the general practitioner's surgery. In addition, since the National Health Strategy in 1990, there are a range of structures and initiatives within the broad spectrum of health services implemented to facilitate and enhance health promotion activity in these settings. We will examine how these settings can be so used.

In Australia for the period 2001–02 there were 1025 acute care hospitals, 724 of which were public hospitals and 301 private hospitals, and 22 public psychiatric hospitals (AIHW 2004, p. 287). There was a rise from 131 351 beds in nursing homes and hostels in 1994 to 140 000 combined beds in 1998, the latter providing a minimal level of health care and long-term accommodation for young disabled people and older people (AIHW 2000, p. 282). In addition, there are a wide range of community health services provided directly to individuals, such as ambulatory care, including services in the home (such as Home and Community Care, a Commonwealth/state-funded initiative), domiciliary nursing and outreach services. Some of these broadly described 'community health services' include sexual health services, family planning organisations, women's health services, child health centres, alcohol and other drug treatment services, dental services and school health nurses. Some of these services—child health centres, for example—are government funded; others are provided through private health care practitioners, such as domiciliary nursing services. People employed in health occupations in 2001 constituted almost 5 per cent (450 711) of employed Australians (AIHW 2004a). Total health services expenditure in Australia was $66.6 billion in 2001–02, more than one-third of that, or 35.4 per cent, was spent on hospital services (AIHW 2004a).

The wide geographical distribution of primary health care and hospital facilities, and the large number of people who use them each year, means that they can be powerful models for promoting the health of individuals who attend them, and their local communities. As service providers, employers, producers/consumers and researchers, health care services have a range of opportunities in which to provide leadership in promoting health (Nutbeam et al. 1993b).

At first view, health promotion appears at odds with the curative tradition of acute care hospitals and other health care settings where, most often, the presentation of illness is a focus—for example, patients presenting in a general practitioner's office. Nonetheless, opportunistic health promotion activity is occurring increasingly in such settings, both within Australia and internationally. Infrastructure support is also being provided through government primary health care policies, joint hospital and community health initiatives, the establishment in Australia of Divisions of General Practice, and community health centre service integration. This chapter highlights recent developments in promoting health in health care settings.

SOCIO-HISTORICAL DEVELOPMENTS IN HEALTH CARE IN AUSTRALIA

Colonial Australia's services for the sick began inauspiciously with the pitching of several tents on the west of Sydney Cove after the First Fleet arrived in 1788. This was followed by the arrival from England of a prefabricated hospital in 1790 (O'Connor 1991). Later, Governor Macquarie began a building project designed to provide the colony with 'a spacious, elegant and indispensably necessary building' (Historical Records of New South Wales, 1892–1901). Considerable controversy was generated by the terms of the contract, and disapproval of Macquarie's use of rum as a means of paying the contractors came from the Colonial Office in London. Sydney's general hospital was completed in 1817, the first major hospital to service the colony.

Although the hospital was an imposing structure, initially the facilities and quality of care were poor. The kitchen had to be converted into a mortuary, which resulted in patients doing their own cooking in the wards. Both colonists and convicts were treated in the hospital, there was no segregation of the sexes, patients were locked in the wards at night without access to any attendants and all lavatories were outside the building (Gibbin 1932).

Between 1819 and 1836, a noticeable improvement in treatment and facilities at the general hospital occurred because of the appointment of a principal surgeon, John Bowman, who introduced a new administration. By 1836, the Colonial Medical Service was assimilated into the military establishment, thus placing all convict and military medical services under the Army Hospital Regulations. In 1848 a board of directors took over the hospital when the remaining convicts were transported to Van Diemen's Land; the hospital was renamed the Sydney Infirmary and Dispensary.

In the early years of settlement, the majority of the population were convicts, and medical services and treatment facilities were principally concerned with keeping the convicts alive and in a fit state for work (O'Connor 1991). As the colony matured and diversified, the free colonists realised that there was a need for shelter and medical services for the poor, aged and infirm. To meet that need the Benevolent Society of New South Wales was established in 1818; up to 70 per cent of its income was provided by the colonial government.

The initial government responsibility for the provision of medical facilities and medical care for the colonists changed and expanded to meet the needs of an increasing population, through the provision of private medical facilities and treatment. The government provided for the mentally ill outside the Colonial Medical Service. The third element in this health care structure was 'benevolence', which was considered by the government as the responsibility of the community (O'Connor 1991).

These events formed the beginnings of the complex and costly jigsaw of Australian health care delivery. Financing health care can be a source of tension between the federal and state governments, between political parties, and among professional groups of health care providers. McKeown (1976) argued that health care has played a relatively small role in determining the health of society. In regard to promoting health in the population at large, McKeown's thesis is that organisational and therapeutic effectiveness have been overshadowed by lifestyle and environmental factors (Harper et al. 1994, p. 57). Yet health care expenditure, health care organisation and delivery, and access to medical and hospital services still dominate much of the discussion about health care. The debate in the late 1990s about tax rebate incentives for individuals to purchase private health insurance is indicative of the myriad options, and the appropriate mix of public and private responsibilities for health expenditure priorities. According to the state government, Queensland has a good health system; however more money needs to be invested because of population growth and ageing. An extra $6.367 billion has been allocated to Queensland Health over the five years 2005–06 to 2010–11. The extra money will cover:

- increased remuneration for doctors;
- additional funding for hospital services, for example, emergency departments and intensive care;
- additional funding for priority delivery areas, for example, cardiac, cancer, mental health, Indigenous health and workforce training;
- additional funding to address overdue hospital maintenance and capital works;
- extra staff, including doctors, nurses, allied health professionals (Queensland Government 2005a).

It is not surprising, then, that attention has been drawn to the need to examine health promotion and health care services, given the expenditure on such services in the health care system and the evidence, until recently, of limited focused and supported health promotion in that sector.

Primary health care is one approach that combines health care delivery with principles of participation, community development and health promotion. It is a 'philosophy permeating the entire health system, a strategy for organising health care and a level of care and a set of activities' (WHO 1982). Primary health care can mean a first level of medical care (Baum 1998). However, the spirit of the World Health Organization's 'Health For All' document—the Alma-Ata Declaration of 1978 (WHO/UNICEF 1978)—was much broader than that. Primary health care is about a first level of service—in other words, the first entry point where people access services, such as at a local chemist. It is also a specific approach to health care. This latter approach to health care embraces resource distribution, community participation, a focus on prevention, and a broad approach to addressing health problems such as education, housing and food supply.

PRIMARY HEALTH CARE—ITS PLACE IN AUSTRALIAN HEALTH CARE

As a public policy approach to health, primary health care seeks to shift substantial resources to the first level of the health system, to operate directly with people in their social context and to have local involvement in decision-making (National Centre for Epidemiology and Population Health 1992). Thus, primary health care as a public policy offers a promising shift in the future from a technocratic, cure-focused and increasingly specialised health system with diminishing returns, to a new and growing emphasis on health promotion (Baum & Labonte 1992; Fry & Baum 1992; Baum 2004).

Primary health care is both a level of service provision and an approach to health care (WHO/UNICEF 1978). The approach involves a multi-disciplinary method of working, community involvement in the organisation of health care, an emphasis on equitable distribution of resources and outcomes, and responsiveness to local health needs. In addition, it draws on sectors outside the health system where relevant (Baum 2004).

The Alma-Ata Declaration on Primary Health Care (WHO/UNICEF 1978) defined primary health care for policy-makers in many settings.

Broadly, the term refers to health services with which people first come into contact. These services include general practitioners (GPs), local pharmacists, community and child health services, and self-help groups. Parents caring for children and people working in care for the aged, disabled or chronically ill are providing primary health care (Queensland Health 1993a). Primary health care includes essential health services for care of common problems, as well as health promotion and illness prevention. The three pillars of primary health care are equity, participation and intersectoral action (Baum 2004).

Owen and Lennie (1992) nominate four components of primary health care as practised in Australia today:

- a private, for-profit component—GPs, pharmacists, dentists, 'alternative practitioners';
- a public component—community health centres, child and school health services, hospital outpatient services, home help, home nursing, and so on;
- a non-government, non-profit component—family planning associations, church organisations;
- a domestic component—carers in the home, individual self-care.

Owen and Lennie (1992) argue that community health centres embrace each of these components in their delivery of integrated care and promotion of community health. The role of community health centres was discussed in Chapter 7.

To sum up, primary health care operates at the local or regional level and attempts to improve the health of the community through a variety of strategies and services. It emphasises:

- building self-reliance at a personal and community level;
- supporting community participation in health care programs and in health development;
- intersectoral collaboration in working towards environments that are supportive of health and in which 'healthy choices are the easier choices';
- integration of health services to facilitate continuity of care and efficiency in resources used;
- special attention to high-risk and vulnerable groups, as a precondition for equity in health outcomes and health care access;
- appropriate technology.

So, what are the differences and commonalities in the terms 'public health' and 'primary health care'? This conceptual relationship is often unclear. *Primary Health Care in South Australia: A discussion paper* contended that:

> the goal of health equity is common to both, as is social action, and both include the prevention of ill health—the difference tends to be the level at which each is focused. Public health is concerned with state, national and international work with an emphasis on healthy public policy; primary care services can be construed as important operational arms of public health policies and strategies. (South Australian Health Commission 1988b, p. 17)

In Queensland, the principles of primary health care were adopted in a 1993 Primary Health Care Policy that aimed to improve the health of the Queensland population (Queensland Health 1993a). Primary health care strategies as outlined above formed a whole-of-government primary health care plan for the state. Quality of care, accountability, research, education and training, evaluation and monitoring are also included in this document (Queensland Health 1993a).

Translating the philosophy of primary health care and its policy frameworks into action has been achieved through a number of strategic initiatives in health care delivery in Australia. Integration of health care is seen as a major priority by all levels of government in Australia and internationally. In 1999, the Australian Health Ministers' Conference (AHMC) agreed that integration of care would be a primary focus within the Australian health care system. This focus is articulated in the Australian Health Care Agreement 1998–2003 (Commonwealth Department of Health and Ageing 2004), the National Public Health Partnership (NPHP 1997) and the Review of the General Practice Strategy (Commonwealth Department of Health and Aged Care 1998).

STRATEGIES FOR PRIMARY HEALTH CARE IN ACTION

Challenges remain in implementing integrated health services, in terms of the priorities of health promotion and illness prevention within such a framework. Dwyer (2000) raises these challenges in a discussion of 'single purpose' programs, such as tobacco control and injury prevention. There have been population health gains in such single purpose programs, yet for each of these program areas there are potentially multiple health outcomes and determinants. Harnessing cooperative and collaborative approaches through integrated delivery systems and across settings and sub-populations presents new challenges for health promotion and illness prevention. Moreover, in the current discussions about models and planning, the potential for health promotion to improve population health needs to be securely on the agenda.

The evidence base indicates that primary health care has a significant role in reducing health inequities, however the data regarding the most advantageous types of interventions, and the appropriate contexts, is limited (HIRC PHC Network 2004). Accordingly, it is essential that more research be performed to address these questions (HIRC PHC Network 2004). In 2004, one of the recommendations of the national roundtable on primary health care was to improve research capacity in primary health care (HIRC PHC Network 2004).

For health systems that depend more on primary health care and general practice (compared to those more reliant on specialist care), there are benefits in terms of enhanced equity, more appropriate use of services, enhanced user satisfaction, improved access to care with the associated lower morbidity and mortality, and reduced cost (WHO/Regional Office for Europe's Health Evidence Network 2004).

PATIENT EDUCATION—A FOCUS FOR HEALTH PROMOTION

Traditional forms of health promotion in hospital settings have included patient education, employee health and safety programs, and the provision of preventive and screening services to the local community. Promotion of health for patients has always been implicit in any patient care given, yet the expansion of patient education to include broader strategies than individual instruction about medication, for example, has been evident in a series of initiatives in hospitals throughout Australia. Enhancing the knowledge of GPs in health counselling and health education has also been proposed (National Health Strategy 1993b).

Patient education affords many opportunities to improve the health of people who have a defined health problem, or in some cases to slow the rate of deterioration—for example, in the case of arthritis. Patient education has been defined by Lorig et al. as 'any set of planned, educational activities designed to improve patients' health behaviors, health status, or both' (2001, p. xiii). Patient education can occur in hospitals, in non-government organisations, community health centres, workplaces and community settings. Patient education can occur on a one-to-one basis or in small or large groups.

Patient education has been an area of health promotion that hospitals have been involved in most successfully. It can encompass broader education towards health, linking hospital-based workers with people in other settings such as community agencies and community health centres (National Health Strategy 1993b, p. 137B8). Patient education has become more complex as, increasingly, patients are engaged in managing their own health conditions. The three distinguishing features of such a self-management model are: dealing with the consequences of disease—illness, not just the physiological disease; being concerned with problem-solving, decision-making and patient confidence, rather than prescription and adherence; and placing patients and health professionals in partnership relationships—the continual patient/health professional communication (Lorig & Associates 2001, p. xiv). Holman and Lorig (2000) attribute importance to this because chronic diseases are the principal health problem of our times. With chronic disease, the patient's life is irreversibly changed, with variations in treatments and uncertain outcomes.

There is now evidence of the effectiveness of patient education where a number of approaches are utilised. Three approaches are the self-management education model for chronic disease, professionally led group education, and management via electronic communication.

The aim of the self-management education model is to have patients manage their chronic disease. One particular study of arthritis self-management (Lorig et al. 1993) focused on the continuous use of medication, behaviour change, pain control, adjusting to social and workplace dislocations, and emotional coping. Patients experienced reduced symptoms, improved physical activity and significantly less need for medical treatment. An important element for participants is learning from each other, with the benefit of growth in confidence in their ability to cope with their disease. In a more recent study to evaluate the effectiveness of a self-management program for a heterogeneous group of chronic disease patients, Lorig et al. (1999) found improved health behaviours and health status compared with usual care. It also resulted in fewer hospitalisations and days of hospitalisation (Lorig et al. 1999).

Self-management initiatives have been extensively researched, and Wagner's (1998) model has been universally accepted as a guide to contemporary chronic disease management. The model has since been expanded and is outlined below (further information may be found on the Improving Chronic Illness Care website, www.improvingchroniccare.org):

1. **Mobilise community resources to meet needs of patients**
    - Encourage patients to participate in effective community programs.
    - Form partnerships with community organisations to support and develop interventions that fill gaps in needed services.
    - Advocate for policies to improve patient care.

2. **Create a culture, organisation and mechanisms which promote safe, high-quality care**
    - Visibly support improvement at all levels of the organisation, beginning with the senior leader.
    - Promote effective improvement strategies aimed at comprehensive system change.
    - Encourage open and systematic handling of errors and quality problems to improve care.
    - Provide incentives based on quality of care.
    - Develop agreements that facilitate care coordination within and across organisations.

3. **Empower and prepare patients to manage their health and health care**
    - Emphasise the patient's central role in managing their own health.
    - Use effective self-management support strategies that include assessment, goal-setting, action planning, problem-solving and follow-up.
    - Organise internal and community resources to provide ongoing self-management support to patients.

4. **Assure the delivery of effective, efficient clinical care and self-management support**
    - Define roles and distribute tasks among team members.
    - Use planned interactions to support evidence-based care.
    - Provide clinical case management services for patients with complex needs.

- Ensure regular follow-up by the care team.
- Give care that patients understand and that fits with their cultural background.

5. **Promote clinical care that is consistent with scientific evidence and patient preferences**
   - Embed evidence-based guidelines into daily clinical practice.
   - Share evidence-based guidelines and information with patients to encourage their participation.
   - Use proven provider education methods.
   - Integrate specialist expertise and primary care.

6. **Organise patient and population data to facilitate efficient and effective care**
   - Provide timely reminders for providers and patients.
   - Identify relevant sub-populations for proactive care.
   - Facilitate individual patient care planning.
   - Share information with patients and providers to coordinate care.
   - Monitor performance of practice team and care system (Improving Chronic Illness Care 2006).

Group patient education has been successfully trialled. With agendas largely set by patients, health professionals facilitate structured discussions about issues concerning their chronic conditions (Beck et al. 1997). Participants have experienced increased quality of life, much slower decline in activities of daily living, greater satisfaction and reduced use of medical services. This form of group education has been a central theme in patient education and one that is most often used by health promoters from a variety of professional backgrounds.

With increasing availability of electronic communication, it is possible to manage chronic disease via the telephone or other electronic means. (See Chapter 7 for a discussion on virtual communities.) Rural and remote patients can be reached in such a manner, particularly if there is continuity between the patient and health professional (Holman & Lorig 2000). Telephone management has been shown to reduce costs and improve the health status of participants (Simon et al. 2000). The following case study illustrates the utilisation of a computerised telephone system for behaviour change and chronic disease management.

INTERACTIVE TECHNOLOGY: TELEPHONE-LINKED-CARE

A team of investigators from Queensland University of Technology (QUT), in collaboration with researchers from Boston University in the United States, conducted usability trials of an American designed computerised telephone system for behaviour change and chronic disease management. The system, called Telephone-Linked-Care (TLC) (Friedman 1998; Pinto et al. 2002), was designed and extensively evaluated by researchers from Boston University and other American institutions over fifteen years. It operates as an at-home monitor, educator and counsellor. It interviews users by using pre-recorded messages and questions, and listening to the answers—it recognises speech over the phone. The system records the answers and uses these data to provide feedback and tailor conversations, not only during the current session but also during future phone calls by the same user. Participants call TLC weekly from their regular telephone or mobile phone.

The team performed an initial pilot trial to assess the usability/acceptability of TLC for physical activity promotion after its adaptation to the Australian context. It was conducted with individuals from the general population and volunteers living with a chronic disease. It showed good acceptability levels with positive satisfaction ratings and adherence to call schedules. It also identified issues related to transferring such a program from the American to the Australian context, due to differences in language, socio-cultural and environmental factors, health systems and accepted health guidelines.

The same researchers are developing an Australian adaptation of a TLC program for diabetes self-management support and clinical monitoring. This program will be evaluated in a usability pilot trial to be followed by a randomised controlled trial. One of the fundamentals of diabetes management is to assist people to gain skills and confidence in the management of their condition, and this system aims to assist people with type 2 diabetes to adopt or maintain the key diabetes self-care behaviours such as blood glucose monitoring, nutrition, physical activity, foot care, and medication and appointment adherence. It is not intended to replace practitioners; rather, it provides a valuable tool in the overall treatment of a patient. This approach is compatible with contemporary efforts to facilitate improved self-care and patient empowerment and is of particular relevance for people who currently have poor access to traditional health services because of geography or time constraints. The system also has the potential to improve communication amongst health professionals and with patients because of the automatic summary and alert reports it can send out. Other advantages include consistent fidelity of implementation at low cost; easy access at any time of the day or night, as frequently as required or requested by a patient; and usage can be monitored and sub-optimal use enhanced.

The pilot studies, funded by the Diabetes Australia Research Trust and QUT, will determine the extent to which this approach to health care is accepted by the Australian community.

Source: Professor Brian Oldenburg, Dr Dominique Bird and Professor Robert Friedman

As you can see, there is a demonstrated and increasing evidence base for patient education. In each of the above models, there is a role for health promoters in cooperative planning with patients. The *Ottawa Charter for Health Promotion* (WHO 1986a) utilises the term 'enable'. Patient education is about 'enabling' health and self-management opportunities for those with chronic and acute health conditions.

Lorig and Associates (2001) suggested that many health professionals are attracted to the idea of patient education yet are often frustrated in their attempts to be effective with their programs. The authors outlined some of the common difficulties in patient education and provided tips on why people do not attend patient education programs, be they in hospitals or community settings. They suggested ways of enhancing success, including ideas about how and to whom to 'market' one's program (Lorig & Associates 2001).

Some of the strongest allies in this marketing approach are other health professionals. Work collaboratively to gain their support, not only in the creation of your program but also in the job of promoting it. Second, in marketing your program to your patients, make sure its title is not off-putting and that it has a positive ring to it. 'Self-help for the elderly', for example, is not particularly appealing, but 'Growing younger and healthier' might be (Lorig & Associates 2001, p. 149). Use of the media, newspapers and an accessible venue are important in establishing any program. Lorig suggested using focus groups to assist in planning an effective program, especially for people who are hard to reach, as well as scouring community resources for assistance with publicity, the distribution of materials, venues and financial assistance. Lorig and Associates (2001) provide a number of tools for planning patient education programs. These include patient needs assessment, questions for patients, and measures to evaluate patient education programs. These are practical aids for health promoters working in this increasingly important area (Lorig & Associates 2001).

The links between health care services and their communities have an increasingly important role in promoting health among patients. The empowerment continuum outlined in Chapter 7 is a tool that can assist you in patient education and advocacy endeavours.

HEALTH PROMOTION IN GENERAL PRACTICE

Traditionally, GPs have concentrated their practice on individual health with the GP managing the illnesses and care of patients on a one-to-one basis. The document *The Future of General Practice* (National Health Strategy 1992c, p. 83) recognised an expanded role for the GP in health promotion. Five specific strategies were proposed to encourage GPs to be more active in health promotion:

- supporting opportunistic health promotion (see below);
- improving education and information dissemination to GPs about health promotion;
- increasing and improving the use of record systems in general practice for the purpose of health promotion;
- making health targets more relevant to general practice, including involving GPs in local planning and clearly defining who is responsible for specific health promotion activities;
- providing support for GPs who want to be involved in population health promotion.

Let's examine these points one by one. Opportunistic health promotion involves encouraging the patient to identify risk factors. As Ellis and Leeder (1991) said, 'the opportunity to introduce appropriate preventive action to 80 million health consultations a year is too good to waste' (National Health Strategy 1992c, p. 84). The need to improve general practitioners' knowledge of health promotion derives from, among other things, surveys of GPs in which instances of inadequate drug and alcohol knowledge were identified. In the area of record systems, recall and reminder arrangements can be used to engage general practitioners in contributing to a database on health needs. Such systems work in Victoria for pap smear detection. Involving GPs in local regional authorities and on community health centre boards might broaden their approach to health promotion. The question of what role GPs would have in working towards health targets would have to be negotiated with local authorities. GPs' involvement in population health promotion would mean—besides their linking with local health authorities in order to develop workable models of service delivery—their working in multidisciplinary teams with other professionals.

CHANGES IN GENERAL PRACTICE

Changes in general practice in Australia were proposed by three organisations since the 1990 seminar Towards Evaluation in General Practice: A workshop on general practice (National Health Strategy 1992c, p. 72). They were the Commonwealth Department of Health and Human Services, the Royal Australian College of General Practitioners and the Australian Medical Association (see McGrath 1994). McGrath argued that it is difficult to determine the extent to which broad international movements such as primary health care, health promotion, ecology of health and the new public health have influenced decisions on changes in general practice. However, several initiatives have played a role in the growing integration of health promotion into general practice. The focus of general practice, accordingly, is being shifted towards a concern for the wellbeing of populations of people (McGrath 1994).

The introduction of Divisions of General Practice (DGP) throughout Australia has been offered as the basis for bringing health promotion into general practice. The first divisions were established in 1992 in Tasmania and in central Sydney (National Health Strategy 1992c, p. 108). Divisions of General Practice have two main aims: to increase communication among GPs in a geographical area; and to improve dialogue between GPs and other health professionals, hospitals, regional health authorities and non-government organisations.

An example of this is the Teams of Two project, which is a partnership between the Alliance of NSW Divisions and Centre for Mental Health, NSW Health (Milson & Pick 2004), to develop and support a cooperative learning program (NSW Health 2005). The program was officially launched in July 2003 at a statewide facilitation skills workshop for GPs, area mental health service clinicians and divisional representatives (Berry 2006). The project extends earlier work performed to improve collaboration between general practice and mental health services (NSW Health 2005).

One of the main goals was to reorient mental health services to recognise general practice as a vital component of the mental health care system (Milson & Pick 2004). The original objectives were:

- to increase mutual understanding of general practitioners' and mental health services' clinical and organisational roles;
- to increase training and support for general practitioners and mental health services;
- to strengthen existing local service links between general practitioners and mental health services;
- to increase awareness of local pathways to mental health care;
- to develop partnerships in mental health care with other relevant organisations (Milson & Pick 2004).

Participants engage in problem-solving activities aimed at enhancing clinical skills and exploring the GP/mental health service relationships in the provision of mental health care (NSW Health 2005). A joint learning environment is the setting for discussion and problem-solving and uses customised material (such as case studies), developed under the Teams of Two joint learning initiative (Milson & Pick 2004). Referral, feedback, collaborative case management, and ongoing communication to ensure the effective management of people experiencing chronic or acute mental health problems are common issues that are considered and discussed in the case scenarios (Milson & Pick 2004).

The workshops bring together small groups of GPs and mental health professionals and, depending on the topic chosen, may include professionals from drug and alcohol services and aged care assessment teams. Seven workshop modules have been developed under three broad areas:

- physical health/mental health
- acute mental health presentations
- depression in older people (Milson & Pick 2004; NSW Health 2005).

A formal evaluation of the program commenced in 2004. At the end of June 2004, 40 workshops had been held across the state and 45 more were planned for the following months. A total of 28 out of 38 New South Wales divisions were involved at this time. As of March 2005, 1400 GPs and other health workers had participated in the Teams of Two project (NSW Health 2005). Participants highlighted the benefit of networking and meeting face to face (Milson & Pick 2004). The initiative has provided a forum for problem-solving and the discussion of best practice, and appears to have improved awareness regarding work practices (Milson & Pick 2004). Teams of Two has demonstrated the capacity to contribute to improvements in knowledge, perspectives and practices (Berry 2006).

The program continues with the next stage of the Teams of Two initiative, which commenced in 2006. This phase of the project aims to encourage partnerships between general practice and public mental health and drug and alcohol services in New South Wales, in order to provide better care to patients who have a comorbid substance use and mental health disorder (Berry 2006).

It was suggested by the authors of *Pathways to Better Health* (National Health Strategy 1993b, p. 123) that general practice can play an important role in health promotion, because GPs conduct more health consultations than do other professional groups, are geographically dispersed and practise preventive and curative services. Furthermore, GPs are familiar to community members, possess credibility and have the respect of the community. They provide a cost-effective service and cater for a diverse patient population.

McGrath (1994) argued that, despite the characteristics of GPs which facilitate their involvement in health promotion, there are a number of factors that *prevent* their effective participation. GPs, as members of the medical profession, work within a biomedical model of health, they have limited training in preventive techniques and in communication skills, and they have doubts about the effectiveness of health promotion and the ethics of treating people who are well (McGrath 1994).

Despite the major challenges associated with involving general practice in health promotion, the development of DGP creates the potential for GPs to become further involved in fostering community health. In fact, several authors have commented on the role of the GP within an integrated primary health system. Appleby et al. (1999) identified a number of barriers to the integration of general practice in primary health care. These included disputes between the different levels of government and their services; the manner in which the GP's role is currently defined; and the system of GP remuneration. Some suggestions for improvement included the expansion of the role of the DGP and general practitioner remuneration, more links to hospitals, and a focus on information technology to link service providers. Since the formation of the DGP fourteen years ago, 94 to 95 per cent of GPs are now members of a local Division of General Practice (Hutton 2005; ADGP 2006). According to Hutton (2005) the DGP have been particularly successful in improving immunisation coverage and building information technology capacity in general practice.

In 1998, the Australian Divisions of General Practice (ADGP) was established, following an Australian Government General Practice Strategy Review recommendation that a national organisation of divisions be funded. The ADGP represents 118 Divisions of General Practice and seven state-based organisations across Australia. The ADGP aims to promote the health and wellbeing of Australians through DGP, and its current programs include:

- Enhanced divisional quality use of medicines—developed in the context of the National Medicines Policy to improve the quality use of medicines in the community.
- Chronic disease management (CDM)—in general practice this involves appropriate prevention, early identification and best practice management strategies.
- Lifescripts—supports the Divisions Network and general practice to build on prevention activities in the areas of smoking, nutrition, alcohol, physical activity and weight management.
- MindMatters plus General Practice Initiative—seeks to increase the capacity of demonstration schools, together with their local community, to provide support for students with high mental health needs.
- National General Practice Immunisation Program—aims to improve the quality of vaccination services provided by general practice, with the overall goal of improving immunisation rates Australia-wide.

- National Primary Mental Health Care Initiative—supports GPs in the provision of quality mental health care (ADGP 2006).

Further developments have occurred to focus the attention of GPs in Australia on population health and primary health care. This emphasis stems from a focus within funding patterns and the recent attention on integration, chronic and complex care, and rural, remote and Indigenous health (Queensland Divisions of General Practice 2000). The General Practice Strategy Review Report's (Commonwealth Department of Health and Aged Care 1998) recommendations drew attention to the expanded role of GPs to address public health problems. In addition, this focus for general practice was emphasised in a Commonwealth Department of Health and Aged Care report in 2000. The clarification of the role of the GP within these expanded concepts and the elucidation of definitions was the focus of a workshop in Brisbane in July 2000. The Enhanced Primary Care (EPC)/Population Health Workshop aimed to provide a process for discussing definitional issues and their application in general practice. The EPC Package was announced in the 1999–2000 budget as a way of improving the health care and wellbeing of older Australians and those with chronic and complex care needs. The program provides a framework for a multidisciplinary approach to health, and now includes:

- health assessments for people aged 75 and over (55 and over for Indigenous Australians, in recognition of their specific health needs);
- a health check every two years for Indigenous Australians aged between fifteen and 54;
- comprehensive medical assessments for residents of residential aged care facilities;
- multidisciplinary care planning;
- multidisciplinary case conferencing;
- multidisciplinary discharge care planning and case conferencing.

In 2004, people with chronic conditions and complicated care needs being managed by their GP under an EPC care plan also became eligible for certain allied health services, including Aboriginal health workers, audiologists, chiropractors, chiropodists, dieticians, mental health workers, occupational therapists, osteopaths, physiotherapists, podiatrists, psychologists, speech pathologists and diabetes educators (Commonwealth Department of Health and Ageing 2005).

HEALTH-PROMOTING HOSPITALS

The emergence of the concept of health-promoting hospitals (HPH) is closely linked with the emergence of the new public health and the central role of health promotion in contemporary public health practice. The WHO's description of health promotion supports the notion of the application of health promotion in a range of settings, including hospitals:

> At a general level, health promotion has come to represent a unifying concept for those who recognise the need for change in the ways and conditions of living in order to promote health. Health promotion represents a mediating strategy between people and their environments, synthesising personal choice and social responsibility in health to create a healthier future. (WHO 1986b)

Commencing in 1988, the HPH project was founded on the aims of the Ljubljana Charter on Reforming Health Care (WHO 1996b) and the Vienna Recommendations on Health Promoting Hospitals (WHO 1997c), in addition to the Ottawa Charter (WHO 1986a). The recommendations are guidelines for effecting change in the treatment-oriented culture of hospitals into one that encourages health promotion, disease prevention and rehabilitation (WHO/Regional Office for Europe 2005b).

At a WHO business meeting in 1991, the concept of health-promoting hospitals was formalised in the Budapest Declaration. The Declaration established an international network of health-promoting hospitals. It identified four possible levels of commitment to the project: participation as an accepted model hospital; affiliation as a potential model hospital; temporary affiliation of relevant individual projects; and networking with interested people (Gorey 1994). The content and aims of the Budapest Declaration incorporate the action steps of the Ottawa Charter and place those steps within the hospital environment. For example, the health-promoting hospital should:

- develop a common corporate identity within the hospital which embraces the aims of the health-promoting hospital;
- encourage an active and participatory role for patients according to their special health potential;

- create healthy working conditions for all hospital staff;
- maintain and promote collaboration between community-based health promotion initiatives and local government bodies.

The International Network of Health Promoting Hospitals was founded in 1993. After twelve years, the network had spread to more than 700 hospitals in over twenty countries (WHO/Regional Office for Europe 2005b), and initiated many 'Models of Good Practice', including comprehensive 'Pilot Hospital Projects' in eleven European countries. The World Health Organization has published a series of proceedings from international health-promoting hospitals' conferences held in Europe over the past few years (Pelikan 2000). The series contains discussions on the quality, effectiveness and sustainability of health-promoting hospital projects.

Health promotion programs in health care settings have considerable potential, as hospitals employ between 1 and 3 per cent of the health care workforce and expend from 40 to 70 per cent of national health care budgets. These settings have particular physical, chemical, biological and psychosocial risk factors (WHO/Regional Office for Europe 2005b). Furthermore, a large proportion of hospital admissions are related to unhealthy lifestyles, hence the potential for cost savings is considerable if patients can be persuaded to adhere to current recommendations regarding smoking, alcohol, nutrition and physical activity (Lonvig 2004).

Clearly, hospitals are not the key agencies for health promotion. Nevertheless:

- as institutions with a large number of workers and service users, they can reach a large section of the population (personnel, patients and relatives);
- as centres of modern medicine, research and education that accumulate much knowledge and experience, they can influence professional practice in other centres and social groups; and
- as producers of large amounts of waste, they can contribute to the reduction of environmental pollution and, as large-scale consumers, they can favour healthy products and environmental safety. (WHO/Regional Office for Europe 2005b)

There are a number of ways in which hospitals can be health-promoting environments: protecting the physical environment; providing suitable facilities; caring for the wellbeing of users and employees; and promoting the health of users and employees (Whitehead 2004; WHO/Regional Office for Europe 2005b). However, as Gorey (1994) pointed out, intellectual acceptance and policy formulation do not always translate into action. The reasons for the paucity of health promotion within hospitals are both diverse and complex; health promotion may not be considered as a legitimate role or priority for hospitals (Wright et al. 2002; Johnson & Nolan 2004; Whitehead 2004; WHO/Regional Office for Europe 2005b). Limited resources also contribute to the limited application of health promotion models in hospitals (Whitehead 2004). In addition, evaluation of health promotion initiatives in hospitals is often limited (Whitehead 2004), and therefore the evidence base for the efficacy of such programs is deficient.

Stanton et al. (1996), in their examination of health promotion activities in Queensland public hospitals, found that barriers included a lack of finance, lack of interest by relevant stakeholders and a lack of appropriate programs, training and patient receptivity. Success in facilitating health promotion programs in hospitals will need to include a change in the environment—in particular, the views of medical superintendents. The combination of attitude change and availability of a motivated person, such as a health promotion officer, would be needed to produce an increase in the level of health promotion in public hospitals (Stanton et al. 1996). Moreover, hospitals should realise that health promotion involves more than 'putting up posters' (Playdon 1997, p. 18), and that the health of patients and staff, as well as the wider community of which the hospital is part, are a fundamental part of the hospital mandate (Playdon 1997; Cullen 2002; Wright et al. 2002).

The breadth and depth of opportunities for health promotion in health care settings, utilising a holistic approach, draw on a number of elements of the health-promoting hospital concept. The range of strategies is outlined in the following box. As you can see, there are a number of ways in which health care settings can play a role in developing healthy environments and health-promoting opportunities for staff, patients and the community. It must be remembered that hospitals and health care settings have high status in the community and are thought to be credible institutions in relation to health (Tones 1995). Because of this credibility, opportunities exist to link health promotion to staff, patients and the community these settings serve.

HEALTH CARE SETTINGS AND HEALTH PROMOTION

1. Physical environment

How can the physical environment be protected?
- Use measures to reduce air, soil and water pollution.
- Manage waste effectively.
- Select energy-efficient transport systems and use gas, water and electricity efficiently.

What strategies could be used?
- Recycle supplies in order to reduce the use of non-renewable resources and to contribute to broader recycling efforts in the community.
- Employ best practice in waste minimisation.
- Employ best practice in use of electricity, gas and other fuels.

2. Built environment

How can building design protect and promote the health and safety of service users and employees?
- Ensure ready access to people with limited mobility.
- Ensure that facilities are physically comfortable and welcoming.
- Provide facilities for group education.
- Protect all people from exposure to chemicals, radiation or other hazards.
- Provide secure parking areas.
- Use non-slip floor covering which minimises noise levels.

What strategies could be used?
- The Australian Community Health Association, the Council on Healthcare Standards and the Commonwealth Department of Health conduct accreditation programs to achieve and maintain high-quality services and standards of care.
- Matters such as wheelchair access, secure parking areas and fire safety are included.

3. Social environment

How can the health care setting care for the social and psychological wellbeing of users and employees?
- The quality of the social environment is important in promoting health, by encouraging a sense of belonging and social contact.
- For employees, work satisfaction is important.
- Quality of care and consumer awareness are primary goals.

What strategies could be used?
- For service users, care and sensitivity with which treatment is delivered are important to their recovery.
- Social and psychological aspects of caring for people in contact with, or who work in, health services are important factors in promoting health.

4. Health-promoting environment

How can the health care setting promote the health of users and employees?
- Health services have a direct role to play in actively promoting the health of users and employees.

What strategies could be used?
- Health services could work with local communities to increase the range of options for physical and recreational activity available to community members.

Source: Nutbeam et al. (1993b)

A number of examples exist in Australia where the health-promoting hospital concept has been put in place. In 1989, WHO/UNICEF published a joint statement that set a global standard for maternity services. This became known as Baby Friendly. WHO/UNICEF have developed a comprehensive set of guidelines for the maternity setting, titled Ten Steps to Successful Breastfeeding, listing practical ways in which hospitals can actively support the promotion of infant health through breastfeeding. In Australia, workshops have been organised and a national database developed in order to implement these guidelines. 'Baby-friendly hospitals' are being established throughout the country.

At St Vincent's Hospital in Melbourne, with the assistance of change agents from VicHealth, the organisational culture changed by involving staff in the planning and design of new staff facilities, including a bistro and exercise facilities. In Queensland, the Green Hospital Award Scheme encouraged hospitals throughout the state to implement policies and practices that reduce their impact on the environment and encourage a supportive social and physical environment for staff and patients (Gorey 1994). In Adelaide, the Flinders Medical Centre became affiliated with the WHO network of health-promoting hospitals in 1994 (Playdon 1997). Health promotion staff located at the hospital have initiated a number of projects; these include the linkage of the community with self-help groups for cardiac rehabilitation programs, and ensuring access to nutritious food for hospital workers. Also in Adelaide, the Centre for Health Promotion of the Women's and Children's Hospital collaborates with other organisations in order to enhance women and children's health by: developing and delivering health promotion programs for the community; improving the hospital's capacity to promote health; and supporting community-based services in health promotion and disease prevention.

The centre is responsible for a number of initiatives including: the provision of health promotion leadership across the Children, Youth and Women's Health Service; supporting health promotion as part of first-class clinical care in acute and primary health care services; and developing strategies promoting healthy pregnancy, breastfeeding and healthy weight for children (Women's & Children's Hospital 2006).

In Brisbane, the Royal Women's Hospital established a day-care centre for staff in 1994. This has been expanded for use by staff at the three hospitals in the complex: the Royal Women's, Royal Brisbane and Royal Children's hospitals. The Lady Ramsay Child Care Centre caters for the needs of working parents within the complex (Hayes 2000). Each of these examples demonstrate similarities and differences in approach—from creating healthy environments for staff and rewarding a 'green' hospital, to extending hospital–community links in cardiac rehabilitation and focusing on staff needs through the provision of a child care centre.

In 2002, the Latrobe Regional Hospital in Victoria became a member of the International Network of Health Promoting Hospitals. In mid 2004, two working groups were established: the Health Promoting Hospitals

Working Group (HPHWG) and the Workplace Health Promotion Working Group. Current activities of the Health Promoting Hospitals Project include:

- Workplace Health Promotion activities—including strength training, massage therapy, Rural Health Week initiatives, Ride to Work Day;
- 'The Healthiest Gippsland', a mural being developed by Latrobe City schools for the Gippsland Cancer Care Centre (Latrobe Regional Hospital 2005).

There are still challenges facing health care settings in moving from their traditional role and taking up new opportunities. Clearly, the overriding challenge is still in 'translating the creative vision of Health Promoting Hospitals into pragmatic action' (Gorey 1994, p. 219). These examples illustrate the imaginative links hospitals can make in creating partnerships for health promotion to meet community needs.

REVIEW

Health care delivery in Australia is changing rapidly, with new integrated roles for health care services and the communities they serve. The role of the general practitioner as a community health resource is also changing to be part of this new agenda in population health. Health promotion and illness prevention initiatives have occurred traditionally in hospitals, or in community health centres through patient education. General practitioners have provided opportunistic health promotion for patients in their surgeries. More recently, primary health care has been translated into a number of integrated health care system-wide initiatives. These draw the health sector in partnership with community organisations to address health issues. With a focus on healthy public policies in a variety of settings—for instance, schools, the workplace and communities—health-promoting hospitals are being developed. The International Network of Health Promoting Hospitals through the WHO Regional Office is one initiative that captures the total hospital environment as a setting for a broad range of health promotion activity. Such activity can focus on health promotion programs to create health within the hospital for employees, patients and local communities. With the reality of increased scrutiny on the health sector, health promotion practitioners can be leaders in originating health opportunities through creative partnerships in their practice in the health care setting, with patients and with their local communities. Conversely, for practitioners working in schools and communities, creative links to the hospital expand the integrated base of health promotion practice.

REVISION

Consider the main issues addressed in this chapter. Review each point in light of your understanding of health promotion in health care settings, primary health care and general practice.

1. *What forces will have an impact on health care delivery in Australia now and in the future? What are the implications for health promotion in health care delivery?*
2. *Define primary health care, and the key components of a primary health care policy. Identify primary health care strategies and cite examples of how they are practised.*
3. *In what range of health care settings are health promotion strategies practised?*
4. *What is the role of the general practitioner in health promotion?*
5. *What strategies are recommended to enhance this role?*
6. *How can patient education be reinforced in health care settings?*
7. *Do you know of health promotion programs in health care settings in your own city or community?*
8. *What are creative health promotion opportunities for linking your local hospital with its community?*

11

Promoting health in rural and remote communities

- *Defining rural, regional and remote*
- *Rural and remote areas and health status*
- *Rural attitudes to health and health care*
- *Rural health policy*
- *Health promotion in rural communities*
- *Models for use in implementing health promotion*

Australia is very much an urban society, with about 66 per cent of Australians living in major population centres—specifically, centres with more than 250 000 people (Australian Institute of Health and Welfare (AIHW) 2004a). This chapter, however, is concerned with health promotion among the nearly 7 million people who live outside of these major population centres, in regional, rural and remote Australia (AIHW 2004a).

What do we know about the health status of rural Australians? In fact, what do we know about who they are, where they live, how they live, and the economic and occupational characteristics of rural and remote communities? What is a rural or remote community? How are 'rural', 'regional' and 'remote' defined? These questions are important ones for us to consider before we can discuss the role of health promotion in rural communities throughout Australia.

DEFINING RURAL, REGIONAL AND REMOTE

Defining a rural, regional or remote community has always been difficult, as has defining the terms 'rural', 'regional' and 'remote'. Should we simply consider the distinction between rural, regional and remote, and urban, as being extremes on a continuum? This is not a useful distinction, as there is no point along the continuum from large agglomerations to small clusters of scattered dwellings where urbanity disappears and rurality appears. Attempts to distinguish rural, regional or remote from urban have varied according to focus. This could include geographical criteria (such as distance from urban centres); demographic or social criteria (including population size, population density, community attitudes and lifestyle); or economic criteria (such as type and intensity of land use, and occupational structures) (Humphreys & Weinand 1989, p. 258; AIHW 1998). Most of the more recent attempts to define, classify and/or rank rurality have used a combination of population size, distance from major towns/services, and population density (Reid & Solomon 1992, p. 26; AIHW 1998).

In 1990, the Department of Community Services and Health used population size and density by Statistical Local Area (SLA) to classify areas into five broad subdivisions: 'urban', 'rural major', 'rural other', 'remote major' and 'remote other' (Buckley & Gray 1993). Reid and Solomon (1992) used a classification system based on the population size of the locality, the characteristics of the SLA in which the locality was situated, and the distance of the locality from a hospital. Using this classification, the area and the population were classified as 'large area/large population', 'large area/small population', 'small area/large population' and 'small area/small population'. The areas were further categorised according to their distance from another hospital. In 1994, the Department of Primary Industries and Energy and the then Department of Human Services and Health developed a classification system entitled the Rural, Remote and Metropolitan Area classification (RRMA). This system has seven categories: 'capital cities', 'other metropolitan centres', 'large rural centres', 'small rural centres', 'other rural areas', 'remote centres' and 'other remote'. The Australian Institute of Health and Welfare (AIHW) updated this classification system in 1997 to cater for the changes in the geographical boundaries used in the 1996 census by the Australian Bureau of Statistics (ABS). In 1999, the Commonwealth Department of Health and Aged Care released the Accessibility/Remoteness Index of Australia (ARIA); this was developed in order to provide a standard classification, and continuous measure of remoteness, for the whole of the country. It replaced the RRMA (Commonwealth Department of Health and Aged Care 1999). ARIA index values range from 0 (most accessible/least remote) to 12 (least accessible/ most remote), and are based on distance to four categories of service centre (AIHW 2004c). ARIA Plus ranges from 0 to 15, which represents a position's remoteness, based on the road distance to five categories of service centre (ABS 2003b; AIHW 2004c).

The ABS developed the Australian Standard Geographical Classification (ASGC) to allow quantitative comparisons between 'city' and 'country' in Australia (ABS 2003b). This classification makes use of ARIA Plus methodology as the underlying measure of remoteness. The difference between 'city' and 'country' is their physical remoteness from goods and services. The ASGC divides Australia into six broad regions called remoteness areas: 'major cities of Australia', 'inner regional Australia', 'outer regional Australia', 'remote Australia', and 'very remote Australia' (ABS 2003b). The sixth area, 'migratory', comprises 'off-shore', 'shipping' and 'migratory Collector's Districts' (AIHW 2004c).

There are, however, a range of other issues which impact on the definition of 'rural' or 'remote' and that need to be considered, because the essential elements of the rural–urban difference are those that impact on health-related behaviour, and not just the size of the population being considered. We do know there is considerable diversity among rural Australians. For instance, some live close to major urban centres, while others are extremely remote from even small population centres. Diversity is also evident in demographic, ethnic, economic and occupational characteristics. Given this diversity, it is not surprising that health status varies among rural and remote Australians, ranging from a level equal to or better than that of urban Australians, to the unacceptable levels of health of rural and remote Indigenous Australians (AIHW 2004a).

In a national workshop for rural health workers held in 1991, participants discussed definitions of 'rural' and 'remote', describing 'rural' as a multidimensional term incorporating accessibility and level of service and involving, for the health worker, a sense of professional isolation. One of the important aspects in drawing distinctions between 'urban', 'rural' and 'remote' is the 'self-definition of the population'. Some localities may be classified as rural or remote using population size or geographical location, but the residents may not consider themselves as rural or remote nor, for that matter, isolated (Centre for Rural Social Research 1992, p. 5). Remote areas are typically defined in terms of distance and perceptions about the people; those living in remote areas are seen to exhibit hardiness and self-sufficiency (Centre for Rural Social Research 1992, p. 6).

In attempting to define 'rural', it has been argued that we need to separate it from 'agricultural', because 'in most senses—economically, occupationally, socially, culturally—rural has been comprehensively "urbanised", e.g. telecommunications, media and the frequently cited "global village"' (Humphreys 2000).

Internationally, and in Australia, the last fifteen years have seen an increasing interest and research into rural health. Frequently, 'rural' and 'remote' are used collectively, for example, 'rural and remote health', alternately, 'remote health' is assumed to be included when there is any discussion of 'rural health', with no recognition that there may be differences between the two (Wakerman 2004). According to Wakerman (2004), remote health should be considered a separate discipline to 'rural health' as such definitions impact on policy development, planning and resource allocation. Furthermore, the clarity of the meaning of 'remote' is significant for methodological issues, and with the growing use of the expression by diverse interest groups, a shared understanding would be constructive (Wakerman 2004).

Too often we have accepted that the health concerns of rural/remote people are unlike those of the urban population—but can this assumption be justified? There is certainly diversity in the characteristics of rural and remote communities throughout Australia. This diversity is reflected in geographical location, culture, economics and occupational status. Given this diversity, there will inevitably be a wide range of health needs in rural and remote areas and limitations on people's access to services across the spectrum from health promotion to treatment and rehabilitation. Furthermore, these health needs have tended, in the past, to be addressed through piecemeal efforts variously managed by federal, state and territory governments, and local authorities.

In 1990 the then Department of Health, Housing and Community Services launched its Rural Health Support, Education and Training initiative (Rural Health Research and Education Program 1992). At the first National Rural Health Conference in Toowoomba in 1991, a national rural health strategy was produced. In addition, the National Rural Health Alliance (NRHA) was established; its mission was '. . . to promote the provision of high quality, accessible and appropriate health care in rural and remote areas of Australia through partnerships between health consumers and providers' (Reid & Solomon 1992, p. 41).

A range of other activities have taken place which support and extend these initial developments. The establishment of a national Indigenous health strategy addressed the health needs of Indigenous people living in rural and remote areas (see Chapter 8). The Australian government also developed a multipurpose service to facilitate funding and ensure that a more flexible range of services were available to rural and remote communities (Reid & Solomon 1992). Furthermore, most state health departments have established rural health units. Rural health matters are also serviced by a number of other agencies and organisations, such as the Farmsafe Australia project. In 1998, the AIHW produced the first report to focus on the health of Australians living in rural and remote areas. Furthermore, the National Rural Health Alliance (NRHA) produced a report in 1999, entitled *Healthy Horizons: A framework for improving the health of rural, regional and remote Australians*, as a joint initiative of the National Rural Health Policy Forum and the NRHA. This framework was designed to provide direction for Commonwealth, state and territory governments in developing strategies and allocating resources to improve the health and wellbeing of people in rural, regional and remote Australia. The National Health and Medical Research Council's (NHMRC) Rural Health Research Committee collated information about rural health research with the objectives of developing a strategy and agenda for rural health research, and developing mechanisms for translating research into policy and action to improve health in rural and remote communities (NHMRC 1998).

It is evident from our discussion that any definition of 'rural' and 'remote', in the context of health issues and health care, needs to consider the perceptions of rural people about their own 'rurality'. Health promoters working in rural and remote communities should be aware of their clients' perceptions of their own circumstances and lifestyle, in addition to using the more quantitative data available on the nature and scope of such communities.

RURAL AND REMOTE AREAS AND HEALTH STATUS

In recent years, the focus on the health of populations living in rural, regional and remote areas has increased markedly at a national and international level. Canada, the United Kingdom, continental Europe and the United States all have national and regional policies and plans to guide the development of the health, social and community services in their rural communities (NRHA 1999).

Australia is experiencing a resurgence in interest and development in rural, regional and remote areas. The first National Rural Health Conference, held in Toowoomba in 1991, highlighted the need to develop guidelines by which to assess the health needs of rural Australians. The report called for an approach that would achieve:

> . . . a broad understanding of the variations in needs between different sorts of communities and the development of specific criteria or indicators to enable health planners and community representatives in each community to identify quickly, easily and accurately the range of services and resources needed. (Proceedings of the First National Rural Health Conference 1992, p. 20)

Understanding the health needs of rural Australians is as important to health promoters as it is to health planners and community representatives. A myth long held by many Australians is that people who live in the country experience less illness and are generally healthier than those who live in urban areas. Rural life is often seen as 'unproblematic, free from social problems and stresses' (Wong 1990; Humphreys et al. 1993; NRHA 1999). This pre-Second World War view of rural life remains a common vision of rural Australia for many urban people. The reality is that rural Australia has undergone dramatic changes in the last five decades and those changes continue to impact on rural life. Rural communities are often characterised by unemployment and poverty, by a shift of the labour market (school leavers and older labour) from inland areas to the coast, and by the removal of government and non-government services to larger centres. The consequent decline of small country towns reflects the changing nature of rural Australia (AIHW 1998). Blainey (1983) referred to the 'tyranny of distance' both within Australia and between Australia and other countries. In rural communities, many families truly experience that tyranny through their lack of access to essential services and education and health resources, particularly mental health services (Reid & Solomon 1992, p. 16; AIHW 1998). In a recent study of the association between socioeconomic status (SES) and general practitioner (GP) utilisation across SLAs that differed in their geographic remoteness, Turrell et al. (2004) found that in remote/very remote SLAs people most in need of GP services are least likely to receive them. However, not all rural Australians suffer inequity in service access. For some, local access to services is better than that of their urban counterparts—although most rural people will experience some inequity in access to specialist services (AIHW 1998).

Health inevitably becomes a concern when rural communities increasingly experience poverty, high levels of unemployment, ageing of the population, and economic problems such as the major economic downturn of the past thirty years, the restriction of overseas markets, consolidation of properties, fluctuating interest rates and the collapse of small business (NRHA 1999). The health status of rural and remote Australians is poorer than for urban people, and this difference is reflected in higher mortality rates, higher rates of hospitalisation and reduced use of some services (AIHW 2004a).

Farm related morbidity and mortality is a significant problem for rural and remote Australians. Morbidity and mortality rates are higher for male farmers than for the Australian male population overall. This is a result of both the higher injury rate and from other aspects of farming (Fragar & Franklin 2000). For the period 1990–93, the age standardised mortality rate for male farmers aged between fifteen and 65 years was 39 per cent higher than that of the general working male population (Fragar & Franklin 2000). There are approximately 150 people killed each year on farms as a result of accidental injuries, with tractor rollover and run-over accidents being a significant risk area (Fragar & Franklin 2000). The higher morbidity and mortality for males is also affected by higher suicide rates, higher rates of some cancers and higher rates of traffic accidents (Fragar & Franklin 2000). In response to the high farm-related injury rates, the Rural Industries Research and Development Corporation (RIRDC) launched its farm occupational health and safety program in 1990, to provide guidance for research and development (RIRDC 2002). The objectives for the period 2002–06 were:

- to increase the adoption of safe systems of work on farms;
- to develop the information and systems to ensure the health and safety of persons transporting, handling, applying and otherwise affected by agricultural and veterinary chemicals;
- to complete on-farm safety management packages for all major commodities including horticultural industries, and encourage their incorporation into broader farm management packages;
- to update and further develop training material and delivery modes more likely to be taken up by farmers;

- to maintain, support and utilise the collection of data on farm health and safety issues (RIRDC 2002).

The more remote regions are characterised by higher proportions of Indigenous Australians who often have complex health problems (AIHW 2004a), and problems associated with participation by males in high-risk behaviours leading to injury-related hospitalisation and death (NRHA 1999, vol. II, p. 8). The Indigenous population contributes substantially to the health differentials for mortality between urban and remote populations with regards to diabetes, homicide, suicide and coronary heart disease (NRHA 1999; AIHW 2004a). In broad epidemiological terms, it is possible to identify long-standing health problems occurring in the rural sector. Family violence and stress-related illnesses, heart attacks, ulcers and alcoholism have increased, as has the incidence of suicide (AIHW 2005b).

Research and government reports, such as the 2001 National Health Survey (ABS 2002c) and the 1997 Survey of Mental Health and Wellbeing of Adults (ABS 1998b) have highlighted the extent of mental illness in rural communities throughout Australia. Based on ABS analysis of data from these surveys, people in regional areas were as likely to report affective or anxiety disorders, substance abuse and psychological distress as those in major cities. However, the data suggest that, compared with those in major cities, depression was 1.4 times as prevalent for 45–64 year olds from inner regional areas, and 0.4 times as prevalent among those 65 years and over from outer regional areas; males in outer regional areas were 0.73 times as likely to report anxiety; and substance abuse disorders in 18–24-year-old women from regional areas was twice as prevalent as their counterparts in major cities (AIHW 2005b). In particular, difficulties in providing treatment for mental health problems in country areas have been seen to be associated with geographical isolation, attitudes of rural people towards mental health, concerns about confidentiality, and the lack of resources provided to services with a high proportion of relatively inexperienced staff (Yellowless & Hemming 1992, p. 153; AIHW 1998; NRHA 1999).

Rural communities report an above-average incidence of accidents and injuries, and prevalence of respiratory diseases (AIHW 2005b). Evidence suggests that low levels of health information are common among people living in rural communities (AIHW 1998).

Data from the ABS 1995 and 2001 National Health Surveys was analysed by the AIHW by rural, regional and remote areas. Generally, the prevalence of excess weight rises with increasing rurality and remoteness, and the prevalence of smoking is markedly higher in remote areas than in other areas (AIHW 2005b). In addition, Peach et al. (1998) note that diseases strongly associated with diet and smoking were statistically significantly higher in remote areas. Programs, research and policies that address the socioeconomic disadvantages of living in rural, regional and remote areas are likely to lead to a greater understanding of, and reduction in, mortality (NRHA 1999).

An examination of rural health concerns demonstrates an important role for health promotion, as the research literature suggests a relationship between occupation, lifestyle and poor health in rural, regional and remote populations in Australia. However, as we have seen throughout this book, focusing solely on the individual and on lifestyle changes in health-compromising behaviours will not reduce morbidity patterns. Structural, social and economic changes must go hand in hand with lifestyle changes. The challenge for health promoters is to advocate for the latter while helping to develop the former.

RURAL ATTITUDES TO HEALTH AND HEALTH CARE

Data on the attitudes of rural communities to health and health care are scarce. However, over the past fifteen years a number of studies addressing health concerns, service provision, health promotion, and health and safety programs have highlighted characteristics of rural communities.

Humphreys and Weinand (1989) indicated that attitudes of rural dwellers to health and to the use of health care services varied significantly from those of urban residents. Rural dwellers were found to be more self-reliant and independent even in the face of obvious ill health or disability. Such independence was evident in higher levels of self-treatment and self-medication. Humphreys et al. (1993) reported that the changing nature of rural communities and the economic and social changes facing them have had a profound effect on their attitudes and beliefs about their 'rurality' and their needs. Moreover, we know from a wide range of research that, without access to the fundamental benefits of life, health issues are less likely to be identified as a priority in rural communities. For example, in a study of rural residents' characteristics and the issues of concern to them, Bourke (2001) found that health was rated the third most important issue after unemployment and the economy. Humphreys et al. (1997) reported that males living in rural and remote areas visit their GP less than males living in capital cities. In addition, many rural residents accept injury and illness as part of normal life and therefore many do not seek help for chronic conditions. Ultimately, healthy lifestyle change means very little without commensurate attention to social and economic needs (AIHW 1998).

In contrast, Bramston et al. (2000) found no significant differences in Queensland women's perceptions of their quality of life and emotional distress across rural, remote and urban settings. They believe that the specific individual contexts within the rural, remote and urban settings need to be integrated into research methodologies, as formerly there has been too much prominence placed on the rural–urban divide (Bramston et al. 2000).

RURAL HEALTH POLICY

Humphreys and Weinand (1989, p. 271) argued for a shift in policy focus away from 'after-the-event treatment and care' towards more preventive measures that incorporate health care education and counselling. The Rural Health Task Force noted in its interim report in 1990 that to meet the health needs of rural communities it may be necessary to reorient health services with a greater emphasis upon a primary health care approach, particularly its health promotion and preventive health care aspects. The report also recommended a multidisciplinary approach to meet the needs of rural communities (Australian Health Ministers' Advisory Council 1990, pp. 5, 7).

Originating from the first National Rural Health Conference in 1991, the National Rural Health Strategy (Department of Health, Housing and Community Services 1991a) placed rural health and health care firmly on the political agenda (see Chapter 3 for a discussion of the National Health Strategy). The initiative was partially in response to government recognition that rural Australians had different health needs to those of their urban counterparts (Wass 1994). The establishment of a national body to direct and coordinate rural health policy and practice was recommended (Department of Health, Housing and Community Services 1991a). The strategy also addressed a number of related issues:

- research into the particular needs of rural dwellers and approaches to address those needs;

- support and education for rural health workers;
- problems of access and equity with respect to health services, health information and education experienced by rural dwellers;
- promotion of health for people living in rural communities;
- effective health planning to meet the needs of groups with special needs.

Endorsed in 1994, the National Rural Health Strategy outlined actions governments and health organisations could take to improve the health services, workforce and health status of Australians in rural, regional and remote areas. However, Wass argued that the National Rural Health Strategy and implementation of the policy have both failed to take a primary health care approach to the health needs of people living in rural communities. Furthermore, she argued that up until the mid 1990s there had been only limited action to promote the health of rural Australians (1994, p. 24).

At conferences held in 1997 on issues affecting the health of rural, regional and remote Australia, the need for a new national focus on the reforms required was highlighted. In response, a framework was produced to guide the development of health programs and services in rural, regional and remote Australia, and provide direction to governments and guidance to communities. Its vision, principles and goals are based on a primary health care approach and the views of a wide range of stakeholders (NRHA 1999). The vision for the health of rural, regional and remote Australians states that 'people in rural, regional and remote Australia will be as healthy as other Australians and have the skills and capacity to maintain healthy communities' (NRHA 1999, vol. I, p. 3). Seven interdependent goals have been established to focus national activity and planning on issues of high priority for the health of rural, regional and remote Australians. While these goals are ambitious, the framework has been set in place, and key issues identified, for advancing the health of rural, regional and remote Australians. The goals, and some of the strategies to improve the health and wellbeing of rural and remote Australians under these goals, are:

1. **Improve highest priorities first**
   The highest health priorities are primarily those of the National Health Priority Areas (NHPA); however, particular diseases and risk factors,

which are disproportionate in rural, regional and remote areas, are also targeted. Of the seven NHPA, diabetes and injury prevention and control are particularly significant in non-metropolitan areas (NRHA 2002b).

2. **Improve the health of Aboriginal and Torres Strait Islander peoples living in rural, regional and remote Australia**

This goal recognises the excessive burden of disease and chronic illness experienced by Indigenous Australians, and highlights the importance of respect for culture, community control and holistic approaches (NRHA 2002b). An important action towards achieving this goal is the endorsement and signing by Commonwealth, state and territory governments of the *National Strategic Framework for Aboriginal and Torres Strait Islander Health: Framework for action by governments* (NATSIHC 2003).

3. **Undertake research and provide better information about rural, regional and remote Australians**

The research capacity of rural, regional and remote Australia has increased significantly over the past few years, primarily because of the development of university departments of rural health and rural clinical schools (NRHA 2002b).

4. **Develop flexible and coordinated services**

Such services aim to support approaches to the prevention and treatment of disease that incorporate community-controlled and community-identified initiatives; one example of a flexible model of service delivery is the Regional Health Services Program (NRHA 2002b).

5. **Maintain a skilled and responsive health workforce**

Commonwealth, state and territory governments have invested in the recruitment and retention of health professionals in rural and remote services. Programs include temporary solutions, such as the employment of overseas-trained doctors to provide crucial medical coverage, and more enduring measures, such as programs to encourage rural students to consider the health professions as possible career paths (NRHA 2002b).

6. **Develop needs-based flexible funding arrangements for rural, regional and remote Australia**

In some Indigenous communities, standard funding systems such as Medicare and the Pharmaceutical Benefits Scheme (PBS) often do not achieve the anticipated outcomes. In the Northern Territory, through the Primary Health Care Access Program, Medicare and PBS funding is distributed from a central fund according to the needs of the population (NRHA 2002b).

7. **Achieve recognition of rural, regional and remote health as an important component of the Australian health system**
   Increasingly, it is recognised that rural, regional and remote Australians have poorer health status on many indicators and inferior access to services, and therefore have a valid claim to a larger proportion of health care resources. People in non-metropolitan areas are keen to participate in the preparation and development of any federal, state and local initiatives (NRHA 2002b).

The focus of the publication *Healthy Horizons* is the seven national goals; however, it also recommends some key principles to direct the implementation of the goals in an approach appropriate to the individual situation of different communities. Any group hoping to contribute to improving the health of rural, regional and remote communities should be guided by these principles (NRHA 2002b).

Another initiative occurred late in 1999 when the Regional Australia Summit was held in Canberra. The summit covered demographic changes, natural resource management, government, business, technological and community developments in rural and regional communities. The workshops were based on twelve areas of significance for regional Australia, one of which was health (Humphreys 2000). The summit noted that regional Australia is currently characterised by:

- the poorer health status of its residents compared with their metropolitan counterparts;
- the appalling health status of Aboriginal and Torres Strait Islander communities;
- the excessive mortality and morbidity within groups such as the agricultural and mining workforce;
- the disproportionate disadvantage confronting older people in small rural and remote communities.

The summit's health workshop then identified the following five priority areas for action.

- The needs and considerations of rural and remote communities need to be recognised with respect to health education and training, standards and competencies, governance, service delivery and resource allocation.
- Access to health care services must be improved and consumer empowerment maximised by the removal of geographical, cultural and socioeconomic barriers.
- Health services designed around community size, make-up and stated health needs should be provided through a health workforce trained to deliver such services.
- Resource allocation that is equitable in terms of health needs relative to the urban population must be ensured.
- It must be ensured that all parties take account of the social and economic determinants of health, including the wide range of national economic and social policies (Humphreys 2000, p. 54).

According to Humphreys, the ultimate success of the Regional Australia Summit will be determined by the extent to which the health, wellbeing and prosperity of rural, remote and regional Australians have been improved, and existing problems addressed (2000, p. 55).

The eighth National Rural Health Conference, held in Alice Springs in March 2005, had as its key focus remote area health, along with Indigenous health and wellbeing. The conference delegates recognised that the health status of people in remote and rural areas could best be enhanced by a better grasp of the social, ecological and financial determinants of people's health and the importance of intersectoral relationships. However, this necessitates an enhanced understanding and assessment of these multifaceted systems and associations. In addition, there was an accord that simply increasing the size of the workforce would not solve the considerable rural and remote health workforce problems. The delegates considered that the manner in which the health workforce is utilised is as important as workforce recruitment. Thus, some of the functions currently undertaken by particular professions could be efficiently incorporated into the roles of other groups, and strategies to develop various professional groups—such as nurse practitioners, community midwives and therapy assistants—would be worthwhile (NRHA 2005). With the overarching goal of parity in health status for people in rural and remote areas by 2020, the conference delegates considered that the welfare of people in rural and remote Australia could be improved and maintained by the implementation of the following ten recommendations:

1. Ensure health needs, not service availability, drives investment in health, particularly in relation to Medicare.
2. Focus on helping Indigenous mothers and children.
3. Provide fair transport and accommodation allowances for sick people and their carers in remote and rural areas.
4. Review the alcohol taxation system to reduce harm from alcohol.
5. Develop a cross-sectoral project on human and environmental well-being in remote settlements.
6. Ensure better infrastructure to support health in remote and rural areas.
7. Have inter-professional education for health students.
8. Develop a better coordinated strategic research on health in remote and rural areas.
9. Ensure organisations check their approaches to thinking and working in remote and rural health.
10. Use the conference's ideas! (NRHA 2005, p. 3)

HEALTH PROMOTION IN RURAL COMMUNITIES

Implementing health promotion and illness prevention strategies in an isolated community often engenders high levels of frustration. Inadequate resources and sporadic back-up services (McMurray 1993, p. 45), inappropriate constraints set by regulatory provisions (National Centre for Epidemiology and Population Health 1992) and a lack of understanding of primary health care on the part of some administrative bodies often hamper the process (NRHA 1999, vol. I).

As we have seen in this chapter, the pattern of mortality and morbidity in rural Australia suggests an important role for health promotion in country areas. Humphreys et al. (1993) examined the sources of health-related information seen to be most valued by rural residents and the range of variables influencing that valuation. The authors pointed to the overwhelming importance of the general practitioner and the pharmacist in the provision of preventive health information for all rural people (p. 149). Furthermore, they recommended closer integration between health promoters and rural general practitioners (Humphreys et al. 1997). The results of their study suggested that, for rural people, acquiring information about preventive measures is most likely, in the first instance, to depend on visiting a general practitioner. Given that many rural residents visit their general practitioner principally for curative treatment, and that many live some distance from a general practitioner, they are more likely than their urban counterparts to suffer from a lack of information on preventive measures. The survey respondents reported a relatively low preference for radio and television as a source of information. This is disturbing, given the fact that these media are readily available to most rural residents. By contrast, magazines, newspapers and health pamphlets are generally more highly valued (Humphreys et al. 1993, p. 155). The authors recommended more research on the effectiveness of existing programs and the role of information at certain stages of the 'adoption' process.

More recent research (NRHA 1999) supporting research done in the late 1980s suggested that a better balance between curative and preventive services is required in rural communities if the inequities in health status are to be ameliorated (Humphreys & Weinand 1989; AIHW 1998; NRHA 1999). Community-based health promotion interventions—usually addressing a specific health issue or cluster of issues such as cervical screening or heart health or injury prevention projects—have taken place in rural communities in Australia. The Anti-Cancer Council of Victoria has undertaken region-based campaigns to increase cervical screening in rural Victoria (Hirst et al. 1990; Cockburn et al. 1991). Health promotion strategies associated with these campaigns have included:

- awareness and education sessions with women's groups
- workplace activities, including information and education opportunities
- service provider involvement
- provision of screening services
- community education
- media activities.

While results have achieved the primary objective of attracting older and mostly unscreened women into screening programs (AIHW 1998), researchers caution that 'reaching the most at-risk populations takes time, intersectoral cooperation and clearly defined messages' (Cockburn et al. 1991, p. 34; AIHW 1998). These issues are still relevant in the 21st century.

As we noted earlier in this chapter, many of the occupations in rural, regional and remote regions, such as mining and farming, have higher rates of injury than other occupations (AIHW 1998; Fragar & Franklin 2000).

Over the four-year period from 1989–92 there were 587 fatalities (Franklin et al. 2000). Strategies designed to address rural injuries include the National Farmsafe program to coordinate injury prevention. And the publication *Goals and Targets for Australia's Health in the Year 2000 and Beyond* included the following aim: 'To reduce the differences in morbidity and work-related mortality rates between rural and urban populations' (Nutbeam et al. 1993b, p. 63). The target was 'to reduce work-related deaths on farms by 20 per cent by the year 2000'.

The first national conference to address the issues of farm health and safety was held in New South Wales in 1988. The conference provided health promotion practitioners and occupational health and safety experts with the opportunity to discuss a range of programs from all over the world. Later, the National Ministerial Advisory Group on Farm Safety was established. This group contained a broad membership and represented the key players in the process, including the Australian Workers Union, the Country Women's Association, the National Farmers Federation, Worksafe Australia and the Rural Training Council of Australia. The advisory group developed a draft strategy for farm occupational health and safety, which was subsequently adopted at the national level (Farmsafe '88 1989).

The aim of the program was to develop a national framework for community-driven occupational health and safety projects and to and promote farm safety (Clarke & Wolfenden 1991). Strategies were established in five broad areas:

- development of Farmsafe Action Groups and resource and support networks (all involving local organisations);
- education and training for key participants, such as farm people and rural schoolchildren;
- a data collection and analysis system to provide evidence on the nature and extent of the problems, to allow priority setting, and to ensure ongoing research, monitoring and evaluation;
- a national information resource;
- a review of existing legislation in the states and territories.

Farmsafe committees have been established in most states, and most are located within the occupational health and safety units of state governments. The Farmsafe movement is a classic example of the Ottawa Charter in practice, focusing as it does on the three principles of health improvement:

advocacy for health; adequate resources to enable all people to assume their fullest potential; and mediation by professional groups and health personnel between all parties involved (Clarke & Wolfenden 1991, p. 20).

In 1993 a farm injury prevention initiative called the Giddy Goanna Project was initiated by the Oakey/Crows Nest Farm Safety Action Group in Queensland, in response to concerns about high levels of morbidity and mortality, especially for children, in the rural environment (see the following case study). Rates of injury death in Australia steadily increase according to the degree of spatial isolation of the population. National mortality data for the period 1990–92 depict a steady increase in the rates of unintentional injury death with decreasing size of the population centres. Injury in the rural environment also tends to be more severe. Children are strongly represented in the injury mortality statistics; in fact, injury is the leading cause of death in children aged one to fourteen years. The association between injury and population density is also reflected in younger age groups, with children from remote areas having more than twice the risk of dying from injury as children from metropolitan areas. The following case study illustrates a comprehensive approach to the prevention of injury in rural families and, in particular, rural children.

THE GIDDY GOANNA CHILD HEALTH AND SAFETY PROGRAM

The Giddy Goanna project was initially conducted by the Southern Queensland Rural Division of General Practice (SQRDGP). In 1995, Giddy Goanna Ltd, a non-profit company, took over the operation of the project to allow it to continue beyond the short-term nature of project funding. The project commenced as a farm safety project, but due to its success widened its coverage to encompass a wide range of health and safety issues, making Giddy Goanna relevant for all children. Giddy Goanna is primarily aimed at children aged 3 to 6 years, but has a much wider appeal, with interest from children aged 2 to 9 years. This makes the development of content for the programs very challenging.

The Giddy Goanna project aims to improve the health, safety and wellbeing of children and their families throughout Australia and the world; its objectives are:

- to identify areas of need, using statistics and expert opinion;
- to produce high-quality entertaining resources that effectively educate children and their families;
- to involve parents, teachers, health/safety workers and relevant others in the child's health/safety education process;
- to make the program/resources accessible to children of all cultures, geographic locations and socioeconomic status;
- to increase families' knowledge of risks inherent in their child's environment;
- to involve parents in child safety health promotion activities;
- to develop an economically successful and self-sustaining program, so more programs can be developed and distributed for children.

The original Giddy Goanna strategy involved the production and sale of a series of high-quality puzzle booklets. Giddy Goanna is a child character who is fun-loving, adventurous and safety-conscious. In the books he is joined by three Careless Cousins, who often forget the safe way to do things, and Father Goanna, who is involved with grown-up issues such as mowing the lawn and the use of chainsaws and tractors. The booklets were followed by a mail-based Kids Club and field-day style, farm-based safety demonstrations for primary schoolchildren.

Evaluation of the booklets and demonstration days has found both strategies have a positive influence upon children's knowledge and attitudes towards farm safety. Despite the lack of formal identification of behaviour change, both evaluations found that parents had observed changes in their children's behaviour subsequent to reading the booklets or attending a demonstration day. Parents were also very supportive of both types of intervention and welcomed the support in teaching and reinforcing safety issues.

Evaluation also found there is difficulty with programs trying to address a broad age range. For example, while younger children found some of the activities difficult or confusing, some of the older children did not find them sufficiently challenging. A similar situation occurred with the demonstration days, with most of the intervention effect occurring with younger children. Booklets and characters may need to be designed for specific segments of the target age group.

Many parents and community leaders also felt that the two project strategies should be accompanied by complementary resources for parents and schools, thus promoting cooperation and support from a variety of sources and an increased likelihood of positive outcomes.

Since evaluation there have been further story and puzzle booklets addressing mainstream safety issues, and demonstration days held in an urban format. Both innovations are designed to broaden the popular and successful strategies from a specifically rural focus into a safety project with more general application in the wider community.

In 2004, the project strategies were revised. Demonstration days and Kids Club activities were both effective but expensive to continue in a low funding environment. In 2005, Giddy Goanna released a DVD, music CD, a live show to tour primary schools throughout Australia, a classroom activities pack and Giddy's sixth book. In development are a range of other products which include a television series, an email-based Kids Club, interactive games for X-Box/Playstation/Gameboy platforms, and further books, DVDs and CDs. For more information about the Giddy Goanna program, visit the website at www.giddygoanna.org.

Source: Peter Anderson, Lecturer, School of Public Health, Queensland University of Technology and Pam Brown, Giddy Goanna Ltd

Wolfenden et al. (1991) described a community-based program in child injury prevention in a small rural community in New South Wales. The program followed the tenets of the Ottawa Charter by aiming to integrate community action and professional health promotion practice. A local intersectoral planning group was established; extensive local injury data were collected and a wide range of resource materials was produced. A manual for injury prevention workers was produced for eventual distribution throughout Australia—one of the main outcomes of the project was the data gathered on the process of health promotion in a local rural community.

Community-based approaches that gain active and intersectoral support early in the process are essential for success. They allow health promoters to access local resources and draw on existing community activities. Wolfenden et al. (1991) reported that local data and locally developed materials are essential in engaging the interest of participants. The rural child injury prevention project is a good example of diffusion of an innovation in circumstances in which the habits and attitudes of the target population are a prime consideration—in this case, being traditionally 'late adopters' of change (Humphreys et al. 1993).

The work of the Central Western Region of New South Wales in promoting health and safety on the farm (Wilson 1990) had similar implications for health promotion initiatives in rural communities: encouraging local farm people to recognise the issues and allowing them to define solutions. Again, intersectoral collaboration and local involvement proved essential for success.

Inclusion of injury prevention and health promotion in the school curriculum and the involvement of schoolchildren are important components of both a comprehensive approach to rural health and specific efforts to promote health and safety in rural communities. The case study below used effective intersectoral collaboration and successfully addressed the expressed needs of the community for which the intervention was designed.

COMMUNITY PUBLIC HEALTH PLANNING IN RURAL AND REMOTE AREAS

In 1998, communities in rural and remote regions in Queensland identified as exhibiting low health status and disadvantage were invited to participate in the Community Public Health Planning in Rural and Remote Areas Project, in order to address health determinants. Participant communities were funded for three years, and the funds were administered by an appropriate community-based organisation in each community.

The program used a community development approach and was facilitated by project coordinators based in rural centres. The project coordinator assisted communities to define their agendas and develop plans to address identified needs, and supported the development of coalitions to promote the inclusion of marginalised groups or communities where no existing networks or advocates exist.

As the program emphasis was on health determinants, collaboration with a comprehensive range of stakeholders was required at all organisational and community levels. This emphasis aimed to increase the ability of the program to be meaningfully community-driven, allowing strategies which address traditionally 'non-core' health issues, such as employment, education, transport and housing, to be integrated into the program.

Community health is associated with a diverse array of factors, including economic, environmental and social issues. The aim of the project was to collaborate with communities to facilitate an increase in their community capacity to address health determinant issues. These concerns are usually addressed by a range of government sectors, thus it was important to reinforce relationships across and within departments and communities, and ensure communities could acquire the most suitable support for their needs.

Evaluation activities were integrated into project implementation, and sought to measure changes in community capacity, as well as to reinforce and resource the action research cycle (plan, act, observe, reflect and so on) at all implementation levels.

By project completion, it was anticipated that relationships between the communities and other sectors would be developed or strengthened, and health inequities in rural and remote Queensland addressed. Outcomes thus far include:

- improved local ownership and involvement
- reinforcement of knowledge transfer systems
- improved ability of communities to identify issues
- enhanced human, social and intellectual capacity of the population (Coutts et al. 2005).

However, the growth of local networks has slowed; the communities' problem-solving abilities need further development; and information exchange between some networks needs expansion (Coutts et al. 2005).

Source: Sue Smyllie, Project Manager (at the time of this project), Community Public Health Planning in Rural and Remote Areas Project, Queensland Health

MODELS FOR USE IN IMPLEMENTING HEALTH PROMOTION

Some health promotion activities in rural Australia have focused on lifestyle modification, such as exercise, diet or smoking cessation programs. We do have more information now about the differences between rural and urban patterns of health in the Australian population. These differences suggest a role for health promotion, particularly in terms of the tenets of the Ottawa Charter, because of the nature of social, economic and lifestyle factors influencing mortality and morbidity in rural communities. The principles of health promotion for sustainable development discussed in Chapter 3 have relevance here in our consideration of an appropriate model to guide the implementation of health promotion in rural communities. In Canada, some health promoters use a model of integrated (sustainable) rural community development. The model (see Figure 11.1) demonstrates the basic interdependence of social, economic and environmental spheres of human/natural activity in sustaining community life.

Figure 11.1: A model for sustainable rural communities

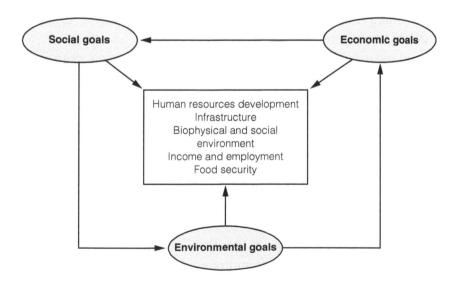

Source: Adapted from Sadler and Jacobs (1990, p. 9)

Each rural community is encouraged to develop settings and establish processes in which members can talk about their community's special circumstances in order to develop their own perspective. For example, what represents rural community sustainability for our community, how do we assess our local issues in an integrated manner, and how do they relate to broader actions? The model defines essential components of rural community life and its sustainability as being:

- **Human resources development.** This includes migration in and out of the community, information technology, communication processes, leadership and education.
- **Infrastructure.** Social and economic infrastructure includes community decision-making processes and networks, the economic base, land use, and planning bodies for economic development. Communication and transport infrastructures are also important.
- **Biophysical and social environment.** The biophysical environment must be developed in a sustainable manner as far as possible. The social environment should be conducive to good quality of life, working conditions and mental health.
- **Income and employment.** Income from farm and non-farm employment is a major issue from both a social and an economic standpoint. For example, how can sustainable employment systems be created in isolated rural communities?
- **Food security.** This includes food production, processing, distribution and consumption. It is a particularly important issue in the case of single parents, children and the elderly.

With this model as an overall development framework, the needs of rural communities can be addressed in a more comprehensive and holistic manner. The research data to date clearly demonstrate that the health of rural communities is closely associated with rural occupations and lifestyle. As we have seen in many other chapters in this book, health promotion interventions designed to meet the needs of the individual without any consideration of the social and economic determinants of health will have a limited long-term impact. Comprehensive intervention models are needed that build upon existing community health promotion and community development activities. Health promoters working in rural communities need to strive for intersectoral collaboration in their work in order to ensure the maximum use of resources and available expertise.

Examples of large-scale research and demonstration health promotion programs in rural settings in Australia have been reported. Van Beurden et al. (1991) examined the transfer and adoption of a cholesterol intervention from the Pawtucket Heart Health Program in urban areas of the United States to a rural setting in Australia. The research is particularly valuable in its recommendation (1991, p. 182) that adopters of programs developed elsewhere first ask themselves five principal questions:

- What is the setting of the intervention in geographical, social, political, policy and organisational terms?
- How should the intervention function within this setting, and what are its resource requirements?
- Is the intervention appropriate to the adopter's goals in full or in part?
- How should the adopter modify the local setting to allow the successful transfer of all components essential to the program?
- How should the adopter tailor the program itself to suit the local setting?

Unlike the sustainable development model for rural communities discussed above, this model focuses more on 'traditional' community health promotion interventions. Nevertheless, a health promoter wishing to adopt an innovative program developed overseas or elsewhere within Australia can apply the model and its questions in the pilot and implementation phases. Van Beurden et al. (1991) suggest that program adoption can be managed successfully provided the health promoter recognises the problems inherent in such a transfer and acts accordingly. For example, some change in health policy and organisational structure may be necessary in one's region, which may require a considerable process of advocacy and negotiation with key decision-makers (van Beurden et al. 1991, p. 189).

Research findings over the past fifteen years support the notion that health promotion programs using the tenets of the Ottawa Charter—that is, those that advocate for health and safety, provide resources to enable action to occur and work on collaborative action—are more likely to achieve success (Wilson 1990; van Beurden et al. 1991; Wolfenden et al. 1991; NRHA 1999).

Indeed, meeting the special needs of rural communities for health promotion and illness prevention involves a commitment on the part of the health promoter to act as a mediator between all the parties concerned.

REVIEW

In this chapter, we examined the concepts of 'rural' and 'remote', and advocated a definition that recognises the needs and perceptions of rural and remote area people themselves. The research literature suggests that rural people experience patterns of health and illness different from those of their urban counterparts. A number of health promotion initiatives have emerged over the past two decades, which have been designed to address rural problems.

Rural communities are experiencing social and economic change at a rapid rate, and there are inequities in access to services for people living in both rural and remote communities. Reducing these inequities involves more than the provision of education and information about health. It involves policy commitment on the part of government agencies and a willingness to tackle the difficult question of resource distribution and service provision.

Evidence from contemporary health promotion programs in rural communities suggests that following the tenets of the Ottawa Charter and engaging the community in defining their needs and participating in the process will mean health and safety objectives are more likely to be achieved.

REVISION

Consider the main issues addressed in this chapter. Review each of these points in light of your understanding of the health needs of rural people, the differences between rural, remote and urban settings, and the nature of health promotion in rural communities.

1. *How might health promotion strategies differ in rural and remote communities from those in urban communities?*

2. *Identify and explain the differences in health status between rural and urban Australians, particularly as they affect the development and implementation of health promotion interventions.*
3. *Consider the important dimensions of rural and remote communities affecting the development and implementation of health promotion strategies.*
4. *Analyse the range of health promotion opportunities in rural and remote communities in relation to the concepts and principles of the new public health.*
5. *Critically examine the case studies of health promotion initiatives in rural communities.*

Glossary

Advocacy (for health) Refers to working for political, regulatory or organisational change on behalf of a particular interest group or population (Green & Kreuter 1999). 'Such action may be taken by and/or on behalf of individuals and groups to create *living conditions* which are conducive to *health* and the achievement of healthy *lifestyles*' [emphasis added] (WHO 1998).

Alliance 'An alliance for health promotion is a *partnership* between two or more parties that pursue a set of agreed upon goals in *health promotion*' (WHO 1998).

Cardiovascular disease Any disease of the heart or blood vessels, including heart attack, angina, stroke and peripheral vascular disease (AIHW 2002a).

Chronic disease The Australian chronic disease framework focuses on non-communicable diseases only, CVD (coronary heart disease and stroke), diabetes, some cancers and respiratory disease (chronic obstructive pulmonary disease and asthma), and mental health problems and/or depression. Chronic diseases typically have complicated causality and several risk factors, in addition to a long latency phase and little likelihood of cure (NPHP 2001).

Community While typically viewed in geographical terms, 'community' must also be identified on the basis of shared interests or characteristics, such as ethnicity, sexual orientation or occupation.

Community capacity '. . . the characteristics of communities that affect their ability to identify, mobilise, and address social and public health outcomes' (McLeroy 1998 cited in Goodman et al. 1998, p. 259). While various definitions emphasise different aspects of community capacity, some of the shared characteristics comprise resources (financial, human and social capital), leadership, participation and relationships (Chaskin 2001).

Community development The process whereby people's awareness of the conditions affecting their health and quality of life is developed, and whereby they are ultimately empowered with the skills needed to take control of and improve those conditions in their community. From a health promoter's point of view, it is the process of helping communities to identify issues of concern and facilitating their efforts to bring about change.

Community empowerment Improvement in or of the capacity of a community to identify, respond to and resolve its problems.

Community health promotion The community defines the issues; collaborative relationships are negotiated between the community and the health promoter in terms of the role of the health promoter and the expectations of both parties; and program goals and success criteria are negotiated.

Community organisation Linking of community groups and structures and the residents over common issues; helping them with organisational efforts to bring about change.

Community participation Involvement of people in programs and processes relating to their health. The term is sometimes used to refer to involvement of people in health promotion activities. Others use it to refer to involvement of people in wider decisions relating to health.

Coronary heart disease (CHD) Heart attack and angina (chest pain). Also known as ischaemic heart disease (AIHW 2002a).

Decision-makers Individuals who make decisions about policy and the allocation of resources (both human and material) for existing and future programs. They usually include administrators and representatives of government or funding bodies.

Ecological public health Emphasises the common ground between achieving health and sustainable development. To be able to sustain the environment in which we live is central to our continuing existence. This concept includes making our cities less polluted and more energy efficient, with more emphasis on recycling, reducing consumption and becoming more self-sufficient in food production.

Ecology Study of the web of relationships among the behaviours of individuals and populations and their social and physical environments (Green & Kreuter 1999).

Effectiveness The ability of an intervention or strategy to achieve its intended effect in the setting in which it is implemented.

Efficacy This term usually relates to the question, 'can the intervention or strategy work?'

Efficiency The effectiveness of a program in relation to its costs. Costs can be measured in terms of dollars or resources but can also include adverse effects of the intervention on individuals or the community as a whole.

Empowerment The capacity to define, analyse and act upon problems in one's life and living conditions.

Enabling factors Any characteristic of an individual, a group or the environment that is conducive to positive health behaviour or conditions (or, depending on the context, to conditions that lead to ill health).

Evaluation The process by which we judge the worth or value of something.

Formative evaluation Evaluation for improving the program as it is being implemented (Hawe et al. 1990).

Goal The desired long-term outcome of a health intervention.

Haemophilus influenzae (Hib) A life-threatening bacterial infection which, prior to the advent of immunisation in 1993, was one of the most common causes of meningitis in young children. It can also cause epiglottitis, pneumonia, joint infection and cellulitis.

Health behaviour The combination of knowledge, practices and attitudes that together contribute to motivate the actions we take regarding health. These behaviours may promote good health or, if harmful, be a determinant of disease (WHO 2005b).

Health belief A statement, idea or sense, which may be explicit or implied, that is accepted by an individual or group and as such may motivate behaviour related to health.

Health education The provision of learning experiences which encourage voluntary modifications of behaviour that are conducive to health.

Health-promoting hospital A hospital that has a corporate culture offering an active and participatory role for patients, creates healthy working conditions for staff, and maintains and promotes collaboration between community-based initiatives, local government and the hospital.

Health-promoting school One that is continuously improving its capacity as a healthy setting for living, learning and working (WHO 1997a).

Health promotion The process of encouraging and enabling individuals and communities to increase their control over the determinants of health and thereby improve their health. Health promotion represents a mediating strategy between people and their environments, combining personal choice and social responsibility for health to create a healthier future (WHO 1986a).

Health protection Enforced regulation of human behaviour to protect individual and community health.

Health status The state of physical, mental and emotional health of an individual or community.

Healthy public policy Seeks to create a social, economic and physical environment that assists and encourages people to make healthy choices in lifestyle.

Herd immunity The whole population is protected, including non-immune people, because there are sufficient immune individuals to preclude the survival of the infectious agent within that population.

Impact evaluation Concerned with the immediate effects of a program, i.e. its effects on those factors that contribute to or cause the health problem (Hawe et al. 1990).

Incidence The number of new cases (of a disease, condition or event) occurring during a given period (AIHW 2002a).

Intersectoral collaboration A combination of interorganisational, cooperative and synergistic working alliances (Butterfoss et al. 1993). 'A recognized relationship between part or parts of different sectors of society which has been formed to take action on an issue to achieve *health outcomes* or *intermediate health outcomes* in a way which is more effective, efficient or sustainable than might be achieved by the *health sector* acting alone' [emphasis added] (WHO 1998).

Management Involves tasks and discipline and people. Denotes both a function and the people who discharge it.

Needs assessment The initial stage in the planning of a health intervention; it involves the identification of priority health issues, from the perspective of the target group, for making the intervention more effective.

Network A largely informal 'structure' or process that enables the health worker to draw on the range of expertise and abilities of contacts in the network.

New public health Refers to developments in which general policy replaced individual behaviour as the centre of attention, and in which the older 'lifestyle approach' was replaced by the notion of enhancement of life skills. Has regained the political base it had during the 'sanitary revolution' and now emphasises the socioeconomic factors that impinge on people. Has rejoined its environmental base, with a focus on social systems in which people live (McPherson 1992).

Outcome evaluation Measures whether a program has achieved its goal (e.g. has the problem been alleviated). Concerned with longer-term effects than those addressed in *impact evaluation* (Hawe et al. 1990).

Population health 'Population health is distinct from clinical interventions in that it places emphasis on whole populations and takes actions that will change collective health ... determinants of population health are usually different from those of the health of individuals' (Baum 2004, pp. 531–2).

Predisposing factor Any characteristic that predisposes an individual, a community or an element of the environment towards behaviour or conditions related to health; includes beliefs, attitudes and factors such as socioeconomic status.

Prevalence The number or proportion (of cases, instances etc.) present in a population at a given time (AIHW 2002a).

Preventive medicine The application of scientific knowledge regarding causation and the natural history of disease, enabling discrete medical interventions to be made in order to prevent the onset or stall the progress of illness.

Primary health care The local or community level of the health care system; an approach to health care more generally and a broad policy model for health planning. Operates directly with people in their social context, seeks local involvement in decision-making and encourages the giving of higher priority to people's views.

Process evaluation First element of evaluation, determines to what extent a program has been implemented as planned (Hawe et al. 1990).

Program A grouping of resources, both human and financial, for the purpose of performing activities, all of which fall within definable boundaries (the latter help to enable the activities of the program to be evaluated).

Public health The efforts organised by society to protect, promote and restore the public's health. It is the combination of sciences, skills and beliefs that are directed to the maintenance and improvement of all people through collective or social actions (Last 1997).

Remote Places geographically isolated from public amenities, community services, acute hospital facilities and (usually) medical practitioners (Kreger 1991).

Risk factors 'Social, economic or biological status, behaviours or environments which are associated with or cause increased susceptibility to a specific disease, ill health, or injury' (WHO 1998).

Rural A multidimensional term incorporating accessibility and level of service. Population size, geographical location, distance from services and 'self-definition' of the population can be used to define rural.

School health A holistic view of health: utilises all educational opportunities to encourage health, within and outside the school; strives to harmonise the health messages from various sources that influence students; empowers children and youth to promote conditions supportive of health.

Self-care/help/management Individuals (and their carers) using their own resources and abilities to manage their condition supported by professionals (Department of Health, England 2005).

Self-help groups Small groups of consumers, whose membership is voluntary, who want to bring about desired social and/or personal change (Katz & Bender 1976).

Site/setting The physical or organisational context in which a program is implemented, for example a school, a workplace, a hospital.

Social capital The processes and conditions among people and organisations that lead to accomplishing a goal of mutual social benefit, usually characterised by four interrelated constructs: trust, cooperation, civic engagement and reciprocity (Green & Kreuter 1999). 'Social capital represents the degree of social cohesion which exists in communities. It refers to the processes between people which establish networks, norms, and social trust, and facilitate coordination and cooperation for mutual benefit' (WHO 1998).

Social indicator A variable that is directly measurable and used as an indication of the wellbeing of individuals in a community—for example, income levels, educational attainment and life expectancy.

Social marketing The application of marketing concepts and techniques to the marketing of various socially beneficial ideas or causes instead of products or services in a commercial sense.

Stakeholder An individual or entity with a substantial involvement in an activity or project—for example, a decision-maker, a member of the client group or a program developer.

Strategic management Involves defining an organisation's mission and overseeing its development through to the implementation phase.

Strategic planning Involves translating an organisation's mission into specific strategies; concludes at the stage of selecting one or more strategies.

Strategy A coherent set of approaches used (in health promotion) to achieve a desired change in enabling or reinforcing factors.

Target group Those members of a group or community for whom a health goal is devised and the health intervention carried out.

Workplace health promotion Educational, organisational or economic activities in the workplace designed to improve the health of workers and therefore the community at large. This type of health promotion involves worker and management participation on a voluntary basis in the implementation of jointly agreed programs that utilise the workplace as a setting for promoting better health (National Steering Committee on Health Promotion in the Workplace 1989).

Bibliography

Ackermann, A. 1997, 'Defining the health promoting school', in D. Colquhoun, K. Goltz and M. Sheehan (eds), *The Health Promoting School*, Harcourt, Brace and Company, Sydney, pp. 27–52.

Alcorso, J. and Schofield, T. 1991, *The National Non-English Speaking Background Women's Health Strategy*, AGPS, Canberra.

Alinsky, S. 1969, *Reveille for Radicals*, University of Chicago Press, Chicago.

——1972, *Rules for Radicals*, University of Chicago Press, Chicago.

Anderson, D.F. 1990–91, 'Workplace action for health', *Health Promotion Canada*, vol. 29, no. 3, pp. 13–14.

Appleby, N.J., Dunt, D., Southern, D.M. and Young, D. 1999, 'General practice integration in Australia—primary health services provider and consumer perceptions of barrier and solution', *Australian Family Physician*, vol. 28, no. 8, pp. 858–63.

Arnstein, S. 1969, 'A ladder of citizen participation', *Journal of the American Planning Association*, vol. 35, no. 4, July, pp. 216–24.

——1971, 'Eight rungs on the ladder of citizen participation', in S.E. Cahn and B.A. Passett (eds), *Citizen Participation: Effecting Community Change*, Prager, London, pp. 216–25.

Ashton, J., Grey, P. and Barnard, K. 1986, 'Healthy Cities, WHO's new public health initiative', *Health Promotion*, vol. 1, pp. 319–24.

Ashton, J. and Seymour, J. 1988, *The New Public Health*, Open University Press, London.

——1990, *The New Public Health*, 2nd edn, Open University Press, Milton Keynes.

AusAID (Australian Agency for International Development), viewed 17 January 2005, <http://<.ausaid.gov.au/hottopics/topic.cfm?Id=9562_2054_7529_7688_4864#toll>

Australasian College of Occupational Medicine (ACOM) 1990, *Health Promotion in Industry*, 2nd edn, Melbourne.

Australian Bureau of Statistics (ABS) 1992, *National Health Survey*, Summary Report, ABS, Canberra.

——1994, *National Aboriginal and Torres Strait Islander Survey 1994: Health of Indigenous Australians*, ABS, Canberra.

——1997, *Causes of Death Australia 1996*, ABS cat. no. 3303.0, AGPS, Canberra.

——1998a, *Population projections 1997 to 2051*, ABS cat. no. 3222.0, ABS, Canberra.

——1998b, *National Survey of Mental Health and Wellbeing of Adults 1997*, Monograph Series Number 5.

——1999, *The Health and Welfare of Australia's Aboriginal and Torres Strait Islander Peoples*, ABS, Canberra.

——2002a, *Population Distribution, Indigenous Australians*, cat. no. 4705.0, ABS, Canberra.

——2002b, *National Health Survey: Aboriginal and Torres Strait Islander Results, Australia, 2001*, cat. no. 4715.0, ABS, Canberra.

——2002c, National Health Survey.

——2003a, 2001 Census Basic Community Profile and Snapshot.

——2003b, ASGC Remoteness Classification: Purpose and use *(Census Paper No. 03/01)*, viewed 23 May 2005, <www.abs.gov.au/websitedbs/D3110122.NSF/0/f9c96fb635cce780ca256d420005dc02/$FILE/Remoteness_Paper_text_final.pdf>

——2006, National Health Survey.

Australian Bureau of Statistics and the Australian Institute of Health and Welfare (ABS & AIHW) 2003, *The health and welfare of Australia's Aboriginal and Torres Strait Islander Peoples*, ABS cat. no. 4704.0, AIHW cat. no. IHW 6, ABS, Canberra.

——2005, *The health and welfare of Australia's Aboriginal and Torres Strait Islander Peoples*, ABS cat. no. 4704.0, AIHW cat. no. IHW14, ABS, Canberra.

Australian Divisions of General Practice (ADGP) 2006, viewed 20 February 2006, <www.adgp.com.au/site/index.cfm?display=8>

Australian Government 2005, *Building a healthy, active Australia*, viewed 23 January 2006, <www.healthyactive.gov.au/news_whatweredoing.htm#health>

Australian Health Ministers' Advisory Council Rural Health Care Task Force 1990, *Preliminary Report to the Australian Health Ministers' Advisory Council*, Canberra.

Australian Health Ministers' Advisory Council Standing Committee on Aboriginal and Torres Strait Islander Health 2002, *Aboriginal and Torres Strait Islander Health Workforce National Strategic Framework*, AHMAC, Canberra.

Australian Health Ministers' Advisory Council Working Party on Child and Youth Health 1994, *The Health of Young Australians: A draft policy paper*, AGPS, Canberra.

Australian Health Promoting Schools Association (AHPSA) 2000, 'A national framework for health promoting schools' (2000–2003).

——2005, viewed 6 March 2005, <www.ahpsa.org.au/about.html>

Australian Institute of Health (AIH) 1990, *Australia's Health 1990*, the second biennial health report of the Australian Institute of Health, AGPS, Canberra.

Australian Institute of Health and Welfare (AIHW) 1992, *Australia's Health 1992*, the third biennial health report of the Australian Institute of Health and Welfare, AGPS, Canberra.

——1994, *Australia's Health 1994*, the fourth biennial health report of the Australian Institute of Health and Welfare, AGPS, Canberra.

——1998, *Australia's Health 1998*, the sixth biennial health report of the Australian Institute of Health and Welfare, AGPS, Canberra.

——2000, *Australia's Health 2000*, the seventh biennial health report of the Australian Institute of Health and Welfare, AGPS, Canberra.

——2002a, *Chronic Diseases and associated risk factors in Australia, 2001*, AIHW cat. no. PHE 33, AIHW, Canberra.

——2002b, 2001 National Drug Strategy Household Survey: first results. Drug Statistics Series No. 9, AIHW cat. no. PHE 35, AIHW, Canberra.

——2002c, *Australia's children: Their health and wellbeing 2002*, AIHW cat. no. PHE 36, AIHW, Canberra.

——2002d, *Australian health inequalities: 1 birthplace*, authored by M. Singh and M. de Looper, Bulletin no. 2, AIHW cat. no. AUS 27, AIHW, Canberra.

——2002e, *Australia's health 2002*, the eighth biennial health report of the Australian Institute of Health and Welfare, AIHW, Canberra.

——2003, *Australia's Young People: Their health and wellbeing 2003*, cat. no. PHE 50, AIHW, Canberra.

——2004a, *Australia's Health 2004*, the ninth biennial health report of the Australian Institute of Health and Welfare, AGPS, Canberra.

——2004b, *Australia's mothers and babies 2002*, AIHW cat. no. PER 28, AIHW National Perinatal Statistics Unit (Perinatal Statistics Series No. 15), Sydney.

——2004c, *Rural, Regional and Remote Health: A guide to remoteness classifications*, AIHW cat. no. PHE 53, AIHW, Canberra.

——2004d, *Heart, stroke and vascular diseases—Australian facts 2004*, AIHW cat. no. CVD 27, AIHW and National Heart Foundation of Australia (Cardiovascular Disease Series No. 22), Canberra.

——2004e, *National Drug Strategy Household Survey: Detailed findings*, Drug Statistics Series Number 16, cat. no. PHE 66, AIHW, Canberra.

——2005a, *Australian hospital statistics 2003–04*, cat. no. HSE 37 (Health Services Series no. 23), AIHW, Canberra.

——2005b, Rural, Regional and Remote Health: Indicators of health, cat. no. PHE 59 (Rural Health Series no. 5), AIHW, Canberra.

——2005c, *Australian Hospital Statistics 2003–04*, AIHW, Canberra.

——2005d, *Expenditures on Health for Aboriginal and Torres Strait Islander People, 2001–02*, cat. no. HWE–30, AIHW, Canberra.

——2005e, *Diabetes in Culturally and Linguistically Diverse Australians: Identification of communities at high risk*, authored by A.M. Thow and A-M. Waters, cat. no. CVD 30, AIHW, Canberra.

——2005f, AIHW, viewed 27 January 2005, <www.aihw.gov.au/international/>

——2005g, *Statistics on drug use in Australia 2004*, cat. no. PHE 62 (Drug Statistics Series No. 15), AIHW, Canberra.

Australian Institute of Health and Welfare and Commonwealth Department of Health and Family Services (AIHW & COH&F) 1997, *First report on National Health Priority Areas 1996*, cat. no. PHE 1, AIHW and DHFS, Canberra.

Awofeso, N. 2003, 'The Healthy Cities approach—reflections on a framework for improving global health', *Bulletin of the World Health Organization*, vol. 83, no. 3, pp. 222–3.

Baranowski, T., Perry, C.L. and Parcel, G.S. 1997, 'How individuals, environments and health behavior interact', in K. Glanz, F.M. Lewis and B.K. Rimer (eds), *Health Behavior and Health Education: Theory, research and practice*, Jossey-Bass, San Francisco.

Barber, B. 1996, *Jihad vs. McWorld-Trade*, Ballantine Books, New York.

Barney, J. and Hesterly, W. 2006, *Strategic Management and Competitive Advantage: Concepts*, Pearson, NJ & London.

Bartholomew, L.K., Parcel, G.S. and Kok, G. 1998, 'Intervention mapping: A process for designing theory- and evidence-based health education programs', *Health Education and Behavior*, vol. 25, pp. 545–63.

Bartholomew, L.K., Parcel, G.S., Kok, G. and Gottlieb, N. 2001, *Intervention Mapping: Designing theory- and evidence-based health promotion programs*, Mayfield Publishing Co., Mountain View, CA.

Baum, F. 1992a, 'Moving targets: Evaluating community development', keynote address presented at Fourth Annual Health Promotion Research Conference, Australian Public Health Association Health Promotion Special Interest Group, Adelaide, 16–18 February.

——1992b, 'Healthy Cities and change: Social movement or bureaucratic tool?', *Health Promotion International*, vol. 8, no. 1, pp. 31–40.

——1998, *The New Public Health: An Australian perspective*, Oxford University Press, Melbourne.

——1999, 'The role of social capital in health promotion: Australian perspectives', *Health Promotion Journal of Australia*, vol. 9, no. 3, pp. 171–8.

——2004, *The New Public Health* [electronic resource], 2nd edn, Oxford University Press, Melbourne.

Baum, F. and Labonte, R. 1992, course notes, Flinders University, South Australia.

Baum, F.E. and Keleher, H. 2002, 'Public health', *Medical Journal of Australia*, vol. 176, p. 36.

Beaglehole, R., Bonita, R., Horton, R., Adams, O. and McKee, M. 2004, 'Public health in the new era: improving health through collective action', *The Lancet*, vol. 363, no. 9426, pp. 2084–6.

Beck, A., Scott, J., Williams, P., Robertson, B., Jackson, D., Gade, G. and Cowan, P. 1997, 'A randomized trial of group outpatient visits for chronically ill older HMO members: The cooperative health care clinic', *Journal of the American Geriatric Society*, vol. 45, pp. 543–9.

Beer, M., Eisenstat, R.A. and Spector, B. 1990, 'Why change programs don't produce change', *Harvard Business Review*, November–December, pp. 158–9.

Bellingham, R. 1990, 'Debunking the myth of individual health promotion', *Occupational Medicine: State of the art reviews*, vol. 5, no. 4, pp. 665–75.

Bellingham, K. 1991, 'Integrating health promotion with occupational health and safety objectives', *Occupational Health Magazine*, August, pp. 5–6.

Bennett, S.A. 1996, 'Socioeconomic trends in death from coronary heart disease and stroke among Australian men, 1970–1993', *International Journal of Epidemiology*, no. 25, pp. 266–75.

Bensberg, M. 2004, 'Can organisational behaviour lend a health-promoting hand?', *Health Promotion Journal of Australia*, vol. 15, pp. 109–13.

Berney, L. 1992, 'The Industrial Injury Prevention Project', *Journal of Occupational Health and Safety, Australia and New Zealand*, vol. 8, no. 4, pp. 123–5.

Berry, K. 2006, 'Drug and Alcohol and Mental Health Comorbidity Module', *PARCupdate*, vol. 3, no. 1, viewed 7 March 2006, <www.parc.net.au/PARC UpdateFeb06.htm>

Better Health Commission 1986, *Looking Forward to Better Health*, vols 1, 2 and 3, AGPS, Canberra.

——1994, *Better Health Outcomes for Australians: National goals, targets and strategies for better health outcomes into the next century*, Commonwealth Department of Human Services and Health, Canberra.

van Beurden, E., James, R. and Henrickson, D. 1991, 'Implementation of a large scale community based health promotion campaign with a limited budget', *Health Promotion Journal of Australia*, vol. 1, pp. 35–9.

Blainey, G. 1983, *The Tyranny of Distance: How distance shaped Australia's history*, Sun Books, Melbourne.

Blanchard, A. and Horan, T. 1998, 'Virtual communities and social capital', *Social Science Computer Review*, vol. 16, pp. 293–307.

Bloom, N., Kretschmer, T. and Van Reenen, J. 2006, 'Work–life balance, management practices and productivity', Centre for Economic Performance, The London School of Economics and Political Science.

Board of Studies NSW 1999, *Personal Development, Health and Physical Education, Stage 6 Syllabus*, Board of Studies, NSW, viewed 2 March 2005, <www.board ofstudies.nsw.edu.au/syllabus99/syllabus2000lista.html>

Booker, V., Robinson, J., Kay, B., Najera, L. and Stewart, G. 1997, 'Changes in empowerment: Effects of participation in a lay health promotion program', *Health Education and Behavior*, vol. 24, no. 4, pp. 452–64.

Booth, M.L. and Samdal, O. 1997, 'Health-promoting schools in Australia: Models and measurement', *Australian and New Zealand Journal of Public Health*, vol. 21, no. 4, pp. 365–70.

Bourke, L. 2001, 'Australian rural consumers' perceptions of health issues', *Australian Journal of Rural Health*, vol. 9, no. 1, pp. 1–6.

Bramley, D., Hebert, P., Rod Jackson, R. and Chassin, M. 2004, 'Indigenous disparities in disease-specific mortality, a crosscountry comparison: New Zealand, Australia, Canada, and the United States', *The New Zealand Medical Journal*, vol. 117, no. 1207, viewed 22 July 2005, <www.nzma.org.nz/journal/117–1207/1215/content.pdf>

Bramston, P., Rogers-Clark, C., Hegney, D. and Bishop, J. 2000, 'Gender roles and geographic location as predictors of emotional distress in Australian women', *Australian Journal of Rural Health*, vol. 8, pp. 154–60.

Breckon, D.J. 1997, *Managing Health Promotion Programs: Leadership skills for the 21st Century*, Aspen Publishers, Baltimore, MD.

Breucker, G. 2004, *Towards Healthy Organisations in Europe: From utopia to real practice*, BKK Federal Association, Essen, Germany European Network for Workplace Health Promotion, viewed 2 June 2005, <www.enwhp.org/download/Towards%20Healthy%20Organisations%20in%20Europe.doc>

Bridgman, P. and Davis, G. 2000, *The Australian Policy Handbook*, 2nd edn, Allen & Unwin, Sydney.

Brown, V.A. 1992, 'Health care policies, health policies, or policies for health', in H. Gardner (ed.), *Health Policy*, Churchill Livingstone, Melbourne.

Brown, V.A., Ritchie, J.E. and Rotem, A. 1992, 'Health promotion and environmental management: A partnership for the future', *Health Promotion International*, vol. 7, no. 3, pp. 219–30.

Buckley, P. and Gray, G. 1993, *Across the Spinifex: Registered nurses working in rural and remote South Australia*, Flinders University of South Australia, School of Nursing, Adelaide.

Butler, P. and Cass, S. 1993, *Case Studies in Community Development*, Centre for Development and Innovation in Health, Blackburn, Vic.

Butterfoss, F.D., Goodman, R.M. and Wandersman, A. 1993, 'Community coalitions for prevention and health promotion', *Health Education Research: Theory and practice*, vol. 8, no. 3, pp. 315–30.

Calgary Health Region, viewed 24 November 2005, <www.calgaryhealthregion.ca/hecomm/pubpolicy/faces.htm> (adapted from the Health Promotion Framework developed by Hamilton, N. and Bhatti, T. 1996, *Population Health Promotion: An integrated model of population health and health promotion*, Health Promotion Development Division, Ottawa.)

Carson, B.E. and Bailie, R. 2004, 'National health workforce in discrete Indigenous communities', *Australian and New Zealand Journal of Public Health*, vol. 28, no. 3, pp. 235–45.

Cass, A., Cunningham, J., Snelling, P., Wang, Z. and Hoy, W. 2004, 'Exploring the pathways leading from disadvantage to end-stage renal disease for Indigenous Australians', *Social Science & Medicine*, vol. 58, no. 4, pp. 767–85.

Catford, J. 1991, Editorial, 'Primary environmental care: An ecological strategy for health', *Health Promotion International*, vol. 6, no. 4, pp. 239–40.

——1994, 'Strategic management in health promotion', workshop presented at the School of Public Health, Queensland University of Technology, Brisbane, 6 June.

——2004, 'Health promotion: Origins, obstacles and opportunities', in H. Keleher and B. Murphy (eds), *Understanding Health: A determinants approach*, Oxford University Press, Oxford.

Centers for Disease Control and Prevention (CDC) 1999, *Framework for Program Evaluation in Public Health*, MMWR 1999, 48 (no. RR–11), pp. 1–40.

——2000, Evaluation Working Group, 'Practical evaluation of public health programs', viewed 20 September 2005, <www.cdc.gov/eval/workbook.PDF>

——2005a, National Center for Chronic Disease Prevention and Health Promotion, 'Coordinated School Health Programs' (CSHP), viewed 31 January 2005, <www.cdc.gov/HealthyYouth/CSHP/index.htm>

——2005b, Centers for Disease Control and Prevention, 'Moving into Action: Promoting heart-healthy and stroke-free communities (employers)', US Department of Health and Human Services, Atlanta, GA.

Center of Excellence in Disaster Management and Humanitarian Assistance (COEDMHA), viewed 17 January 2005, <http://coe-dmha.org/Tsunami/Tsu013005.htm>

Centre for Rural Social Research 1992, *Better Rural Health: Guidelines for education and training programs for rural health workers*, Charles Sturt University, Wagga Wagga.

Chang, J. 2004, 'Balancing act', *Sales and Marketing Management*, vol. 156, no. 2, p. 16.

Channon, M. 1993, 'Review of goals and targets for Australia's health in the year 2000 and beyond', *Consumers' Health Forum of Australia*, no. 25, May.

Chapman, S. and Lupton, D. 1994, *The Fight for Public Health: Principles and Practice of Media Advocacy*, British Medical Journal Publishing Group, Sydney.

Charlton, R. 1993, 'Should lifestyle and health promotion of the workforce be employer responsibilities?', *Journal of Occupational Health and Safety Australia and New Zealand*, vol. 9, no. 6, pp. 585–9.

Chaskin, R.J. 2001, 'Building community capacity: A definitional framework and case studies from a comprehensive community initiative', *Urban Affairs Review*, vol. 36, no. 3, pp. 291–323.

Chen, J. and Kennedy, C.M. 2001, 'Television viewing and children's health', *JSPN*, vol. 6, no. 1, pp. 35–8.

Child, J. 2005, *Organization: Contemporary principles and practice*, Blackwell, Malden, MA.

Chu, C., Breucker, G., Harris, N., Stitzel, A., Gan, X., Gu, X. and Dwyer, S. 2000, 'Health promoting workplaces: International settings development', *Health Promotion International*, vol. 15, no. 2, pp. 155–67.

Chu, C., Driscoll, T. and Dwyer, S. 1997, 'The health promoting workplace: An integrative perspective', *Australian and New Zealand Journal of Public Health*, vol. 21, no. 4, pp. 377–85.

Chu, C. and Dwyer, S. 2002, 'Employer role in integrative workplace health management: A new model in progress', *Disease Management & Health Outcomes*, vol. 10, no. 3, pp. 175–86.

Chu, C. and Forrester, C. 1992, *Workplace Health Promotion in Queensland*, Queensland Health, Better Health Program, Brisbane.

Clarke, L. and Wolfenden, K. 1991, 'Community organisation to reduce injury on Australian farms', *Health Promotion Journal of Australia*, vol. 1, no. 2, pp. 17–22.

Clay, E. 2005, *Making Sense of the Indian Ocean Tsunami*, Overseas Development Institute, viewed 17 January 2005, <www.odi.org.uk/tsunami.html>

Cockburn, J., White, V.M., Hirst, S. and Hill, D. 1991, 'Response of older rural women to a cervical screening campaign', *Health Promotion Journal of Australia*, vol. 1, no. 1, pp. 29–34.

Cohen, S. and Syme, L. 1985, 'Issues in the study and application of social support', in S. Cohen and L. Syme (eds), *Social Support and Health*, Academic Press, Los Angeles.

Colby-Rivkin, M. and Hoopman, M. 1991, *Moving Beyond Risk to Resiliency*, Minneapolis Public Schools, Minneapolis.

Colquhoun, D., Goltz, K. and Sheehan, M. (eds) 1997, *The Health Promoting School. Policy: Programmes and practice in Australia*, Harcourt, Brace and Company, Sydney.

Commonwealth Department of Community Services and Health 1989, *National Better Health Program, Strategic Plan 1989–90 to 1991–92*, AGPS, Canberra.

Commonwealth Department of Health 2004, National Tobacco Legislation Chart, Summary of Existing Legislation.

Commonwealth Department of Health and Aged Care 1998, *Review of the General Practice Strategy*, General Practice Branch, Health Services Division, Canberra.

——2000a, *General Practice in Australia: 2000*, General Practice Branch, Health Services Division, Canberra.

——2000b, *National HIV/AIDS Strategy 1999–2000 to 2003–2004*, Health Services Division, Canberra.

——2003, *Returns on Investment in Public Health: An epidemiological and economic analysis*, Population Health Division, Canberra.

——2004, *National Heart, Stroke and Vascular Health Strategies Group*, National Strategy for Heart, Stroke And Vascular Health In Australia, Canberra, viewed 7 July 2005, <www.seniors.gov.au./internet/wcms/publishing.nsf/Content health-pq-cardio-pubs-strathsvh03.htm/$FILE/strategy.pdf>

Commonwealth Department of Health and Aged Care and the National Key Centre for Social Applications of Geographical Information Systems (GISCA) at the University of Adelaide 1999, 'Measuring Remoteness: Accessibility/remoteness index of Australia' (ARIA), occasional papers: new series no. 6.

Commonwealth Department of Health and Ageing 2003, *Cost-Benefit Analysis of Proposed New Health Warnings on Tobacco Products*, report prepared by Applied Economics for Commonwealth Department of Health and Ageing, viewed 24 August 2005, <www.treasury.gov.au/documents/790/PDF/Cost_Benefit_Analysis.pdf>

——2004, viewed 17 August 2005, <www.health.gov.au>

——2005a, *Enhanced Primary Care Program*, viewed 7 June 2005, <www.health.gov.au/epc>

——2005b, *National HIV/AIDS Strategy 2005–2008: Revitalising Australia's Response*, Health & Ageing, Canberra.

——2005c, 'Health Priorities', viewed 17 August 2005, <www.health.gov.au/internet/wcms/publishing.nsf/content/health%20priorities-1>

Commonwealth of Australia 2002, *National Strategy for an Ageing Australia: An older Australia, challenges and opportunities for all*, Health & Ageing, Canberra.

Coonan, W., Owen, N. and Mendoza, J. 1990, 'Australia: Perspectives in school health', *Journal of School Health*, vol. 60, no. 7, pp. 301–7.

Coutts, J., Roberts, K., Frost, F. and Coutts, A. 2005, *The Role of Extension in Building Capacity: What works, and why*, Rural Industries Research and Development Corporation, Barton, ACT.

Couzos, S. and Murray, R. for the Kimberley Aboriginal Medical Services Council 2003, *Aboriginal Primary Health Care: An evidence-based approach*, 2nd edn, Oxford University Press, Melbourne.

Cullen, A. 2002, 'Health promotion in the changing face of the hospital landscape', *Collegian*, vol. 9, no. 1, pp. 41–2.

Curtin University of Technology 2005, viewed 16 February 2006, <http://lifestyle.curtin.edu.au/index.cfm>

Dahlgren, G. and Whitehead, M. 1992, *Policies and Strategies to Promote Equity in Health*, World Health Organization, Copenhagen.

Davis, A. and George, J. 1998, *States of Health: Health and illness in Australia*, 3rd edn, Harper & Row, Sydney.

Denner, B. 2001, 'Rural workplace health promotion', paper presented at the 6th National Rural Health Conference, Canberra, 4–7 March 2001.

Department of Health, England 2005, viewed 3 November 2005,

Department of Health, Housing and Community Services 1991a, *National Rural Health Strategy*, AGPS, Canberra.

——1991b, *Researching Women's Health: An issues paper*, AGPS, Canberra.

——1993, *Towards Health For All and Health Promotion: The evaluation of the National Better Health Program*, AGPS, Canberra.

Department of Human Services and Health 1995, *The Health of Young Australians: A national health policy for children and young people*, AGPS, Canberra.

Deschesnes, M., Martin, C. and Jomphe Hill, A. 2003, 'Comprehensive approaches to school health promotion: How to achieve broader implementation?', *Health Promotion International*, vol. 18, no. 4, pp. 387–95.

Dewe, P., Leiter, M. and Cox, T. (eds) 2000, *Coping, Health and Organizations*, Taylor and Francis, London.

Dhillon, H.S. and Philip, L. 1992–93, 'Health in education for all: Enabling school-age children and adults for healthy living', *Hygie*, vol. XI, pp. 17–23.

Dooner, B. 1990–91, 'Achieving a healthier workplace', *Health Promotion Canada*, vol. 29, no. 3, winter, pp. 2–6, 24.

Dorrell, K. 2001, 'Myth of work–life balance', *Benefits Canada*, vol. 25, no. 9, p. 21.

Dow, C. and Gardiner-Garden, J. 1998, 'Indigenous affairs in Australia, New Zealand, Canada, United States of America, Norway and Sweden', Social Policy Group, Paliamentary Library, background paper 15 1997–98, viewed 31 August 2005, <www.aph.gov.au/library/pubs/bp/1997–98/98bp15.htm>

Drucker, P.F. 1990, *Managing the Non-Profit Organisation: Practices and principles*, Butterworth-Heinemann, Oxford.

——1991, 'The new productivity challenge', *Harvard Business Review*, November–December, pp. 69–79.

Duhl, L. 2003, untitled, in Tibbetts, J. 'Spheres of influence, building civic health', *Environmental Health Perspectives*, vol. 111, no. 7.

Dunphy, D. and Griffiths, A. 1998, *The Sustainable Corporation: Organisational renewal in Australia*, Allen & Unwin, Sydney.

Dutton, T., Turrell, G. and Oldenburg, B. 2005, *Measuring socioeconomic position in population health monitoring and health research*, Health Inequalities Monitoring Series No. 3, Queensland University of Technology, Brisbane.

Dwyer, S. 1997, 'Improving delivery of a health-promoting-environments program: Experiences from Queensland Health', *Australian and New Zealand Journal of Public Health*, vol. 21, no. 4, pp. 398–402.

——2000, 'Integrating public health: Exploring models of local practice', Dissertation for Master of Public Health, Queensland University of Technology, Brisbane.

Edye, B., Mandryk, J., Frommer, M., Healey, S. and Ferguson, D. 1989, 'Evaluation of a worksite program for the modification of cardio-vascular risk factors', *Medical Journal of Australia*, vol. 150, pp. 574–81.

Egger, G., Spark, R. and Donovan, R. 2005, *Health Promotion, Strategies and Methods*, 2nd edn, McGraw-Hill, Sydney.

Engelhardt, H.T. 1981, 'The concepts of health and disease', in A.L. Caplan, H.T. Engelhardt and J.J. McCartney (eds), *Concepts of Health and Disease: Interdisciplinary perspectives*, Addison-Wesley, Reading, Mass.

Erben, R., Franzkowiak, K. and Wenzel, E. 1999, 'People empowerment vs. social capital: From health promotion to social marketing', *Health Promotion Journal of Australia*, vol. 9, no. 3, pp. 179–82.

Erben, R., International Union for Health Promotion and Education, Regional Office for the South West Pacific, 1998–2000, viewed 7 September 2005, <www.ldb.org/iuhpe/brisb_98.htm>

Esterman, A.J. and Ben-Tovim, D.I. 2002, 'The Australian coordinated care trials: Success or failure?', *Medical Journal of Australia*, vol. 177, no. 9, pp. 469–70.

Etzioni, A. and Etzioni, O. 1997, 'Communities: Virtual vs. real', *Science*, Issue 5324, vol. 277, July, p. 18.

Everingham, R. and Woodward, S. 1991, *Tobacco Litigation: The case against passive smoking*, Legal Books, Sydney.

Evers, K.E., Cummins, C.O., Prochaska, J.O. and Prochaska, J.M. 2005, 'Online health behavior and disease management programs: Are we ready for them? Are they ready for us?', *Journal of Medical Internet Research*, vol. 7, no. 3, p. e27.

Ewles, I. and Simnett, L. 1995, *Promoting Health: A practical guide*, 3rd edn, Scutari, London.

——2003, *Promoting Health: A practical guide*, 5th edn, Baillière Tindall, New York.

Farmsafe '88 1989, Papers and Proceedings of the Farmsafe '88 Conference, University of New England, Armidale, NSW, 26–29 June.

Farquhar, J.W., Fortmann, S.P., Flora, J.A., Taylor, C.B., Haskell, W.L., Williams, P.T., Maccoby, N. and Wood, P.D. 1990, 'Effects of community-wide education on cardiovascular risk factors: The Stanford Five-City Project', *Journal of the American Medical Association*, vol. 264, pp. 359–65.

Farquhar, J.W., Lefebvre, C. and Blackburn, H. 1985, 'The Stanford Five-City Project: An overview', in J.D. Matarazzo et al. (eds), *Behavioral Health: A handbook of health education and disease prevention*, Wiley, New York.

Farr, T. 1994, Senior Lecturer, Occupational Health and Safety, School of Public Health, Queensland University of Technology, Brisbane, personal correspondence.

Fejo, L. 1994, 'The Strong Women, Strong Babies, Strong Culture Program', *Aboriginal and Islander Health Worker Journal*, vol. 18, no. (6), p. 16.

——1997, 'Strong Women, Strong Babies, Strong Culture Program', AAHPP and PHA (HPSIG) Ninth National Health Promotion Conference, Abstracts, 18–20 May 1997, Darwin, p. 24.

Foucault, M. 1979, *Discipline and Punish: The birth of the prison*, Peregrine Books, Middlesex.

Fragar, L. and Franklin, R.J. 2000, *The health and safety of Australia's farming communities*, a report prepared for the National Farm Injury Data Centre for the Farm Safety Joint Research Venture, ACAHS and RIRDC, Moree.

Franklin, R., Mitchell, R., Driscoll, T. and Fragar, L. 2000, *Farm-Related Fatalities in Australia, 1989–1992*, ACAHS, NOHSC and RIRDC, Moree.

Franks, H.M. and Cronan, T.A. 2004, 'Social support in women with fibromyalgia: Is quality more important than quantity?', *Journal of Community Psychology*, vol. 32, no. 4, pp. 425–38.

Freeman, P. and Rotem, A. 1999, *Essential Primary Health Care Services for Health Development in Remote Aboriginal Communities in the Northern Territory*, WHO Regional Training Centre for Health Development, University of New South Wales, Sydney.

Freire, P. 1973, *Education for Critical Consciousness*, Seabury Press, New York.

Freudenberg, N., Eng, E., Flay, B., Parcel, G., Roberts, T. and Wallerstein, N. 1995, 'Strengthening individual and community capacity to prevent disease and promote health: In search of relevant theories and principles', *Health Education Quarterly*, vol. 22, no. 3, pp. 290–306.

Friedman, R.H. 1998, 'Automated telephone conversations to assess health behavior and deliver behavioral interventions', *Journal of Medical Systems*, vol. 22, no. 2, pp. 95–102.

Fry, D. and Baum, F. 1992, 'Keywords in community health', in F. Baum and D. Fry (eds), *Community Health: Policy and practice in Australia*, Pluto Press, Sydney, pp. 296–309.

Gandevia, B.H. 1971, 'Occupation and disease in Australia since 1788: Part one', *Bulletin of the Postgraduate Committee in Medicine*, vol. 27, no. 8, pp. 157–97.

Gardner, H. and Barraclough, S. 2004, 'Continuity and change in Australian health policy', in *Health Policy in Australia* [electronic resource], H. Gardner and S. Barraclough (eds), Oxford University Press, South Melbourne.

Garrison, D.R. 1992, 'Critical thinking and self-directed learning in adult education: An analysis of responsibility and control issues', *Adult Education Quarterly*, vol. 42, no. 3, pp. 136–48.

General Practice Consultative Committee 1992, *The Future of General Practice: A strategy for the nineties and beyond*, AMA, Parkes, ACT.

Gibbin, E.J.T. 1932, 'Sydney Hospital', *Sydney Medical Journal*, pp. 69–70.

Gibbon, M., Labonte, R. and Laverack, G. 2002, 'Evaluating community capacity', *Health and Social Care in the Community*, vol. 10, no. 6, pp. 485–91.

Girgis, A., Sanson-Fisher, R., Redman, S. and Schofield, M. 1993, 'The staged approach: Resource allocation in health promotion', *National Health Strategy Issues*, paper no. 7, Pathways to Better Health, National Health Strategy Unit, Melbourne.

Glanz, K., Lewis, F.M. and Rimer, B.K. (eds) 1997, *Health Behavior and Health Education: Theory, research, and practice*, Jossey-Bass, San Francisco.

——2002, *Health Behavior and Health Education: Theory, research, and practice*, 3rd edn, Jossey-Bass, San Francisco.

Glasgow, R.E. 2002, 'Evaluation of theory-based interventions: The RE-AIM model', in K. Glanz, F.M. Lewis and B.K. Rimer (eds), *Health Behavior and Health Education: Theory, research, and practice*, 3rd edn, Jossey-Bass, San Francisco, pp. 530–44.

Glasgow, R.E., Vogt, T.M. and Boles, S.M. 1999, 'Evaluating the public health impact of health promotion interventions: The RE-AIM framework', *American Journal of Public Health*, vol. 89, no. 9, pp. 1322–7.

Goetzel, R., Anderson, D., Whitmer, R., Ozminkowski, R., Dunn, R., Wasserman, J. and the Health Enhancement Research Organization (HERO) Research Committee 1998, 'The relationship between modifiable health risks and health care expenditures: An analysis of the multi-employer HERO health risk and cost database', *Journal of Occupational and Environmental Medicine*, vol. 40, no. 10, pp. 843–54.

Golds, M. 1994, 'Taking programs to the communities', *Aboriginal and Islander Health Worker Journal*, vol. 18, no. 6, pp. 14–16.

Golds, M., King, R., Meiklejohn, B., Campion, S. and Wise, M. 1997, 'Healthy Aboriginal communities', *Australian and New Zealand Journal of Public Health*, vol. 21, no. 4, pp. 386–9.

Gomel, M. and Oldenburg, B. 1990, 'The NSW Ambulance Service Healthy Lifestyle Program: A case study in the evaluation of a health promotion program', *Australian Health Review*, vol. 13, no. 2, pp. 133–8.

Goodman, R.M., Speers, M.A., McLeroy, K., Fawcett, S., Kegler, M., Parker, E., Smith, S.R., Sterling, T.D. and Wallerstein, N. 1998, 'Identifying and defining the dimensions of community capacity to provide a basis for measurement', *Health Education & Behavior*, vol. 25, no. 3, pp. 258–78.

Goodstadt, M.S., Hyndman, B., McQueen, D.V., Potvin, L., Rootman, I. and Springett, J. 2001, 'Evaluation in health promotion: synthesis and recommendations', in I. Rootman, M.S. Goodstadt, B. Hyndman, D.V. McQueen, L. Potvin, J. Springett and Z. Ziglio (eds), *Evaluation in Health Promotion: Principles and perspectives*, WHO Regional Publications, European series, no. 92, World Health Organization, viewed 31 August 2005, <http://prevention-dividend.com/en/tools/Evaluation_in_Health_Promotion.htm>

Gordon, D. 1976, *Health, Sickness and Society*, University of Queensland Press, Brisbane.

Gorey, F. 1994, 'Health promoting hospitals: Process on the road from theory to reality', in C. Chu and R. Simpson (eds), *Ecological Public Health: From vision to practice*, Institute of Applied Environmental Research, Griffith University, Brisbane.

Gottlieb, B. 1983, *Social Support Strategies: Guidelines for mental health practice*, Sage Publications, Beverly Hills, CA.

Gracey, M., Williams, P. and Smith, P. 2000, 'Aboriginal deaths in Western Australia: 1985–89 and 1990–94', *Australian and New Zealand Journal of Public Health*, vol. 24, no. 2, pp. 145–52.

Green L., Richard, L. and Potvin, L. 1996, 'Ecological foundations of health promotion', *American Journal of Health Promotion*, vol. 10, no. 4, pp. 270–81.

Green, L.W. 1986, *Community Health*, Mayfield Press, St Louis.

Green, L.W. and Kreuter, M.W. 1991, *Health Promotion Planning: An Educational and Environmental Approach*, 2nd edn, Mayfield, Mountain View, CA.

——1999, *Health Promotion Planning: An educational and ecological approach*, 3rd edn, Mayfield Publishing Co., Mountain View.

——2005, *Health Program Planning: An educational and ecological approach*, 4th edn, McGraw-Hill, New York.

Green, L.W. and Lewis, F. 1986, *Measurement and Evaluation in Health Education and Health Promotion*, Mayfield, Palo Alto, CA.

Green, L.W. and Ottoson, J.M. 1998, *Community and population health*, 8th edn, WCB/McGraw-Hill, Boston.

Green, L.W., Poland, B.D. and Rootman, I. 2000, 'The settings approach to health promotion', in B.D. Poland, L.W. Green and I. Rootman (eds), *Settings for Health Promotion: Linking theory and practice*, Sage Publications, Thousand Oaks/Newbury Park, CA.

Green, L.W. and Raeburn, J.M. 1988, 'Health promotion. What is it? What will it become?', *Health Promotion*, vol. 3, no. 2, pp. 151–9.

——1990, 'Contemporary developments in health promotion: Definitions and challenges', in A. Bracht (ed.), *Health Promotion at the Community Level*, Sage Publications, Newbury Park, CA.

Gross, P.F., Leeder, S.R. and Lewis, M.J. 2003, 'Australia confronts the challenge of chronic disease', *Medical Journal of Australia*, vol. 179, no. 5, pp. 233–4.

Gross, S.M. and Cinelli, B. 2004, 'Coordinated school health program and dietetics professionals: Partners in promoting healthful eating', *Journal of the American Dietetic Association*, vol. 104, no. 5, p. 793.

Gun, R. 1990, 'The union movement and workplace health promotion', *Health At Work Newsletter*, no. 6, spring, pp. 4–5.

Hanchett, E. 1979, 'General systems theory and the community', *Community Health Assessment: A conceptual tool kit*, John Wiley & Sons, New York.

Hancock, T. 1986, 'Après Lalonde—promoting health in the 1980s', *Health Promotion*, vol. 1, no. 1, pp. 99–100.

Hancock, T. and Duhl, L. 1988, *Promoting Health in the Urban Context*, FADL, Copenhagen.

Harper, A.C., Holman, A., D'Arcy, J. and Dawes, V.P. 1994, *The Health of Populations: An introduction*, 2nd edn, Churchill Livingstone, Melbourne.

Harris, C. and Turner, J. 2005, 'Engaging Aboriginal Elders to create a successful program for the community', *Vascular Health Matters*, vol. 13, pp. 4–5.

Harris, E., Wise, M., Hawe, P. and Nutbeam, D. 1994, *Intersectoral Partnerships for Health*, draft report, AGPS, Canberra.

Harris, M.M. and Fennell, M.L. 1988, 'Perceptions of an employee assistance program and employees' willingness to participate', *Journal of Applied Behavioural Science*, vol. 24, no. 4, pp. 423–38.

Hawe, P. 1994, 'Capturing the meaning of "community" in community intervention evaluation: Some contributions from community psychology', *Health Promotion International*, vol. 9, no. 3, pp. 199–208.

Hawe, P., Degeling, D. and Hall, J. 1990, *Evaluating Health Promotion: A health workers guide*, MacLennan and Petty, Sydney.

Hayes, B. 2000, Lady Ramsay Child Care Centre, Brisbane, personal communication.

Health Education Quarterly 1994, vol. 21, no. 2 (full issue on empowerment and health promotion).

Health Inequalities Research Collaboration, Primary Health Care Network (HIRC PHC Network) 2004, *Action on health inequalities: A primary health care research program*, report of a national roundtable, 24 February 2004, Canberra.

Health and Welfare Canada 1977, *Evaluation Guidelines*, Ontario.

Health Ministers Forum 1994, *Towards a National Health Policy: A discussion paper*, New South Wales Department of Health, Sydney.

Health Promotion International 1986, *Editorial: definitions and terms*, vol. 1, no. 2, p. 73.

Health Promotion Queensland 2000, *Development of a Multi-strategy Health Promotion Intervention in a Model Community: Partners working for healthier communities—Bowen and Collinsville*, Queensland Health, Health Promotion Queensland.

Health Targets and Implementation (Health For All) Committee 1988, *Health For All Australians*, report to the Australian Health Ministers' Advisory Council and the Australian Health Ministers Conference, AGPS, Canberra.

Hirst, S., Mitchell, H. and Medley, G. 1990, 'An evaluation of a campaign to increase cervical cancer screening in rural Victoria', *Community Health Studies*, vol. XIV, no. 3, pp. 263–8.

Historical Records of New South Wales 1892–1901, vol. 1, part 2, *Phillip, 1783–1793*, W. Britton, Government Printer, Sydney.

Hobson, C.J., Delunas, L. and Kesic, D. 2001, 'Compelling evidence of the need for corporate work/life balance initiatives: Results from a national survey of stressful life-events', *Journal of Employment Counseling*, vol. 38, no. 1, pp. 38–44.

Holman, C.D. 1992, 'Something old, something new: Perspectives on five "new" public health movements', *Health Promotion Journal of Australia*, vol. 2, no. 3, pp. 4–11.

Holman, H. and Lorig, L. 2000, 'Patients as partners in managing chronic disease', *British Medical Journal*, vol. 320, issue 7234, pp. 526–8.

Hoy, W.E., Rees, M., Kile, E., Mathews, J.D. and Wang, Z. 1999, 'A new dimension to the Barker hypothesis: Low birthweight and susceptibility to renal disease', *Kidney International*, vol. 56, no. 3, pp. 1072–7.

Humphreys, J.S. 2000, 'Health and the 1999 Regional Australia Summit', *Australian Journal of Rural Health*, no. 8, pp. 52–7.

Humphreys, J.S., Matthews-Cowey, S. and Weinand, H.C. 1997, 'Factors in accessibility of general practice in rural Australia', *Medical Journal of Australia*, no. 166, pp. 577–80.

Humphreys, J.S., Rolley, F. and Weinand, H.C. 1993, 'Evaluating the importance of information sources for preventive health care in rural Australia', *Australian Journal of Public Health*, vol. 17, no. 2, pp. 149–57.

Humphreys, J.S. and Weinand, H.C. 1989, 'Health status and health care in rural Australia: A case study', *Community Health Studies*, vol. XIII, no. 3, pp. 258–75.

Hutton, C. 2005, 'Divisions of General Practice, capacity building and health reform', *Australian Family Physician*, vol. 34, no. 1/2, pp. 64–6.

Improving Chronic Illness Care (ICIC) 2006, viewed 15 March 2006, <www.improvingchroniccare.org/change/model/components.html#citation>

In Touch 2005, 'Health Promotion Competencies for Australia', newsletter of the Public Health Association of Australia Inc., vol. 22, no. 9, pp. 9–10.

International Conference on Engaging Communities (ICEC) 2005, United Nations and the Queensland Government, 14–17 August 2005, Brisbane, viewed 9 February 2006, <www.engagingcommunities2005.org/home.html>

Ippolito-Shepherd, J. 2003, 'Health-promoting schools initiative in the Americas', *UN Chronicle*, vol. 40, pp. 16–18.

Jackson, T., Mitchell, S. and Wright, M. 1989, 'The community development continuum', *Community Health Studies*, vol. XIII, no. 1, pp. 66–73.

Johnson, A. and Baum, F. 2001, 'Health promoting hospitals: A typology of different organizational approaches to health promotion', *Health Promotion International*, vol. 16, no. 3, pp. 281–7.

Johnson, A. and Nolan, J. 2004, 'Health promoting hospitals: Gaining an understanding about collaboration', *Australian Journal of Primary Health*, vol. 10, no. 2, pp. 51–60.

Johnston, T. and Coory, M. 2005, 'Reducing perinatal mortality among Indigenous babies in Queensland: Should the first priority be better primary health care or better access to hospital care during confinement?', *Australia and New Zealand Health Policy*, vol. 2, no. 11, viewed 7 July 2005, <www.anzhealthpolicy.com/content/2/1/11>

Jones, J., Kickbusch, I. and O'Byrne, D. 1995, 'Improving health through schools', *World Health*, March–April, vol. 48, no. 2, pp. 10–12.

Jones, S. 1987, 'Current status of health promotion in the workplace in Australia', paper presented at the Health Promotion in the Workplace Conference, Canberra.

Judd, J., Frankish, C.J. and Moulton, G. 2001, 'Setting standards in the evaluation of community-based health promotion programmes—a unifying approach', *Health Promotion International*, vol. 16, no. 4, pp. 367–80.

Kahan, B. and Goodstadt, M. 2001, 'The interactive domain model of best practices in health promotion: Developing and implementing a best practices approach to health promotion', *Health Promotion Practice*, vol. 2, no. 1, pp. 43–67.

——2005, *IDM Manual: IDM manual for using the interactive domain model approach to best practices in health promotion*, 3rd edn May 2005, Centre for Health Promotion, University of Toronto, Toronto.

Kakabadse, A. 2004, *Working in organisations*, Ashgate, Burlington, VT.

Katz, A. and Bender, E. 1976, *The Strength in Us: Self-help groups in the modern world*, New Viewpoints, New York.

Katz, D.L., O'Connell, M., Yeh, M-C., Nawaz, H., Njike, V., Anderson, L.M., Cory, S. and Dietz, W. 2005, 'Public health strategies for preventing and controlling over-weight and obesity in school and worksite settings: A report on recommendations of the task force on community preventive services', MMWR Recommendations and Reports, vol. 54 (RR10), pp. 1–12.

Kerr, J., Weitkunat, R. and Moretti, M. (eds) 2005, *ABC of Behaviour Change: A guide to successful disease prevention and health promotion*, Elsevier Churchill Livingstone, Edinburgh.

Kickbusch, I. 1986a, 'Health promotion: A global perspective', *Canadian Journal of Public Health*, vol. 77, September–October, pp. 321–6.

——1986b, 'Lifestyles and health', *Social Science and Medicine*, vol. 22, no. 2, pp. 117–24.

——1987, 'Issues in health promotion: Dr Ilona Kickbusch', *Health Promotion*, vol. 1, no. 4, pp. 437–41.

——1988, 'Introduction', in R. Anderson, J.K. Davies, I. Kickbusch, D.V. McQueen and J. Turner (eds), *Health Behaviour Research and Health Promotion*, Oxford Medical Publications, Oxford.

——1989a, editorial, *Health Promotion International*, vol. 1, no. 1, pp. 3–4.

——1989b, 'The new public health', address given to the Queensland branch of the Australian Public Health Association, Brisbane, 5 May.

——1989c, 'Self-care in health promotion', *Social Sciences and Medicine*, vol. 29, no. 2, pp. 125–30.

——1997, 'Health promoting environments: The next step', *Australian and New Zealand Journal of Public Health*, vol. 21, no. 4, pp. 431–4.

——1999, 'Good planets are hard to find', in M. Honari and T. Boleyn, *Health Ecology: Health, culture and human-environment interaction*, Routledge, London & New York.

Kiernan, M.J. 1993, 'The new strategic architecture: Learning to compete in the twenty-first century', *Academy of Management Executive*, vol. 7, no. 1, pp. 7–21.

King, L. 1996, 'An outcomes hierarchy for health promotion: A tool for policy, planning and evaluation', *Health Promotion Journal of Australia*, vol. 6, no. 2, pp. 50–1.

King, L. and Ritchie, J. 1999, 'Promoting health in the Northern Territory: A review', WHO Regional Training Centre for Health Development, University of New South Wales, Sydney.

Kirmayer, L., Simpson, C. and Cargo, M. 2003, 'Healing traditions: Culture, community and mental health promotion with Canadian Aboriginal peoples', *Australasian Psychiatry*, vol. 11, supplement, pp. s15–s23.

Kok, G. 1993, 'Why are so many health promotion programs ineffective?', *Health Promotion Journal of Australia*, vol. 3, no. 2, pp. 12–17.

Kok, G. and Green, L. 1990, 'Research to support health promotion in practice: A plea for increased co-operation', *Health Promotion International*, vol. 5, no. 4, pp. 303–8.

Kolbe, L.J. 2005, 'A framework for school health programs in the 21st century', *Journal of School Health*, vol. 75, issue 6, pp. 226–9.

Kreger, A. 1991, *Report on the National Nursing Consultative Committee Project: Enhancing the role of rural and remote nurses*, Department of Health, Housing and Community Services, Canberra.

Labonte, R. 1991a, 'International perspectives on healthy communities', in *Keeping Ahead: Local government and the community health debate*, Municipal Association of Victoria, Melbourne.

——1991b, *Community Health Empowerment*, Centre for Health Promotion, University of Toronto, Toronto.

——1992a, *Community Health and Empowerment: Notes on the new health promotion practice*, Health Promotion Centre, University of Toronto, Toronto.

——1992b, 'Heart health inequalities in Canada: Models, theory and planning', *Health Promotion International*, vol. 7, no. 2, pp. 119–27.

——1993, 1994, *Health Promotion and Empowerment: Practice frameworks*, Issues in Health Promotion Series, Centre for Health Promotion, University of Toronto, Toronto.

——1999, 'Social capital and community development: Practitioner emptor', *Australian and New Zealand Journal of Public Health*, vol. 3, no. 4, August, pp. 430–3.

——2005, 'Community, community development, and the forming of authentic partnerships: Some critical reflections', in M. Minkler (ed.), *Community Organizing and Community Building for Health*, Rutgers University Press, New Brunswick, NJ.

Labonte, R., Woodard, G., Chad, K. and Laverack, G. 2002, 'Community capacity building; A parallel track for health promotion programs', *Canadian Journal of Public Health*, vol. 93, no. 3, pp. 181–2.

Lalonde, M. 1974, *A New Perspective on the Health of Canadians: A working document*, Information Canada, Ottawa.

Last, J.M. 1983, *A Dictionary of Epidemiology*, Oxford University Press, Oxford.

——1997, *Public Health and Human Ecology*, 2nd edn, Appleton and Lange, Stamford, Connecticut.

Latrobe Regional Hospital 2005, viewed 27 February 2006, <www.lrh.com.au/Announcements_files/HPH.htm>

Lawson, J.S. and Bauman, A.E. 2001, 'Public health Australia: an introduction', 2nd edn, McGraw-Hill, Sydney.

Laverack, G. and Wallerstein, N. 2001, 'Measuring community empowerment: A fresh look at organizational domains', *Health Promotional International*, vol. 16, no. 2, pp. 179–85.

Lean, J. 1987, 'Small business health promotion report', *Journal of Occupational Health and Safety: Australia and New Zealand*, vol. 3, no. 1, pp. 27–34.

de Leeuw, E. 2005, 'Who gets what: Politics, evidence, and health promotion', *Health Promotion International*, vol. 20, no. 3, pp. 211–12.

de Leeuw, E. and Skovgaard, T. 2005, 'Utility-driven evidence for healthy cities: Problems with evidence generation and application', *Social Science & Medicine*, vol. 61, pp. 1331–41.

Legge, D. 1989, 'Towards a politics of health', in H. Gardner (ed.), *The Politics of Health: The Australian experience*, Churchill Livingstone, Melbourne.

——1991, 'Towards a politics of health', in H. Gardner (ed.), *The Politics of Health: The Australian experience*, Churchill Livingstone, Melbourne.

Legge, D. and Wilson, G. 1996, *Best Practice in Primary Health Care*, Centre for Development and Innovation in Health, Melbourne and Commonwealth Department of Health and Family Services, Canberra.

Leonard, D., McDermott, R., O'Dea, K., Rowley, K.G., Pensio, P., Sambo, E., Twist, A., Toolis, R., Lowson, S.K. and Best, J.D. 2002, 'Obesity, diabetes and associated cardiovascular risk factors among Torres Strait Islander people', *Australian and New Zealand Journal of Public Health*, vol. 26, no. 2, pp. 144–9.

Leppo, K. and Vertio, H. 1986, 'Smoking control in Finland: A case study in policy formulation and implementation', *Health Promotion International*, vol. 1, no. 1, pp. 5–16.

Lewin, K. 1951, *Field Theory in Social Science*, Harper & Row, New York.

Lewis, M.J. (ed.) 1989, *Health and Disease in Australia: A history*, AGPS, Canberra.

Lin, V. and Pearse, W. 1990, 'A workforce at risk', in J. Reid and P. Trompf (eds), *The Health of Immigrant Australia*, Harcourt Brace Jovanovich Publishers, Sydney.

Lincoln, Y. 1992, 'Fourth generation evaluation, the paradigm revolution and health promotion', *Canadian Journal of Public Health*, vol. 83, supp. 1, March/April.

Lister-Sharp, D., Chapman, S., Stewart-Brown, S. and Sowden, A. 1999, 'Health promoting schools and health promotion in schools: Two systematic reviews', *Health Technology Assessment*, vol. 3, no. 22, pp. 1–219.

Lloyd, P. 1994, 'Public health and national health policy', *Australian Journal of Public Health*, vol. 18, no. 4, pp. 357–8.

Lomas, J. 1997, 'Social capital and health: Implications for public health and epidemiology', *Social Science and Medicine*, vol. 47, no. 9, pp. 1181–8.

Lonvig, E. 2004, Implementation of a general prevention and health promotion strategy (PHP) at a large hospital: Process and model projects', Proceedings of the 12th International Conference on Health Promoting Hospitals, Moscow, 26–28 May.

Lorig, K. and Associates 2001, *Patient Education: A Practical approach*, 3rd edn, Sage Publications, Thousand Oaks, CA.

Lorig, K.R., Mazonson, P.D. and Holman, H.R. 1993, 'Evidence suggesting that health education for self-management in chronic arthritis has sustained health benefits while reducing health care costs', *Arthritis Rheumatology*, vol. 36, pp. 439–46.

Lorig, K.R., Sobel, D.S., Stewart, A.L., Brown, B.W., Bandura, A., Ritter, P., Gonzalez, V.M., Laurent, D.D. and Holman, H.R. 1999, 'Evidence suggesting that a chronic disease self-management program can improve health status while reducing hospitalization: A randomized trial', *Medical Care*, vol. 37, no. 1, pp. 5–14.

Mackerras, D. 1998, 'Evaluation of the Strong Women, Strong Babies, Strong Culture Program: results for the period 1990–1996 in the three pilot communities', Menzies School of Health Research, Darwin.

——2001, 'Birthweight changes in the pilot phase of the Strong Women, Strong Babies, Strong Culture Program in the Northern Territory', *Australian and New Zealand Journal of Public Health*, vol. 25, no. 1, pp. 34–40.

Macklin, J. 1990, *The National Health Strategy: Setting the agenda for change*, background paper 1, National Health Strategy Unit, Melbourne.

Maes, L. and Lievens, J. 2003, 'Can the school make a difference? A multilevel analysis of adolescent risk and health behaviour', *Social Science & Medicine*, vol. 56, no. 3, pp. 517–29.

Mathew, T. 2004, 'Addressing the epidemic of chronic kidney disease in Australia', *Nephrology*, vol. 9, pp. S109–12.

McArdle, J. 1993, 'Community development', *Resource Manual for Facilitators in Community Development*, Employ Publishing, Windsor, Victoria.

McDonald, S.P. and Russ, G.R. 2003, 'Burden of end-stage renal disease among indigenous peoples in Australia and New Zealand', *Kidney International*, vol. 63, suppl. 83, pp. S123–7.

McGrath, B.P. 1994, 'The development of divisions of general practice in Australia: Implications for ecological public health', in C. Chu and R. Simpson, *Ecological Public Health: From vision to practice*, Institute of Applied Environmental Research, Griffith University, Brisbane.

McKenzie, J.F., Neiger, B.L. and Smeltzer, J.L. 2005, *Planning, Implementing, and Evaluating Health Promotion Programs: A primer*, 4th edn, Pearson/Benjamin Cummings, New York.

McKenzie, J.F. and Smeltzer, J.L. 2001, *Planning, Implementing, and Evaluating Health Promotion Programs: A primer*, 3rd edn, Allan & Bacon, Boston.

McKeown, T. 1976, *The Role of Medicine: Dream, mirage or nemesis*, Nuffield Provincial Hospital Trust, London.

McLennon, V. and Khavarpour, F. 2004, 'Culturally appropriate health promotion: Its meaning and application in Aboriginal communities', *Health Promotion Journal of Australia*, vol. 15, no. 3, pp. 237–9.

McLeroy, K. 1994, 'Community coalitions for health promotion: Summary and further reflections', *Health Education Research Theory and Practice*, vol. 9, no. 1, pp. 1–11.

McMichael, A. 1990, 'Health promotion in the workplace—the national picture', paper presented at the Health Promotion in the Workplace Forum, Royal Exhibition Building Conference Centre, Carlton, Victoria, 21 November.

——1993, editorial, 'Public health in Australia: A personal reflection', *Australian Journal of Public Health*, vol. 17, no. 4, pp. 295–6.

McMurray, A. 1993, *Community Health Nursing: Primary health care in practice*, Churchill Livingstone, Melbourne.

——2003, *Community Health and Wellness: A socioecological approach*, Mosby, Sydney.

McPherson, P.D. 1992, 'Health for all Australians', in H. Gardner, *Health Policy*, Churchill Livingstone, Melbourne.

Medicare Australia (formerly the Health Insurance Commission) 2005, viewed 22 August 2005, <www.medicareaustralia.gov.au/yourhealth/our_services/aacir.htm>

Melhuish, A. 1982, *Work and Health*, Penguin, Harmondsworth, England.

Mendoza, J. 1990, Strategic Planning Made Easy, workshop, Adelaide.

——1993, *Model of Competencies*, School of Public Health, Queensland University of Technology, Brisbane.

——1994, *Draft Participants Manual*, Prevention Programs Unit, Work Cover Corporation, Adelaide.

Milio, N. 1985, 'Commentary: Creating a healthful future', *Community Health Studies*, vol. IX, no. 3, pp. 270–4.

——1996, *Engines of Empowerment: Using information technology to create healthy communities and challenge public policy*, Health Administration Press, Ann Arbor.

——1999, 'Health and political ecology: Public opinion, political ideology, political parties, policies and the press', in M. Honari and T. Boleyn (eds), *Health Ecology: Health, culture and human-environment interaction*, Routledge, London & New York.

——2001, 'Glossary: healthy public policy', *Journal of Epidemiology and Community Health*, vol. 55, pp. 622–3.

Milson, P. and Pick, L. 2004, ' "Teams of Two" Program', *PARCupdate*, no. 12, viewed 28 February 2006, <www.parc.net.au/PARCUpdateJuly04.htm#five>

MindMatters 2005, viewed 13 April 2005, <www.curriculum.edu.au/mindmatters>

Ministerial Council on Drug Strategy 2001, *National Alcohol Strategy: A plan for action 2001 to 2003–04*, AGPS, Canberra.

——2004, *The National Drug Strategy: Australia's integrated framework 2004–2009*, AGPS, Canberra.

Minkler, M. 1990, 'Improving health through community organization', in K. Glanz et al. (eds), *Health Behavior and Health Education: Theory, research, and practice*, Jossey-Boss, San Francisco.

——1997, *Community Organizing and Community Building for Health*, Rutgers University Press, New Brunswick, NJ.

——1999, 'Personal responsibility for health? A review of the arguments and the evidence at century's end', *Health Education and Behavior*, vol. 26, no. 1, February, pp. 121–41.

——2005, *Community organizing and community building for health*, Rutgers University Press, New Brunswick, N.J.

Mittelmark, M.B. 2000, 'What is Health Promotion?', viewed 23 September 2005, <www.iuhpe.org/English/news_other>

Moewaka Barnes, H. 2000, 'Collaboration in community action: A successful partnership between indigenous communities and researchers', *Health Promotion International*, vol. 15, no. 1, pp. 17–25.

Mukoma, W. and Flisher, A.J. 2004, 'Evaluations of health promoting schools: A review of nine studies', *Health Promotion International*, vol. 19, no. 3, pp. 357–68.

Mullins, L.J. 2005, *Management and Organisational Behaviour*, Prentice Hall/Financial Times, Harlow, England & New York.

Mumford, A. 1992, 'Generic competencies: A review of Britain', *Human Resources Monthly*, 12–13 June.

Munoz, E., Power, J.R., Nienhuys, T.G. and Mathews, J.D. 1992, 'Social and environmental factors in 10 Aboriginal communities in the Northern Territory: Relationships to hospital admissions for children', *Medical Journal of Australia*, vol. 156, pp. 629–33.

Murphy, L., Kordyl, P. and Thorne, M. 2004, 'Appreciative inquiry: A method for measuring the impact of a project on the wellbeing of an Indigenous community', *Health Promotion Journal of Australia*, vol. 15, no. 3, pp. 211–14.

Nader, P.R. 1990, 'The concept of "comprehensiveness" in the design and implementation of school health programs', *Journal of School Health*, vol. 60, no. 4, pp. 133–8.

——2000, 'Health promoting schools: Why not in the United States?', *Journal of School Health*, vol. 70, no. 6, p. 247.

National Aboriginal and Torres Strait Islander Health Council (NATSIHC) 2003, *National Strategic Framework for Aboriginal and Torres Strait Islander Health: Framework for action by governments*, viewed 10 January 2005, <www.seniors.gov.au./internet/wcms/publishing.nsf/Content/health-oatsih-pubs-healthstrategy.htm/$FILE/nsfatsihfinal.pdf>

National Aboriginal Health Strategy: An evaluation 1994, AGPS, Canberra.

National Aboriginal Health Strategy (NAHS) Working Party 1989, *A national Aboriginal health strategy*, Department of Aboriginal Affairs, Canberra.

National Centre for Epidemiology and Population Health 1992, 'Improving Australia's health: The role of primary health care', in D.G. Legge et al., *Final Report of the Review of the Role of Primary Health Care in Health Promotion in Australia*, Australian National University, Canberra.

National Commission on the Role of the School and the Community in Improving Adolescent Health 1990, *Code Blue*, National Association of State Boards of Education, Alexandria, VA.

National Coordinating Committee for Health Promotion in the Workplace 1992, *Health At Work Newsletter*, issue no. 13, winter.

National Health and Medical Research Council (NHMRC) 1996, *Promoting the Health of Australians: Case studies of achievements in improving the health of the population*, AGPS, Canberra. (This publication was rescinded on 24 March 2005; rescinded publications are publications that no longer represent the council's position on the matters contained therein. This means that the council no longer endorses, supports or approves these rescinded publications.)

——1998, Rural and Remote Health Project, Rural Health Research Committee, Australian Health Ministers' Advisory Council.

——2003a, *The NHMRC Road Map: A strategic framework for improving Aboriginal and Torres Strait Islander health through research*, The Aboriginal and Torres Strait Islander Research Agenda Working Group (RAWG) of the NHMRC, Canberra.

——2003b, *Values and Ethics: Guidelines for ethical conduct in Aboriginal and Torres Strait Islander health research*, viewed 10 January 2005, <www7.health. gov.au/nhmrc/publications/pdf/e52.pdf>

National Health Priority Action Council 2002, 'Future Directions of the National Health Priority Area Initiative', report to Australian Health Ministers' Advisory Council.

National Health Strategy (NHS) 1990, *Setting the Agenda for Change*, background paper no. 1, National Health Strategy Unit, Melbourne.

——1992a, *Enough to Make You Sick: How income and environment affect health*, research paper no. l, National Health Strategy Unit, Melbourne.

——1992b, *Improving Australia's Rural Health and Aged Services*, background paper no. 11, National Health Strategy Unit, Melbourne.

——1992c, *The Future of General Practice*, issues paper no. 3, National Health Strategy Unit, Melbourne.

——1993a, *Removing Cultural and Language Barriers to Health*, issues paper no. 6, National Health Strategy Unit, Melbourne.

——1993b, *Pathways to Better Health*, issues paper no. 7, National Health Strategy Unit, Melbourne.

National Native Title Tribunal 2000, media release, viewed 3 October 2005, <http://222.nntt.gov.au/nntt/mediarel.ns>

National Occupational Health and Safety Commission (NOHSC) 2004, 'Annual Report 2003–2004', viewed 5 May 2005, <www.worksafe.gov.au/OHS Information/NOHSCPublications/annualreport/2003–2004/>

National Public Health Partnership (NPHP) News 1997, 'Introducing you to the National Public Health Partnership', issue 1, p. 1.

——1999, 'The functions of public health in Australia: Towards a definition', issue 10, p. 1.

——2000, 'Public health functions in Australia: A statement of core functions', viewed 11 January 2005, <www.nphp.gov.au/publications/phpractice/delphi-body.pdf>

——2001, 'Preventing chronic disease: A strategic framework', background paper.

——2005, *Healthy Children: Strengthening promotion and prevention across Australia*, National Public Health Strategic Framework for Children 2005–2008, viewed 3 November 2005, <www.nphp.gov.au/workprog/chip/documents/CHIP Framework14Sept05web.pdf>

National Rural Health Alliance 1999, *Healthy Horizons: A framework for improving the health of rural, regional and remote Australians*, vols I to IV, a joint development of the National Rural Health Policy Forum and the National Rural Health Alliance, for the Health Ministers' Conference.

——2002a, *Healthy Horizons: A framework for improving the health of rural and remote Australians summary of progress across Australia*, a report to the Australian Health Ministers' Advisory Council from the National Rural Health Policy Sub-committee.

——2002b, *Healthy Horizons: A framework for improving the health of rural and remote Australians outlook 2003–2007*, The Australian Health Ministers' Advisory Council's National Rural Health Policy Sub-committee and the National Rural Health Alliance.

——2005, Communiqué and Key Recommendations of the 8th National Rural Health Conference, Alice Springs, National Rural Health Alliance, viewed 29 July 2005, <www.ruralhealth.org.au/nrhapublic/publicdocs/conferences/8thNRHC/Communique%20&%20Key%20Recommendations%20FINAL.pdf>

National Steering Committee on Health Promotion in the Workplace 1989, *Health at Work Information Kit*, National Heart Foundation, Western Australian Division, Nedlands, WA.

Nelson, R.G. 2003, 'Intrauterine determinants of diabetic kidney disease in disadvantaged populations', *Kidney International*, vol. 63, suppl. 83, pp. S13–16.

New South Wales Department of Health 1991, '*We're looking good': an evaluation of the Aboriginal Health Promotions Program, 1986–1990*, New South Wales Department of Health, Sydney.

New South Wales Government Community Builders 2005, *Resources for Safe and Healthy Koori Communities*, viewed 14 February 2006, <www.community builders.nsw.gov.au/building_stronger/safer/shkc.html>

New South Wales Health, Centre for Mental Health, 'Teams of Two initiative', viewed 28 February 2006, <www.health.nsw.gov.au/policy/cmh/gps.html>

Noble, C. and Robson, C. 2005, 'Just how far can healthy schools go?', *Health Education*, vol. 105, no. 3, pp. 161–3.

Northern Territory Government 2004, *Health and Physical Education Learning Area*, viewed 28 March 2005, <www.deet.nt.gov.au/education/ntcf/docs/learning_areas_hpe.pdf>

Norton, B.L., McLeroy, K.R. and Burdine, J.N. 2002, 'Community capacity: Concept, theory, and methods', in R.J. DiClemente, R.A. Crosby and M.C. Kegler (eds), *Emerging Theories in Health Promotion Practice and Research: Strategies for improving public health*, Jossey-Bass, San Francisco.

Nutbeam, D. 1993a, 'Evaluation of two smoking education programs under normal classroom conditions', *British Medical Journal*, vol. 306, pp. 102–7.

——1993b, 'Advocacy and mediation in creating supportive environments for health', *Health Promotion International*, vol. 8, no. 3, pp. 165–6.

——1998, 'A staged model for planning implementation and evaluation of health promotion programs', presentation at the 10th National Health Promotion Conference, Adelaide.

——2000, 'Health literacy as a public health goal: A challenge for contemporary health education and communication strategies into the 21st century', *Health Promotion International*, vol. 15, pp. 259–67.

——2004, 'Getting evidence into policy and practice to address health inequalities', *Health Promotion International*, vol. 19, no. 2, pp. 137–40.

Nutbeam, D. and Harris, E. 2004, *Theory in a nutshell: A practical guide to health promotion theories*, 2nd edn, McGraw-Hill, Sydney.

Nutbeam, D., Smith, C. and Catford, J. 1990, 'Evaluation in health education: A review of possibilities and problems', *Journal of Epidemiology and Community Health*, vol. 44, no. 2, pp. 83–9.

Nutbeam, D., Smith, C., Murphy, S. and Catford, J. 1993a, 'Maintaining evaluation designs in long term community based health promotion programmes: Heartbeat Wales case study', *Journal of Epidemiology and Community Health*, vol. 47, pp. 127–33.

Nutbeam, D., Wise, M., Bauman, A., Harris, E. and Leeder, S. 1993b, *Goals and Targets for Australia's Health in the Year 2000 and Beyond*, AGPS, Canberra.

Nutbeam, D., Wise, M. and Leeder, S. 1993c, 'Achieving Australia's national health goals and targets', *Health Promotion Journal of Australia*, vol. 3, no. 2, pp. 4–11.

O'Brien, J. 1994, 'Political arithmetic or numbers game? Reviewing the 1993 National Preventable Mortality and Morbidity Goals and Targets through a Queensland analysis', unpublished Master of Health Science thesis, School of Public Health, Queensland University of Technology, Brisbane.

O'Connor, M. 1991, 'A socio-historical study of health and medical care in New South Wales from settlement to 1850', unpublished PhD thesis, University of Queensland, Brisbane.

O'Connor-Fleming, M., Parker, E., Higgins, H. and Gould, T. 2006, 'A framework for evaluating health promotion programs', *Health Promotion Journal of Australia*, vol. 17, no. 1, pp. 61–6.

O'Dea, K. 1984, 'Marked improvements in carbohydrate and lipid metabolism in diabetic Australian Aborigines following temporary reversion to a traditional lifestyle', *Diabetes*, vol. 33, pp. 596–603.

O'Dea, K., White, N. and Sinclair, A. 1988, 'An investigation of nutrition-related risk factors in an isolated Aboriginal community in northern Australia: Advantages of a traditionally orientated lifestyle', *Medical Journal of Australia*, vol. 148, pp. 177–80.

O'Donnell, M.P. 1995, 'Design of workplace health promotion programs', 4th edn, *American Journal of Health Promotion*, Rochester Hills, Michigan.

O'Donnell, M.P. and Ainsworth, T. 1984, *Health Promotion in the Workplace*, John Wiley & Sons, New York.

O'Donnell, M.P. and Harris, J.S. 1994, *Health Promotion in the Workplace*, 2nd edn, Delmar Publishers, New York.

Office for Aboriginal and Torres Strait Islander Health (OATSIH) 2005, viewed 10 March 2005, <www.health.gov.au/internet/wcms/publishing.nsf/Content/health-oatsih-what-index.htm>

Oldenburg, B., Glanz, K. and French, M. 1999, 'The application of staging models to the understanding of health behavior change and the promotion of health', *Psychology and Health*, vol. 14, pp. 503–16.

Oldenburg, B. and Harris, D. 1996, 'The worksite as a setting for promoting health and preventing disease', *Homeostasis*, no. 5, pp. 226–32.

Owen, J.M. 2004, 'Evaluation forms: Toward an inclusive framework for evaluation practice', in M.C. Alkin (ed.), *Evaluation Roots: Tracing theorists' views and influences*, Sage Publications, Thousand Oaks, CA.

Owen, N. and Lennie, I. 1992, 'Health for all and community health', in F. Baum, D. Fry and I. Lennie (eds), *Community Health: Policy and practice in Australia*, Pluto Press, Sydney.

Oxenburg, M. 1991, *Increasing Productivity and Profit through Health and Safety*, CCH Australia, Sydney.

Palmer, G.R. and Short, S.D. 1989, *Health Care and Public Policy: An Australian analysis*, Macmillan, Melbourne.

——2000, *Health Care and Public Policy: An Australian analysis*, 3rd edn, Macmillan, Melbourne.

Pan American Health Organization (PAHO) 2000, *Natural Disasters: Protecting the public's health*, Washington, DC.

Paradies, Y. and Cunningham, J. 2002, 'Placing Aboriginal and Torres Strait Islander mortality in an international context', *Australian and New Zealand Journal of Public Health*, vol. 26, no. 1, pp. 11–16.

Parker, E. and Steele, J. 1993, 'Training health promotion professionals in Queensland', paper presented to the Public Health Association of Australia Annual Conference, Sydney, 30 September.

Parkinson, R.C. 1982, *Managing Health Promotion in the Workplace*, Mayfield, Mountain View, CA.

Paton, K., Senguptal, S. and Hassan, L. 2005, 'Settings, systems and organization development: The healthy living and working model', *Health Promotion International*, vol. 20, no. 1, pp. 81–9.

Patrick, K., Intille, S. and Zabinski, M. 2005, 'An ecological framework for cancer communication: Implications for research', *Journal of Medical Internet Research*, vol. 7, no. 3, p. e23, viewed 14 December 2005, <www.jmir.org/2005/3/e23/>

Patton, G.C., Glover, S., Bond, L., Butler, H., Godfrey, C., Di Pietro, G. and Bowes, G. 2000, 'The Gatehouse Project: a systematic approach to mental health promotion in secondary schools', *Australian and New Zealand Journal of Psychiatry*, vol. 34, pp. 586–93.

Pawson, R. and Tilley, N. 1997, *Realistic Evaluation*, Sage Publications, Thousand Oaks, CA.

Peach, H.G., Pearce, D.C. and Farish, S. 1998, 'Age-standardised mortality and proportional mortality analyses of Aboriginal and non-Aboriginal deaths in metropolitan, rural and remote areas', *Australian Journal of Rural Health*, no. 6, pp. 36–41.

Pearce, N. and Smith, G.D. 2003, 'Is social capital the key to inequalities in health?', *American Journal of Public Health*, vol. 93, no. 1, pp. 122–9.

Peck, M.S. 1987, *The Different Drum*, Touchstone, New York.

Pelikan, J.M. (ed.) 2000, *Health Promoting Hospital Series*, Ludwig Boltzmann Institute for the Sociology of Health and Medicine, WHO Collaborating Centre for Hospitals and Health Promotion, World Health Organization, Regional Office for Europe, Copenhagen.

Pelletier, K.R. 1997, 'Clinical and cost outcomes of multifactorial, cardiovascular risk management interventions in worksites: A comprehensive review and analysis', *Journal of Occupational and Environmental Medicine*, vol. 39, no. 12, pp. 1154–9.

Peltomaki, P., Johansson, M., Ahrens, W., Sala, M., Wess, C. et al. 2003, 'Social context for workplace health promotion: Feasibility considerations in Costa Rica, Finland, Germany, Spain and Sweden', *Health Promotion International*, vol. 18, no. 2, pp. 115–26.

Perdiguero, E., Bernabeu, J., Huertas, R. and Rodriguez-Ocaña, E. 2001, 'History of health, a valuable tool in public health', *Journal of Epidemiology and Community Health*, vol. 55, pp. 667–73.

Perkins, D.D. and Zimmerman, M.A. 1995, 'Empowerment theory, research and application', *American Journal of Community Psychology*, vol. 23, no. 5, pp. 569–80.

Perkins, E.R., Simnett, I. and Wright, L. (eds) 1999, *Evidence-based Health Promotion*, John Wiley, Chichester, New York.

Petersen, A.R. 1994, 'Community development in health promotion: Empowerment or regulation?', *Australian Journal of Public Health*, vol. 18, no. 2, pp. 213–17.

Pickett, G. and Hanlon, J.J. 1990, *Public Health: Administration and practice*, 9th edn, Times Mirror/Mosby College Publishing, St Louis.

Pinto, B.M., Friedman, R.H., Marcus, B.H., Kelley, H., Tennstedt, S. and Gillman, M.W. 2002, 'Effects of a computer-based, telephone-counseling system on physical activity', *American Journal of Preventive Medicine*, vol. 23, no. 2, pp. 113–20.

Playdon, M. 1997, 'Promoting health in hospitals', *Australian Nursing Journal*, vol. 4, no. 7, pp. 18–19.

Poland, B.D., Green, L.W. and Rootman, I. 2000, *Settings for health promotion: Linking theory and practice*, Sage Publications, Thousand Oaks, CA.

Pollock, M.B. and Hamburg, M.V. 1985, 'Health education: The basic of the basics', *Health Education*, April/May, pp. 105–9.

Potvin, L., Cargo, M., McComber, A., Delormier, T. and Macaulay, A. 2003, 'Implementing participatory intervention and research in communities: Lessons from the Kahnawake Schools Diabetes Prevention Project in Canada', *Social Science & Medicine*, vol. 56, no. 6, pp. 1295–306.

Proceedings of the First National Rural Health Conference 1992, 'A fair go for rural health', Department of Health, Housing and Community Services, Canberra.

Prochaska, J.O. 2005, 'Stages of change, readiness, and motivation', in J. Kerr, R. Weitkunat and M. Moretti (eds), *ABC of Behaviour Change: A guide to successful disease prevention and health promotion*, Elsevier Churchill Livingstone, Edinburgh.

Prochaska, J.O. and Diclemente, C.C. 2005, 'The transtheoretical approach', in J.C. Norcross and M.R. Goldfried (eds), *Handbook of Psychotherapy Integration*, 2nd edn, Oxford University Press, New York.

Prochaska, J.O., Norcross, J.C. and Diclemente, C.C. 2005, 'Stages of change: Prescriptive guidelines', in G.P. Koocher, J.C. Norcross and S.S. Hill, III (eds), *Psychologists' Desk Reference*, 2nd edn, Oxford University Press, Oxford & New York.

Public Health Association of Australia 1990, *Workforce Issues for Public Health*, report of the Public Health Workforce Study, Canberra.

——1997, Policy Statements 1998, Public Health Association, Canberra.

Puska, P. 1992, 'The North Karelia Project: Nearly 20 years of successful prevention of CVD in Finland', *Hygie*, vol. 11, pp. 33–5.

Putnam, R. 1993, *Making Democracy Work: Civic traditions in modern Italy*, Princeton University Press, Princeton, NJ.

——1995, 'Bowling alone: "America's Declining Social Capital"', *Journal of Democracy*, vol. 6, no. 1, pp. 65–78.

——2004, 'Commentary; "Health by association": some comments', *International Journal of Epidemiology*, vol. 33, no. 4, pp. 667–71.

Queensland Divisions of General Practice 2000, *EPC/Population Health Workshop*, Brisbane, 14–15 July.

Queensland Focus Schools Project, MindMatters 2003, Focus Schools Project Final Report.

Queensland Government 2005a, *Special Fiscal and Economic Statement 2005*, viewed 1 December 2005, <www.budget.qld.gov.au/october2005/statement.html>

——2005b, *Get involved*, viewed 14 February 2006, <www.getinvolved.qld.gov.au/share_your_knowledge/un_conference/brisbanedeclaration.html>

Queensland Health 1990, 'A study of employees' attitudes towards smoking in the workplace and other workforce health issues', research report commissioned by the Health Advancement Branch, submitted by P. Walsh, Kenning, Australia.

——1993a, *A Primary Health Care Policy*, Brisbane.

——1993b, *A Primary Health Care Implementation Plan*, Brisbane.

——1999, *Our Jobs, Our Health, Our Future: Queensland Health Indigenous Workforce Management Strategy*, Brisbane.

——2000, 'Health service integration in Queensland', position statement, Brisbane.

——2002, 'Strategic Policy Framework for Children's and Young People's Health 2002–2007', Brisbane.

——2005a, *Discussion Paper: Strategic policy for Aboriginal and Torres Strait Islander children and young people's health 2005–2010*, Brisbane.

——2005b, *Healthier Multicultural Communities Initiative*, viewed 25 October 2005, <http://203.147.140.236/multicultural/pdf/initiative_sept05.pdf>

Queensland State Steering Committee on Health Promotion in the Workplace 1993, (Draft) Position Statement on Health Promotion in the Workplace, Brisbane.

Queensland Studies Authority 2004, *Physical Education Senior Syllabus*, viewed 28 March 2005, <www.qsa.qld.edu.au/yrs11_12/subjects/pe/syllabus.pdf>

QUT Resilience Project 2005, viewed 25 November 2005, <www.hlth.qut.edu.au/ph/resilience/>

Raeburn, J. and Rootman, I. 1998, *People-centred Health Promotion*, John Wiley, Chichester, New York.

Reardon, J. 1998, 'The hisory and impact of worksite wellness', *Nursing Economics*, May–June, vol. 16, no. 3, pp. 117–25.

Reid, M. and Solomon, S. 1992, *Improving Australia's Rural Health and Aged Care Services*, National Health Strategy background paper no. 11, AGPS, Canberra.

Resnicow, K., Cherry, J. and Cross, D. 1993, 'Ten unanswered questions regarding school health promotion', *Journal of School Health*, vol. 63, no. 4, pp. 171–5.

Rissel, C. and Rowling, L. 2000, 'Intersectoral collaboration for the development of a national framework for health', *Journal of School Health*, vol. 70, no. 6, pp. 248–50.

Robbins, S.P. and Mukerji, D. 1990, *Managing Organizations: New challenges and perspectives*, Prentice Hall, New York.

Rollnick, S., Mason, P. and Butler, C. 1999, *Health Behavior Change: A Guide for practitioners*, Churchill Livingstone, Edinburgh.

Rose, M. and Jackson Pulver, L.R. 2004, 'Aboriginal health workers: Professional qualifications to match their health promotion roles', *Health Promotion Journal of Australia*, vol. 15, no. 3, pp. 240–4.

Rossi, P.H., Freeman, H.E. and Lipsey, M.W. 1999, *Evaluation: A systematic approach*, Sage Publications, Thousand Oaks, CA.

Rotem, A., Walters, J. and Dewdney, J. 1995, 'The public health workforce education and training study', *Australian Journal of Public Health*, vol. 19, no. 5, pp. 437–8.

Rothman, J. 1995, 'Approaches to community intervention', in J. Rothman et al. (eds), *Strategies of Community Intervention*, Peacock, New York.

Rothman, J. and Tropman, J.E. 1987, 'Models of community organization and macro practice: Their mixing and phasing', in F.M. Cox et al. (eds), *Strategies of Community Organization*, 4th edn, Peacock, Itasca, Ill.

Rowling, L. 2002, 'State of the art—Health promoting schools—Evidence: About what? In what form? For whom?', keynote address in J. Ritchie (ed.), *Made in the Future: Conference proceedings of the 14th annual conference of Australia Health Promotion Association*, Sydney.

Rowling, L. and Barr, A. 1997, 'Creating supportive environments', in D. Colquhoun, K. Glotz and M. Sheehan, *The Health Promoting School*, Harcourt, Brace and Company, Sydney, pp. 75–94.

Rowling, L. and Jeffreys, V. 2000, 'Challenges in the development and monitoring of Health Promoting Schools', *Health Education*, vol. 100, no. 3, pp. 117–23.

Rowse, T., Scrimgeour, D., Knight, S. and Thomas, D. 1994, 'Food purchasing behaviour in an Aboriginal community', *Australian Journal of Public Health*, vol. 18, no. 1, pp. 63–7.

Royal Commission into Aboriginal Deaths in Custody 1988, *Interim Report*, AGPS, Canberra.

Ruben, A.R. and Fisher, D.A. 1998, 'The casemix system of hospital funding can further disadvantage Aboriginal children', *Medical Journal of Australia*, vol. 169, pp. S6–10.

Rural Health Research and Education Program 1992, *Australian Rural Health: A national survey of education needs*, University of Wollongong, Wollongong.

Rural Industries Research and Development Corporation 2002, *R & D Plan for Farm Health & Safety 2002–2006*, publication no. 02/041, viewed 20 September 2005, <www.rirdc.gov.au/pub/hcc-fhs.pdf>

Rychetnik, L. and Wise, M. 2004, 'Advocating evidence-based health promotion: Reflections and a way forward', *Health Promotion International*, vol. 19, no. 2, pp. 247–57.

Sadler, B. and Jacobs, P. 1990, 'A key to tomorrow: On the relationship of environmental assessment and sustainable development', in P. Jacobs and B. Sadler (eds), *Sustainable Development and Environmental Assessment: Perspectives on planning for a common future*, Canadian Environmental Assessment Research Council, Canada.

Sallis, J.F. and Owen, N. 2002, 'Ecological models of health behavior', in K. Glanz et al. (eds), *Health Behavior and Health Education: Theory, research, and practice*, 3rd edn, Jossey-Bass, San Francisco.

Saunders, M. 2003, 'Indigenous health, indigenous men: Leadership and other bad medicine', *Aboriginal and Islander Health Worker Journal*, vol. 27, no. 6, pp. 10–13.

Schaffer, R.H. and Thomson, H.A. 1992, 'Successful change programs begin with results', *Harvard Business Review*, January/February, pp. 80–9.

Schon, D. 1995, *Reflective Practitioner: How professionals think in action*, 2nd edn, Arena, Aldershot.

Scott, W.G. 2004, 'Public policy failure in health care', *Journal of American Academy of Business*, vol. 5, no. 1/2, pp. 88–94.

Scrimgeour, D., Rowse, T. and Knight, S. 1994, 'Food purchasing behaviour in an Aboriginal community: 2. Evaluation of an intervention aimed at children', *Australian Journal of Public Health*, vol. 18, no. 1, p. 67.

Sefton, C. and Hawe, P. 2002, NSW Safe Communities Pilot Program Evaluation, final report, University of Sydney, Sydney.

Seligman, M. 1975, *Helplessness: On depression, development and death*, W.H. Freeman, San Francisco.

Setleff, R., Porter, J.E., Malison, M., Frederick, S. and Balderson, T.R. 2003, 'Strengthening the public health workforce: Three CDC programs that prepare managers and leaders for the challenges of the 21st century', *Journal of Public Health Management and Practice*, vol. 9, no. 2, pp. 91–102.

Shephard, M., Allen, G., Barratt, L., Barbara, J., Paizis, K., McLeod, G., Brown, M. and Vanajek, A. 2003, 'Albuminuria in a remote South Australian Aboriginal community: Results of a community-based screening program for renal disease', *Rural and Remote Health* 3 (online), article no. 156, viewed 8 June 2005, <http://rrh.deakin.edu.au/articles/subviewnew.asp?ArticleID=156>

Shilton, T.R., Howat, P., James, R. and Lower, T. 2003, 'Review of competencies for Australian health promotion', *Promotion and Education*, vol. 10, no. 4, pp. 162–71.

Shortt, S.E.D. 2004, 'Making sense of social capital, health and policy', *Health Policy*, vol. 70, pp. 11–22.

Simnett, I. 1995, *Managing Health Promotion: Developing healthy organisations and communities*, John Wiley and Sons, Chichester.

Simon, G.E., Von Korff, M., Rutter, C. and Wagner, E. 2000, 'Randomised trial of monitoring, feedback, and management of care by telephone to improve treatment of depression in primary care', *British Medical Journal*, vol. 7234, no. 320, pp. 550–4.

Simons, L., Whish, P., Marra, B., Jones, A. and Simons, J. 1981, 'Coronary risk factors in a rural community which includes Aborigines: Inverell Heart Disease Prevention Programme', *Australian and New Zealand Journal of Medicine*, vol. 11, pp. 386–90.

Simpson, K. and Freeman, R. 2004, 'Critical health promotion and education—a new research challenge', *Health Education Research*, vol. 19, no. 3, pp. 340–8.

Singh, G.R., and Hoy, W.E. 2003, 'The association between birthweight and current blood pressure: A cross-sectional study in an Australian Aboriginal community', *Medical Journal of Australia*, vol. 179, no. 10, pp. 532–5.

Sloan, R. 1987, 'Workplace health promotion—a commentary on the evolution of a paradigm', *Health Education Quarterly*, vol. 14, no. 2, pp. 181–94.

Smith, M.L. and Glass, V.G. 1987, *Research and Evaluation in Education and the Social Sciences*, Prentice Hall, Englewood Cliffs, NJ.

Smith, R., Spargo, R., Hunter, E., King, R., Correll, J., Craig, I. and Nestel, P. 1992, 'Prevalence of hypertension in Kimberley Aborigines and its relationship to ischaemic heart disease', *Medical Journal of Australia*, vol. 156, p. 566.

Sorensen, G., Emmons, K., Hunt, M.K. and Johnston, D. 1998, 'Implications of the results of community intervention trials', *Annual Review of Public Health*, vol. 19, pp. 379–416.

Sorensen, G., Glasgow, R.E. and Corbett, K. 1990, 'Involving worksites and other organizations', in N. Bracht (ed.), *Health Promotion at the Community Level*, Sage Publications, Newbury Park, CA.

South Australia Department of Education and Children's Services 2004, *R–10 Health and Physical Education, South Australian Curriculum, Standards and Accountability*, (SACSA) framework, viewed 2 March 2005, <www.sacsa. sa.edu.au/splash.asp>

South Australian Health Commission 1988a, *A Social Health Strategy for South Australia*, Adelaide.

——1988b, *Primary Health Care in South Australia: A discussion paper*, Adelaide.

Spark, R., Donovan, R.J. and Howat, P. 1991, 'Promoting health and preventing injury in remote Aboriginal communities: A case study', *Health Promotion Journal of Australia*, vol. 1, no. 2, pp. 10–16.

St Leger, L. 1999, 'The opportunities and effectiveness of the health promoting primary school in improving child health—a review of the claims and evidence', *Health Education Research*, vol. 14, no. 1, pp 51–69.

——2001, 'Schools, health literacy and public health: Possibilities and challenges', *Health Promotion International*, vol. 16, no. 2, pp. 197–205.

——2004, 'What's the place of schools in promoting health? Are we too optimistic?', *Health Promotion International*, vol. 19, no. 4, pp. 405–8.

St Leger, L. and Nutbeam, D. 2000, 'Model for mapping linkages between health and education agencies to improve school health', *Journal of School Health*, vol. 70, no. 2, pp. 45–50.

Stace, D.A. and Dunphy, D.C. 1994, *Beyond the Boundaries: Leading and re-creating the successful enterprise*, McGraw-Hill, Sydney.

——2001, *Beyond the Boundaries: Leading and re-creating the successful enterprise*, 2nd edn, McGraw-Hill, Sydney.

Stacey, R. and Griffin, D. 2006, *Complexity and the Experience of Managing in Public Sector Organizations*, Routledge, New York.

Stake, R. 1983, 'Program evaluation, particularly responsive evaluation', in G. Madaus and M. Scriven (eds), *Evaluation Models: Viewpoints on educational and human services evaluation*, Kluwer-Nijhoff Publishing, Boston.

Stanton, W.R., Balanda, K.P., Gillespie, A.M. and Lowe, J. 1996, 'Barriers to health promotion activities in public hospitals', *Australian and New Zealand Journal of Public Health*, vol. 20, no. 5, pp. 500–4.

Starr, P. 1982, *The Social Transformation of American Medicine*, Basic Books, New York.

Stewart, D., Hardie, M., Sun, J. and Patterson, C. 2005, 'Comprehensive health promotion in primary schools: The "Resilient Children and Community" project', International Conference on Engaging Communities, Brisbane.

Stewart, D., Sun, J., Patterson, C., Lemerle, K. and Hardie, M. 2004, 'Promoting and building resilience in primary school communities: Evidence from a comprehensive "Health Promoting School" approach', *International Journal of Mental Health Promotion*, vol. 6, no. 3, pp. 26–33.

Stewart, K.E., Cianfrini, L.R. and Walker, J.F. 2005, 'Stress, social support and housing are related to health status among HIV-positive persons in the Deep South of the United States', *AIDS Care*, vol. 17, no. 3, pp. 350–8.

Stufflebeam, D. 2003, 'The CIPP Model for Evaluation: An update, a review of the model's development, a checklist to guide implementation', presented at the 2003 Annual Conference of the Oregon Program Evaluators Network (OPEN), Portland, Oregon.

Suchman, E.A. 1967, *Evaluative Research*, Russell Sage Foundation, New York.

Susser, M. 1981, 'Ethical components in the definition of health', in A.L. Caplan et al. (eds), *Concepts of Health and Disease: Interdisciplinary perspectives*, Addison-Wesley, Reading, Mass.

Swayne, L.E., Duncan, W.J. and Ginter, P.M. 2006, *Strategic Management of Health Care Organizations*, Blackwell Publishing, Malden, MA.

Swerissen, H. and Tilgner, L. 2000, 'A workforce survey of health promotion education and training needs in the state of Victoria', *Australian and New Zealand Journal of Public Health*, vol. 24, no. 4, pp. 407–12.

Syme, L. 1996, 'To prevent disease: The need for a new approach', in D. Blane et al. (eds), *Health and Social Organisation*, Routledge, London.

Szreter, S. 1988, 'The importance of social intervention in Britain's mortality decline c.1850–1914: A reinterpretation of the role of public health', *Social History of Medicine*, vol. 1, no. 1, pp. 1–37.

Szreter, S. and Woolcock, M. 2004, 'Health by association: Social capita, social theory, and the political economy of public health', *International Journal of Epidemiology*, vol. 33, pp. 650–67.

Tang, K.C., Ehsani, J.P. and McQueen, D.V. 2003, 'Evidence based health promotion: Recollections, reflections, and reconsiderations', *Journal of Epidemiology and Community Health*, vol. 57, pp. 841–3.

Tasmanian Qualifications Authority (TQA) 2005, viewed 2 March 2005, <www.tqa. tas.gov.au/1074>

Taylor, C. 2005, 'Life in the Balance', *Incentive*, vol. 179, no. 1, pp. 16–19.

Terris, M. 1987, 'Epidemiology and the public health movement', *Journal of Public Health Policy*, vol. 8, no. 3, p. 315.

Tesh, S. 1982, 'Political ideology and public health in the 19th century', *International Journal of Health Services*, vol. 12, no. 2, p. 321.

Theuringer, T. and Missler, M. 2003, 'Brave new working world? Europe needs investment in workplace health promotion—more than ever before', *Promotion & Education*, vol. 10, no. 4, pp. 178–81.

Thompson, J. 1990, 'Program evaluation within a health promotion framework', *Canadian Journal of Public Health*, vol. 83, supp. 1, March/April, p. s67.

Thompson, S. and Gifford, S. 2000, 'Trying to keep a balance: The meaning of health and diabetes in an urban Aboriginal Community', *Social Science and Medicine*, vol. 51, pp. 1457–72.

Thomson, N. 1991, 'A review of Aboriginal Health Status', in J. Reid and P. Trompf (eds), *The Health of Aboriginal Australia*, Harcourt Brace Jovanovich, Sydney.

——2003, *The Health of Indigenous Australians*, Oxford University Press, Melbourne.

Tibbetts, J. 2003, 'Building civic health', *Environmental Health Perspectives*, vol. 111, no. 7, pp. 400–3.

Tones, K. 1995, 'Editorial: The health promoting hospital', *Health Education Research*, vol. 10, no. 2, pp. I–V.

Tones, K. and Green, J. 2004, *Health Promotion: Planning and strategies*, Sage Publications, London.

Toowoomba City Council 2005, *Safe Community Program*, viewed 14 February 2006, <www.toowoomba.qld.gov.au/index.php?option=content&task=view &id=389&Itemid=385>

Tsouros, A.D. (ed.) 1991, *World Health Organisation Healthy Cities Project: A project becomes a movement; Review of progress 1987 to 1990*, FADL Publishers, Copenhagen.

Turrell, G. 2002, 'Reducing socioeconomic health inequalities: Issues of relevance for policy', *NSW Public Health Bulletin*, vol. 13, no. 3, pp. 47–9.

Turrell, G., Oldenburg, B., Harris, E. and Jolley, D. 2004, 'Utilisation of general practitioner services by socio-economic disadvantage and geographic remoteness', *Australian and New Zealand Journal of Public Health*, vol. 28, no. 2, pp. 152–8.

Turrell, G., Oldenburg, B., McGuffog, I. and Dent, R. 1999, *Socioeconomic Determinants of Health: Towards a national research program and a policy and intervention agenda*, Queensland University of Technology, School of Public Health, Ausinfo, Canberra.

Tursan d'Espaignet, E., Measey, M.L., Carnegie, M.A. and Mackerras, D. 2003, 'Monitoring the "Strong Women, Strong Babies, Strong Culture Program": The first eight years', *Journal of Paediatrics and Child Health*, vol. 39, pp. 668–72.

Umoona Kidney Project 2005, viewed 8 June 2005, <http://som.flinders.edu.au/FUSA/Renal/usumm.htm>

United Nations Development Program 2005, *Tsunami Spotlights Long-Term Development Needs*, viewed 17 January 2005, <www.undp.org/bcpr/disred/documents/news/2005/jan/undppr180105.pdf>

United States Department of Health and Human Services 2005, *HealthyPeople 2010*, Office of Disease Prevention and Health Promotion, US Department of Health and Human Services, viewed 25 November 2005, <www.healthypeople.gov/document/html/volume1/12heart.htm>

Usher, R., Bryant, I. and Johnston, R. 1997, *Adult Education and the Postmodern Challenge: Learning beyond the limits*, Routledge, London.

Vega, J. and Irwin, A. 2004, 'Tackling health inequalities: New approaches in public policy', *Bulletin of the World Health Organization*, vol. 82, no. 7, p. 482.

Veith, I. 1982, 'Historical reflections on the changing concepts of disease', in A.L. Caplan et al. (eds), *Concepts of Health and Disease*, Addison-Wesley, Reading, Mass.

Victorian Curriculum and Assessment Authority, State Government of Victoria 2005, *Victorian Essential Learning Standards*, viewed 7 April 2005, <http://vels.vcaa.vic.edu.au/essential/personal/health/>

Voyle, J.A. and Simmons, D. 1999, 'Community development through partnership: Promoting health in an urban indigenous community in New Zealand', *Social Science & Medicine*, vol. 49, pp. 1035–50.

Waddell, C. and Dibley, M. 1986, 'The medicalisation of Aboriginal children: A comparison of lengths of hospital stay of Aboriginal and non-Aboriginal children in Western Australia and the Northern Territory', *Australian Paediatric Journal*, vol. 22, pp. 27–30.

Wagner, E.H. 1998, 'Chronic disease management: What will it take to improve care for chronic illness?', *Effective Clinical Practice*, vol. 1, no. 1, pp. 2–4.

Wagner, E.H., Austin, B.T., Davis, C., Hindmarsh, M., Schaefer, J. and Bonomi, A. 2001, 'Improving chronic illness care: Translating evidence into action', *Health Affairs*, vol. 20, no. 6, pp. 64–78.

Wagner, G.H. 2002, 'Health promoting schools evidence for effectiveness workshops report', *Promotion & Education*, vol. 9, no. 2, pp. 55–61.

Wakerman, J. 2004, 'Defining remote health', *Australian Journal of Rural Health*, vol. 12, pp. 210–14.

Wallerstein, N. and Bernstein, E. 1988, 'Empowerment education: Friere's ideas adapted to health education', *Health Education Quarterly*, vol. 15, no. 4, pp. 379–94.

——1994, 'Introduction to community empowerment, participatory education, and health', *Health Education Quarterly*, vol. 21, no. 2, pp. 141–7.

Walter, C.L. 2005, 'Community building practice: A conceptual framework', in M. Minkler (ed.), *Community Organizing and Community Building for Health*, Rutgers University Press, New Brunswick, NJ & London.

Waltner-Toews, D. 2000, 'The end of medicine: the beginning of health', *Futures*, vol. 32, pp. 655–67.

Wandersman, A., Goodman, R.M. and Butterfoss, F.D. 2005, 'Understanding coalitions and how they operate as organizations', in M. Minkler (ed.), *Community Organizing and Community Building for Health*, Rutgers University Press, New Brunswick, NJ & London.

Warner, K., Wickizer, R., Wolfe, R., Schildroth, J. and Samuelson, M. 1988, 'Economic implications of workplace health promotion programs: Review of the literature', *Journal of Occupational Medicine*, vol. 30, no. 2, pp. 106–12.

Warren, R. 1967, 'The interorganisational field as a focus for investigation', *Administrative Science Quarterly*, December, pp. 396–419.

Wass, A. 1994, *Promoting Health: The primary health care approach*, Harcourt Brace & Company, Sydney.

Weiler, R.M., Pigg Jr, R.M. and McDermott, R.J. 2003, 'Evaluation of the Florida Coordinated School Health Program Pilot Schools Project', *Journal of School Health*, vol. 73, no. 1, pp. 3–8.

Weisbrod, R., Pirie, P. and Bracht, N. 1992, 'Impact of a community health promotion program on existing organisations: The Minnesota Heart Health Program', *Social Science and Medicine*, vol. 34, no. 6, pp. 639–48.

Wenzel, E. 1997, 'A comment on *settings* in health promotion', *Internet Journal of Health Promotion*, viewed 14 March 2005, <www.monash.edu.au/health/IJHP/1997/1>

Western Australia Government Curriculum Council 1998, *Health & Physical Education Learning Area Statement*, viewed 2 March 2005, <www.curriculum.wa.edu.au/pages/framework/framework00.htm>

Whetten, D.A. and Cameron, K.S. 1984, *Developing managerial skills*, Scott, Forestman and Co., Glenview, Illinois.

White, C. 2004, *Strategic Management*, Palgrave Macmillan, Houndmills, England & New York.

Whitehead, D. 2004, 'The European Health Promoting Hospitals (HPH) project: How far on?', *Health Promotion International*, vol. 19, no. 2, pp. 259–67.

——2006, 'Workplace health promotion: The role and responsibility of health care managers', *Journal of Nursing Management*, vol. 14, pp. 59–68.

Whitehead, M. 1995, 'Tackling inequalities: A review of policy initiatives', in M. Benzeval et al. (eds), *Tackling Inequalities in Health: An agenda for action*, King's Fund, London.

Whitehead, M., Dahlgren, G. and Evans, T. 2001, 'Equity and health sector reforms: Can low-income countries escape the medical poverty trap?', *The Lancet*, vol. 358, no. 9284, p. 833.

Willis, E. 1983, *Medical Dominance: The division of labour in Australian healthcare*, Allen & Unwin, Sydney.

Wilson, K. and Rosenberg, M.W. 2002, 'Exploring the determinants of health for First Nations peoples in Canada: Can existing frameworks accommodate traditional activities?', *Social Science & Medicine*, vol. 55, pp. 2017–31.

Wilson, M. 1990, 'Promoting health and safety on the farm', *Australian Health Review*, vol. 13, no. 2, pp. 139–43.

Wilson, M.A. 1996, 'A comprehensive review of the effects of worksite health promotion on health-related outcomes', *American Journal of Health Promotion*, vol. 19, pp. 429–35.

Windshuttle, K. 1980, *Unemployment: A social and political analysis of the economic crisis in Australia*, Penguin, Ringwood, Victoria.

Windsor, R.A., Clark, N., Boyd, N.R., Goodman, R.M. 2004, *Evaluation of Health Promotion, Health Education and Disease Prevention Programs*, 3rd edn, Mayfield Publishing Co., CA.

Winslow, C.E.A. 1920, 'The untilled fields of public health', *Science*, vol. 51, p. 30.

Winter, I. (ed.) 2000, *Social Capital and Public Policy in Australia*, Australian Institute of Family Studies, Melbourne.

Wolfenden, K., Clarke, L., Lower, T. and Murray-Jones, S. 1991, 'Rural child injury prevention—a community-based approach', *Health Promotion Journal of Australia*, vol. 1, no. 2, pp. 23–7.

Women's and Children's Hospital 2006, *Centre for Health Promotion, Women's and Children's Hospital*, North Adelaide, viewed 27 February 2006, <www.wch.sa.gov.au/services/az/other/health_prom/index.html>

Wong, L. 1990, 'Reassessing rural health policy', *Health Issues*, no. 24, pp. 31–4.

Woolcock, M. and Narayan, D. 2000, 'Social capital: Implications for development theory, research, and policy', *World Bank Research Observer*, vol. 15, pp. 225–49.

Woolmer, J., Howat, P. and Sauer, K. 2005, 'Twenty years of workplace health promotion', poster presented at the 36th Public Health Association of Australia Annual Conference 'Successes in Public Health', Perth, viewed 16 March 2006, <http://espace.lis.curtin.edu.au/archive/00000641/>

Worksafe Australia 1993, *Health Promotion in the Workplace Programs: Guidelines for workplaces* (draft), Sydney.

World Bank 1993, *World Development Report*, Oxford University Press, New York.

World Commission on the Environment and Development (WCED) 1987, *Our Common Future*, Oxford University Press, Oxford.

World Health Organization (WHO) 1954, *Expert Committee on Health Education of the Public*, first report of the Expert Committee, World Health Organization Technical Report Series no. 89, Geneva, viewed 14 March 2005, <http://.who.int/bookorders/anglais/detart1.jsp?sesslan=1&codlan=1&codcol=10&codcch=89#>

——1960, *Teacher Preparation for Health Education: Report of a joint WHO/UNESCO Expert Committee*, World Health Organization Technical Report Series no. 193, viewed 14 March 2005, <www.who.int/bookorders/anglais/detart1.jsp?sesslan=1&codlan=1&codcol=10&codcch=193#>

——1966, *Planning for Health Education in Schools*, WHO, Geneva.

——1981, *Global Strategies for Health For All by the Year 2000*, Health For All Series 3, WHO, Geneva.

——1982, *Primary Health Care from Theory to Action*, WHO, Copenhagen.

——1983, *New Approaches to Health Education in Primary Health Care*, WHO, Geneva.

——1986a, *Ottawa Charter for Health Promotion*, WHO, Ottawa.

——1986b, *Targets For Health For All*, WHO, Copenhagen.

——1988, *Adelaide Recommendations on Healthy Public Policy*, Second International Conference on Health Promotion, Adelaide, viewed 1 September 2005, <www.who.int/healthpromotion/conferences/previous/adelaide/en/index1.html>

——1990, *Health in Education For All: Enabling school-age children and adults for healthy living*, WHO Division of Health Education, Geneva.

——1992, *Meeting Global Health Challenges: A position paper on health education*, WHO, Geneva.

——1996a, *Promoting Health Through Schools—The World Health Organization's Global School Health Initiative*, WHO, Geneva.

——1996b, *Ljubljana Charter on Reforming Health Care*, Ljubljana Conference, WHO, Geneva.

——1997a, *Promoting Health through Schools*, report of a WHO Expert Committee on Comprehensive School Health Education and Promotion, Technical Report Series no. 870, WHO, Geneva.

——1997b, *Jakarta Statement on Healthy Workplaces*, Symposium on Healthy Workplaces at the 4th International Conference on Health Promotion, Jakarta.

——1997c, *The Vienna Recommendations on Health Promoting Hospitals* (the Vienna Recommendations were adopted at the 3rd Workshop of National/Regional Health Promoting Hospitals Network Coordinators, Vienna).

——1998, *Health Promotion Glossary*, WHO, Geneva, viewed 14 March 2005, <www.wpro.who.int/hpr/docs/glossary.pdf>

——1999, *Regional Guidelines for Healthy Workplaces*, viewed 16 February 2006, <www.who.int/occupational_health/regions/en/oehwproguidelines.pdf>

——2000, *The Fifth Global Conference on Health Promotion. Health Promotion: Bridging the Equity Gap*, Mexico City, viewed 16 February 2006, <www.who.int/healthpromotion/conferences/previous/mexico/en/hpr_mexico _report_en.pdf>

——2005a, *The Bangkok Charter for Health Promotion in a Globalized World*, Sixth Global Conference on Health Promotion, Bangkok, viewed 16 February 2006, <www.who.int/healthpromotion/conferences/6gchp/hpr_050829_%20BCHP. pdf>

——2005b, *The SuRF Report 2 surveillance of chronic disease risk factors: Country-level data and comparable estimates*, Noncommunicable Diseases and Mental Health World Health Organization, viewed 10 October 2005, <www.who.int/ncd_surveillance/infobase/web/surf2/start.html>

——2005c, viewed 23 January 2005, <www.who.int/hac/crises/international/ asia_tsunami/en/index.html>

——2006a, *The workplace: A priority setting for health promotion*, viewed 16 February 2006, <www.who.int/occupational_health/topics/workplace/en/>

——2006b, *Health promotion: Follow-up to 6th Global Conference on Health Promotion*, viewed 17 February 2006, <www.who.int/gb/ebwha/pdf_files/ EB117/B117_11-en.pdf>

WHO/Regional Office for Europe 1986, 'A discussion document on the concept and principles of health promotion', *Health Promotion*, vol. 1, no. 1, pp. 73–6.

——2005a, *Healthy Cities and urban governance*, viewed 14 December 2005, <www.euro.who.int/healthy-cities>

——2005b, *Health Promoting Hospitals*, viewed 21 June 2005, <www.euro.who.int/ healthpromohosp>

WHO/Regional Office for Europe, the European Commission and the Council of Europe 1998, 'The health promoting school—an investment in education, health and democracy', report of the First Conference of the European Network of Health Promoting Schools, Thessaloniki-Halkidiki, Greece, viewed 14 March 2005, <www.euro.who.int/document/e72971.pdf>

——2002, *Models of Health Promoting Schools in Europe*, Copenhagen, viewed 14 March 2005, <www.euro.who.int/document/e74993.pdf>

WHO/Regional Office for Europe's Health Evidence Network (HEN) 2004, *What are the advantages and disadvantages of restructuring a health care system to be more focused on primary care services?*, viewed 27 February 2006, <www.euro.who.int/document/e82997.pdf>

WHO/Regional Office for the Western Pacific 1999, *Regional Guidelines for the Development of Healthy Workplaces*, WHO, Geneva.

WHO/UNESCO 1986, *Helping a Billion Children Learn About Health*, WHO, Geneva.

WHO/UNESCO/UNICEF 1992, *Comprehensive School Health Education: Suggested guidelines for action*, WHO, Geneva.

WHO/UNICEF 1978, *Alma-Ata 1978, International Conference on Primary Health Care*, Health For All Series 1, WHO, Geneva.

——1989, *Protecting, Promoting and Supporting Breastfeeding: The Special Role of Maternity Service*, WHO, Geneva.

WHO/United Nations Environment Program/Nordic Council of Ministers 1991, *Sundsvall Statement on Supportive Environments for Health*, WHO, Geneva.

World Vision Resource Centre 2005, viewed 23 January 2005, <www.worldvision.com.au/resources/>

Wright, J., Franks, A., Ayres, P., Jones, K., Roberts, T. and Whitty, P. 2002, 'Public health in hospitals: The missing link in health improvement', *Journal of Public Health Medicine*, vol. 24, no. 3, pp. 152–5.

Wyn, J., Cahill, H., Holdsworth, R., Rowling, L. and Carson, S. 2000, 'MindMatters, a whole-school approach promoting mental health and wellbeing', *Australian and New Zealand Journal of Psychiatry*, vol. 34, no. 4, pp. 594–601.

Yellowless, P.M. and Hemming, M. 1992, 'Rural mental health', *Medical Journal of Australia*, vol. 157, pp. 152–4.

Zoller, H.M. 2004, 'Manufacturing health: Employee perspectives on problematic outcomes in a workplace health promotion initiative', *Western Journal of Communication*, vol. 68, no. 3, pp. 278–301.

Useful websites

Aboriginal and Islander Health Worker Journal
   <www.aihwj.com.au>

Asian Development Bank
   Development finance institute committed to cutting poverty in Asia and the
   Pacific region, with 64 member states.
   <www.adb.org>

AusAID (Australian Agency for International Development)
   Australia's overseas aid program to reduce poverty in developing countries.
   <www.ausaid.gov.au>

Australasian Evaluation Society
   <www.aes.asn.au>

Australian Bureau of Statistics
   <www.abs.gov.au>

Australian Divisions of General Practice
   One of Australia's largest representative bodies for general practitioners.
   <www.adgp.com.au>

Australian Health Promoting Schools Association (AHPSA)
   <www.ahpsa.org.au>

Australian Health Promotion Association (and the *Health Promotion Journal of
Australia*)

Australian Indigenous health*info*net
   <www.healthinfonet.ecu.edu.au>

Australian Institute of Health & Welfare (AIHW)
   <www.aihw.gov.au>

Australian Network of Academic Public Health Institutions (ANAPHI)
   <www.anaphi.unsw.edu.au>

Best Practice in Public Health, US Department of Health & Human Services
   Best practices in public health from around the country, to foster an environment of peer learning and collaboration.
   <www.osophs.dhhs.gov/ophs/BestPractice>

Centers for Disease Control and Prevention, US (CDC)
   <www.cdc.gov>

CDC Recommends, Centers for Disease Control and Prevention, US
   A searchable storehouse of documents containing CDC recommendations on a variety of health, prevention and public health practice issues.
   <www.phppo.cdc.gov/cdcrecommends/AdvSearchV.asp>

Cochrane Collaboration
   An international organisation that produces and disseminates systematic reviews of up-to-date health care interventions, to ensure the availability of accurate information.
   <www.cochrane.org>

Cochrane Health Promotion and Public Health Field
   'To promote the conduct, dissemination and utilization of systematic reviews of all health promotion and public health interventions.'
   <www.vichealth.vic.gov.au/cochrane/welcome/index.htm>

Community Toolbox, University of Kansas
   Information on promoting community health and development.
   <http://ctb.ku.edu>

Curtin University of Technology—Healthy Lifestyle Program
   <http://lifestyle.curtin.edu.au>

Department of Health and Ageing
<www.health.gov.au>

Economic Evaluation Database, NHS (NHS EED)
The NHS EED database saves time by collating information; in addition, it provides assessments of the quality of included economic evaluations.
<www.york.ac.uk/inst/crd/crddatabases.htm#NHSEED>

Effective Public Health Practice Project (EPHPP)
An initiative of the Public Health Research, Education and Development Program (PHRED), under the auspices of the Ministry of Health (Canada) and Long-Term Care and the City of Hamilton, Public Health and Community Services.
<www.myhamilton.ca/myhamilton/CityandGovernment/HealthandSocial Services/Research/EPHPP>

Evidence-based health promotion
<www.health.vic.gov.au/healthpromotion/quality/evidence_index.htm>

Evidence for Policy and Practice Information (EPPI) Centre
<http://eppi.ioe.ac.uk/EPPIWeb/home.aspx?Control=Search&SearchDB=rore &page=/hp>

Health Canada
<www.hc-sc.gc.ca>

Health*Insite*
An Australian Government initiative providing up-to-date and quality assessed information on important health topics, such as diabetes, cancer and asthma.
<www.healthinsite.gov.au>

Healthy People 2010 Information Access Project
An online resource of evidence-based strategies related to the Healthy People 2010 objectives, established by the Public Health Foundation, in conjunction with the National Library of Medicine (NLM) and the National Network of Libraries of Medicine (NN/LM).
<www.phf.org/hp2010asst.htm>

Human Rights and Equal Opportunity Commission
<www.hreoc.gov.au/racial_discrimination/face_facts/index.html>

Interactive Domain Model of Best Practices in Health Promotion
<www.bestpractices-healthpromotion.com/index.html>

International Union for Health Promotion and Education (and *Promotion & Education* journal)
<www.iuhpe.nyu.edu>

Medicare Australia
Formerly the Health Insurance Commission
<www.medicareaustralia.gov.au>

National Health and Medical Research Council
<www.nhmrc.gov.au>

National Health Priority Areas (NHPA)
A cooperative initiative of the Commonwealth, state and territory governments, it underscores areas that significantly impact on morbidity and mortality, and have the potential for health improvements.
<www.aihw.gov.au/nhpa/index.cfm>

National Heart Foundation
<www.heartfoundation.com.au>

National Occupational Health and Safety Commission
<www.nohsc.gov.au>

National Public Health Partnership
The NPHP Group is a subcommittee of the Australian Health Ministers' Advisory Council (AHMAC).
<www.dhs.vic.gov.au/nphp>

National Rural Health Alliance

New Zealand Ministry of Health
<www.moh.govt.nz>

Office for Aboriginal and Torres Strait Islander Health (OATSIH)
<www.health.gov.au/internet/wcms/Publishing.nsf/Content/Office+for+
Aboriginal+and+Torres+Strait+Islander+Health+(OATSIH)-1>

Public Health Association of Australia (and the *Australian and New Zealand
Journal of Public Health*)
<www.phaa.net.au>

Queensland Divisions of General Practice (QDGP)
The representative body for divisions of general practice in Queensland, it
promotes the role of general practice in primary health care.
<www.qdgp.org.au>

Queensland Health
<www.health.qld.gov.au>

Rural Industries Research and Development Corporation
Works with rural industries on their research and development needs, including the development, implementation and evaluation of health and safety
programs on farms and in other rural industries.
<www.rirdc.gov.au>

The Evaluation Center, Western Michigan University
<www.wmich.edu/evalctr>

UK Department of Health
<www.dh.gov.uk>

United Nations
<www.un.org/english>

United Nations Development Program
The UN's global development network, an organisation advocating for change
and connecting countries to knowledge, experience and resources to help
people build a better life.

United Nations High Commissioner for Refugees
<www.unhcr.org>

United States Department of Health and Human Services
<www.hhs.gov>

University of Toronto, Department of Public Health Sciences
<www.phs.utoronto.ca>

World Bank
Provides financial and technical assistance to developing countries around the
world, to reduce poverty and improve living standards.
<www.worldbank.org>

World Health Organization
<www.who.int/en>

World Health Organization/Regional Office for Europe
<www.euro.who.int>

World Vision
<www.worldvision.com.au>

Index